Caring for the Coronary Patient

SECOND EDITION

David R. Thompson BSc MA PhD MBA RN FRCN FESC

Professor of Clinical Nursing and Director, Nethersole School of Nursing, Chinese University of Hong Kong, Hong Kong, China

Rosemary A. Webster BSc MSc RN

Senior Nurse for Education and Practice, Cardio-Respiratory Directorate, University Hospitals of Leicester, UK

With additional material by

Tom Quinn MPhil RN FESC

Professor of Cardiac Nursing, School of Health and Social Sciences, Coventry University, Coventry, UK

Foreword by

Professor Dame Jenifer Wilson–Barnett

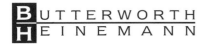

BUTTERWORTH
HEINEMANN

EDINBURGH LONDON NEW YORK OXFORD PHILADELPHIA ST LOUIS SYDNEY TORONTO 2004

NLL13   GNMC   (EGYDM)

BUTTERWORTH-HEINEMANN
An imprint of Elsevier Limited

First edition 1992

ISBN 0 7506 4315 3

British Library Cataloguing in Publication Data
A catalogue record for this book is available from the British Library

Library of Congress Cataloguing in Publication Data
A catalog record for this book is available from the Library of Congress

Notice
Medical knowledge is constantly changing. Standard safety precautions must be
followed, but as new research and clinical experience broaden our knowledge,
changes in treatment and drug therapy may become necessary or appropriate.
Readers are advised to check the most current product information provided by
the manufacturer of each drug to be administered to verify the recommended
dose, the method and duration of administration, and contraindications. It is the
responsibility of the practitioner, relying on experience and knowledge of the
patient, to determine dosages and the best treatment for each individual patient.
Neither the publisher nor the authors assume any liability for any injury and/or
damage to persons or property arising from this publication.

The Publisher

The
Publisher's
policy is to use
**paper manufactured
from sustainable forests**

Printed in China

Contents

Foreword

Given the importance of heart disease for quality of life and cause of death to so many worldwide, this information and excellent text is a great contribution to those who give and need care. Beautifully written and clearly comprehensive this work has increased the availability of knowledge of cardiac function, dysfunction and related illness and related this to an evidence base for care.

In this second edition, almost essentially rewritten from the very successful first edition, the authors manage to offer a comprehensive and useful piece of work. In my opinion, this will improve the information offered to nurses but also to many other disciplines and a wide range of carers. Useful as a reference, revision text or primary source it could be recommended to senior students in healthcare professions as well as practitioners and educators. Although the main policy references use the National Health Service, this could be of international relevance as the majority of information and the rationale for care pertain to all patients and their relatives undergoing coronary care across the globe. Essentially the framework for care, assessment strategies and use of evidence provide an example for others caring for different groups of patients. Discussion on clinical guidelines and the extended role of the nurse provide a modern flavour to the context of care.

In recommending this book to others particular features can be highlighted. The style of interrogation and answers, this dialectical structure offers instant engagement for the reader. Clarity of structure throughout makes search for specific information easy and the logical progression from assessment, diagnosis, interventions or caring processes to evaluation familiar. As a well-referenced text this is equally useful for those working on educational courses or in clinical practice.

Criteria for excellence in any text such as this has been met, including an easy style with substantial depth of information associated with research evidence set in a current environment of care and health care policy. In addition, of particular note, the blend of psychosocial and physical care is perfectly balanced, a refreshing feature often not seen in such volumes provided for this speciality. This has probably been achieved through the author partnership, exploiting their rich clinical and research backgrounds.

Readers are offered a real gift and in these days of multiple sources of information and databases, this book manages to capture a wealth of knowledge and guidance in a relatively compact volume. Coronary care will be enhanced if those responsible access this attractive volume.

Jenifer Wilson-Barnett
BA, MSc, PhD, FRCN, DBE

Preface

The aim of this book is in keeping with the first edition, namely to provide the nurse caring for the acute coronary patient with up-to-date, credible evidence. The focus is still on the caring aspects, which often tend to get overlooked in the increasingly busy and varied 'hi-tec' medical environment of a cardiac care unit, and it remains our intention that the central theme is nursing.

Clearly, since the first edition appeared in 1992, major advances in medicine and technology, in particular, and health care, in general, have taken place. In acute cardiac care, huge changes have occurred, with a rapid and substantial growth in its evidence base and radical changes in its organization and delivery. We have attempted to keep pace with such developments and, hopefully, they are reflected in this new edition. Nevertheless, we have retained the same structure and format and we reiterate that though the book necessitates that areas of care are fragmented into sections and presented in a linear fashion this does not reflect the typical multi-dimensional nature of clinical practice.

This book is not intended to be a treatise on cardiology, nursing or caring but, rather, an aid designed to provide a sound knowledge base for clinically competent nurses who are thoughtful, critical, articulate and compassionate in caring for their patients and families who have experienced an acute coronary event.

Hong Kong, China   D.R.T.
Leicester, UK   R.A.W.
2004

Acknowledgements

It is a pleasure to acknowledge a number of people who helped in the production of this second edition. Catherine Jackson and Morven Dean at Elsevier were helpful and patient throughout the publication process. Professor Tom Quinn thoroughly reviewed the whole text and, in his inimitable way, made many valuable suggestions that improved it. Professor Dame Jenifer Wilson-Barnett again kindly wrote the Foreword.

Chapter 1

Background to the problem

INTRODUCTION

Coronary heart disease (CHD) is the major cause of ill health and premature death in the developed world and although mortality rates continue to fall it is still the single most common cause of death in both men and women in the United Kingdom (UK) (British Heart Foundation (BHF) 2003). One in four men and one in six women die from the disease and in 2000 CHD caused around 125 000 deaths in the UK (BHF 2003).

The main clinical manifestations of CHD are angina and myocardial infarction (MI). These two diagnostic labels used to be considered separately, but now, in the light of developments in diagnostic testing and treatment options, the term acute coronary syndrome (ACS) is applied to a spectrum of CHD ranging from unstable angina to acute myocardial infarction. This is discussed more fully later in the book, but this shift in diagnostic labelling has significant implications for patient information giving, treatment decisions, data collection and the interpretation of audit and research evidence.

DEFINITION

The term coronary heart disease describes the gradual narrowing of the arteries supplying blood to the heart. It is a progressive, degenerative disease which once present contributes to a reduced quality of life and premature death. Narrowing usually occurs as a result of atherosclerosis which is the narrowing and thickening of the arteries due to the development of fibrous tissue and sometimes calcium deposits in the arterial wall and to the development of atheroma (Davies 1987). Atheroma is the build up of fatty material and cholesterol within sections of the arterial wall. However, many more people have coronary atheroma than have CHD, and the mechanisms leading to each of them differ. Functional factors interfering with coronary blood supply are largely responsible for the clinical manifestations of CHD, in the presence of variable degrees of coronary atherosclerosis. The term ischaemic heart disease is also used but tends to refer to coronary heart disease that produces symptoms of ischaemia.

Atherosclerosis in the coronary arteries begins long before the symptoms develop and patients with CHD may be asymptomatic. However, symptoms are often disabling and provoke anxiety. The most common clinical manifestation is chest pain, although talking to those with CHD will serve to highlight how individual and varied symptoms can be.

Diagnostic labels for those with CHD can be confusing for patients and professionals alike and include those given in Table 1.1.

In addition, CHD can lead to disorders of the heart's rhythm (arrhythmias), heart failure and sudden death.

THE COST OF CORONARY HEART DISEASE

Although death rates from CHD have been falling in the UK since the late 1970s, the disease still deprives the economy of people in their most productive years and many young families of their parents. Thus, the costs are enormous; both human (through bereavement, disability and fear) and economic (by premature deaths and retirements, by sickness from work and by increasing demands on the National Health Service).

The experience of suffering an acute cardiac event is almost always frightening and painful, arousing intense distress in the patient and family, especially the spouse. They are confronted with the possibility of death, physical impairment and the experience of suffering a life-threatening crisis. They are likely to be faced with an uncertain future and worry about the patient's ability to resume work, the fulfilment of family obligations and the curtailment of activities that have been important sources of satisfaction and support (Thompson 1990). One study comparing a group of CHD patients with an age and gender matched control group (Lukkarinen and Hentinen 1997) found that those with CHD had a lower quality of life in relation to energy, pain, emotions, sleep and physical exercise as self-assessed on the Nottingham Health Profile quality of life scale (McEwen 1993).

It is estimated that CHD costs the UK economy a total of £10 000 million a year (BMF 2003). This is almost double that for any other single disease for which figures are known.

Overall, there were over 364 000 inpatient cases treated for CHD in National Health Service hospitals in 1999/2000. This represents 4% of all inpatient cases in men and 2% in women (BHF 2003). CHD cost the health care system about £1700 million in 1999. Hospital care accounts for just over half of these costs, the expense of drugs and dispensing them about a third, with only about 1% of such costs being spent on both the prevention of CHD and rehabilitation (Table 1.2).

The escalating cost of CHD is linked to the increased cost of treatments and greater numbers of individuals requiring treatment. Also, management options have widened so that any one individual is likely to have more resources used to diagnose and manage their condition. The results of numerous multicentred randomized controlled trials have added to the evidence base from which clinical decisions on treatment options can be made. This is particularly the case for drug therapy. There were around 130 million prescriptions issued

Table 1.1 Diagnostic labels for those with CHD

Established terms	More recent terms
Stable angina	
Unstable angina	Acute coronary syndrome
Subendocardial MI*	Non-ST segment elevation MI
Non-Q wave MI	
Q-wave MI	ST segment elevation MI

*The terms 'coronary', 'coronary thrombosis' and 'heart attack' are also frequently used, particularly by non-professionals.

for diseases of the circulatory system in England in 2000, about three times as many as were issued in 1981 (BHF 2003) (Figure 1.1).

The amount of coronary artery bypass surgery (CABG) increased fivefold in the 20 years from 1980, almost doubling in the 10 years from 1990.

There are now just under 28 000 operations carried out annually in the UK. There is a similar number of percutaneous transluminal coronary angioplasties (PTCA) performed each year, although rates for both these interventions vary substantially between National Health Service districts (BHF 2003).

GENERAL TRENDS FOR CORONARY HEART DISEASE

Disease statistics can take time to correlate and it is impossible to have an up to the minute picture of any disease process. However, looking at the changes or trends in figures can provide valuable information on factors such as effectiveness of treatments, the impact of risk factors and resource implications. An up-to-date profile of the burden of CHD in the UK can be found in the annual coronary heart disease statistics data base published by the British Heart Foundation.

The high incidence of CHD was observed in Australia, North America and Europe in the early part of the 20th century and reached its peak in the 1960s and 1970s. Trends in cardiovascular disease have been documented by the MONICA project, coordinated by the World Health Organization (Tunstall-Pedoe et al 1994) since the 1980s. This has

Table 1.2 Costs of CHD to the National Health Service and Social care system, 1999, United Kingdom

	£ million	% of total
Primary prevention	12.6	0.7
Primary care	48.8	2.8
Accident and emergency care	16.5	1.0
Outpatient care	33.3	1.9
Inpatient care	917.2	53
Day cases	16.0	0.9
Medication	582.3	33.7
Rehabilitation	28.4	1.6
Community health/social services	74.8	4.3
Total	1729.9	99.9

Source: Liu et al (2002).

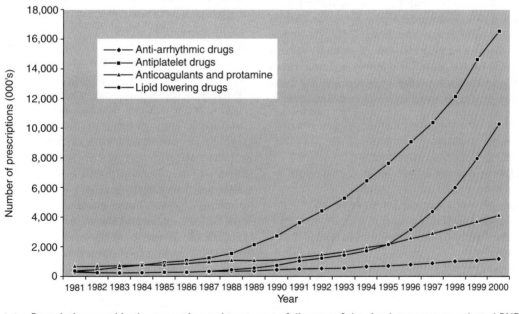

Figure 1.1   Prescriptions used in the prevention and treatment of diseases of the circulatory system, selected BNF paragraphs, 1981–2000, England (from BHF CHD statistics database 2003, fig. 3.1, p. 58).

highlighted that deaths from cardiovascular disease are falling in many populations. In the UK the CHD death rates for adults under 65 years fell 40% in the years from 1988 to 1998 (BHF 2003). The reasons for the widespread fall in mortality are complex, but it is thought that two-thirds of the recorded worldwide reduction can be attributed to a fall in coronary event rate and the remainder a result of reduced case fatality (Tunstall-Pedoe et al 1999). CHD mortality has consistently decreased more than incidence, which has contributed to the increased prevalence of CHD. More people are surviving cardiac events and living longer due to a combination of prevention and medical and surgical treatments (Beaglehole 1999). There has also been an increase in the proportion of CHD admissions for diagnoses other than definite myocardial infarction; possibly a result of changes in admission practices and in the ways in which patients present (Salomaa et al 1999). These factors all have implications for service provision, long-term management and support of individuals and their families.

TARGETS FOR CORONARY HEART DISEASE

The White Paper, 'Saving lives: our healthier nation' (DoH 1999a) attempted to address inequalities in health and significant health issues, including CHD. Chapter 6 of this document puts forward a target of reducing the death rates from CHD and stroke related diseases in people under 75 years by at least two-thirds by the year 2010. It was estimated that this would mean a saving of some 200 000 lives. Proposed strategies to achieve this target included:

- funding for a public education programme for smoking cessation
- banning of tobacco advertising
- targeting areas of known social deprivation known as Health Action Zones
- easier access to services for those with established CHD
- greater equity in access to services across the country
- setting up of a task force to produce a National Service Framework for CHD to set standards and define service models for health provision, disease prevention, diagnosis, treatment, rehabilitation and care.

Table 1.3   Modifiable and non-modifiable risk factors for CHD

Non-modifiable risk factors	Modifiable risk factors
Age	Blood cholesterol
Gender	Tobacco smoking
Ethnicity	High blood pressure
Genetic predisposition	Overweight and obesity
Low birth weight	Diet
Diabetes	Alcohol consumption
Hormonal and	Psychosocial well-being
biochemical factors	Social class
	Geographical distribution

RISK FACTORS AND PRIMARY PREVENTION

Epidemiological studies have sought associations between CHD and physical, biochemical and environmental characteristics of a population or individual. Such characteristics are termed *risk factors*. Individuals, faced with a diagnosis of CHD frequently want to identify why this has happened to them – is it something that they could have avoided? Is there something they can do to prevent a recurrence of the acute event? Identifying a perceived 'cause' can lead to feelings of guilt, blame, hopelessness or resignation. Likewise, not being able to pinpoint a reason for what has happened can result in anger and feelings of 'Why me?'

Risk factors can be divided into those that are modifiable and those that are non-modifiable (Table 1.3). Studies looking at risk factors have consistently shown three potentially modifiable factors to be powerful predictors of CHD: raised cholesterol, cigarette smoking and high blood pressure. The cumulative effect of these three major risk factors accelerates the atherosclerotic process (Figure 1.2). Evidence suggests that CHD is potentially preventable through a healthy lifestyle and appropriate management of raised cholesterol and high blood pressure. There is also reliable research demonstrating that lifestyle changes and appropriate treatments can slow and perhaps even reverse the progression of established CHD.

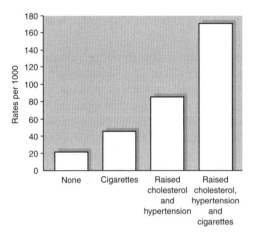

Figure 1.2 Cumulative risk of the three major risk factors on the incidence of a first major coronary event.

Any information and advice about risk factors needs to be given in an individualized and honest manner keeping the significance of known risk factors in perspective. Although there is a positive association between identified risk factors and CHD, it does not mean that any of these risk factors actually cause heart disease. Risk factors may be weak indicators of CHD, for individuals as other mechanisms, only remotely related to the presence of such risk factors, can precipitate the clinical syndromes of the disease. Certainly, there is no basis for comparison between risk factors and the severity or extent of atheroma. It is also naive to compare risk factors in different populations as the mechanisms of disease may differ. While population studies help identify specific significant risk factors for populations, different risk factors may be significant for individuals within that population group. It is important to remember that a significant number of patients presenting with CHD do not have identifiable risk factors, and that standard risk factors explain less than half of the disease.

NON-MODIFIABLE RISK FACTORS

Age

Increasing age adds to the likelihood of having a first and subsequent heart attack. Death rates from CHD also rise steeply with age with mortality doubling over each 5-year period. Death rates have been

falling at a slower rate in the older age groups, for example there was a 45% fall in the death rate for men aged 45–54 in the UK between 1988 and 1998, but the fall for men in the 65–74 age group over the same time frame was only 34% (BHF 2003). Age brings with it increased likelihood of exposure to smoking, the coexistence of hypertension, hyperlipidaemia and diabetes, plus reduced regular exercise. The relative risk of these established risk factors diminishes with age but this is offset by a greater absolute risk. The Framingham study found that cholesterol, blood pressure and smoking were all independent predictors of CHD in males and females up to 94 years of age (Kannel and Larson 1993). Isolated systolic hypertension and large pulse pressure that predominate in the elderly are now recognized as being associated with CHD.

Improvements in health have led to an increased proportion of older and ageing individuals and the success of treatments allows patients with CHD to survive longer. Cardiac rehabilitation and secondary prevention teams are likely to see a significant proportion of older individuals and may question the efficacy of targeting limited resources to this group, although theoretically it is the elderly out of all age groups who have the most to gain. Giving the elderly advice on changing established lifestyles in order to affect modifiable risk factors can be controversial. Clinical trials have, however, shown benefits of lowering both blood cholesterol levels (Heart Protection Study Group 2002) and blood pressure in individuals up to 80 years of age and the majority of the elderly have sufficient remaining life expectancy to warrant vigorous preventative management. The distinction between primary and secondary prevention in the elderly becomes less clear than in the middle aged as the elderly often have advanced pre-symptomatic vascular pathology that imposes a coronary event rate comparable to that of the middle aged who have already sustained a clinical event (Kannel 2002).

Gender

Male mortality rates for CHD are higher than those for females in all age groups, with male rates similar to the female rates of the group 10 years older. This difference has contributed to the perception of CHD as a male problem with the possibility of women being treated differently during the course of their disease. This is despite the fact that twice as many women die from heart and circulatory disease as do from cancer (BHF 2003). Women may present differently and there have been reports of women taking longer to reach hospital and to have CHD diagnosed (Clarke et al 1994) which could reflect the fact that both the individual concerned and those assessing them took longer to suspect a cardiac problem.

The sex difference evens out after the age of 65 when the levels of risk for each sex of dying from CHD converge. This has been attributed to pre-menopausal hormone protection as the menopause heralds an almost threefold rise in the risk of CHD. However, other risk factors such as hypertension, being overweight, reduced regular exercise and raised blood cholesterol and glucose concentrations may be more relevant in women of this age than in men. To date the majority of clinical trials have focused on men and there is a lack of evidence on which to develop management regimens specifically for women.

Ethnicity

An accurate comparison of the occurrence of CHD between countries relies on uniformity in disease classification and reliable data collection. This is not always the case. However, there is consensus that although all ethnic groups have CHD, some have significantly higher rates than others. The link between ethnicity and CHD is complex. For example it is known that migrant groups gradually shift their risk of cardiovascular disease from that of their home country to that of their host country. A number of factors may contribute to the ethnic difference including:

- genetic factors
- a difference in the significance of and response to known risk factors
- environmental factors, e.g. the effect of urbanization and industrialization
- the impact of preventative strategies
- access to medical services
- and for migrant populations – specific characteristics of those who migrate and the

impact of living as an immigrant (e.g. stress, poverty).

In the UK, immigrants from the Indian subcontinent (India, Pakistan and Bangladesh) and their children, as well as political refugees from Kenya and Uganda descended from earlier immigrants from India, are a significant ethnic minority group. It is recognized that they are at increased risk of CHD (McKeigue and Sevak 1994) with mortality rates reported as being approximately 40% higher when compared to the white population (Balarajan 1991). Although the data on actual disease rates are potentially unreliable (Bhopal 2000) and mortality rates are not uniform across all south Asian groups (Bhopal et al 1999), CHD is certainly a significant issue for this population and is likely to become more so as the present comparatively young South Asian population ages. Certainly the death rate in South Asians is not falling as fast as in the rest of the population. South Asians tend to present young and have more widespread coronary artery disease than their white counterparts. They are thought to possess a risk factor profile characterized by high triglycerides, low HDL, glucose intolerance, insulin resistance, abdominal obesity and increased lipoprotein (a) levels (Pinto 1998) and may benefit from a different emphasis to the general population in primary and secondary prevention strategies.

Death rates from CHD for Caribbeans and West Africans are comparatively low. The premature mortality for these groups in England and Wales is reported to be about half the rate of that in the general population for men and about two-thirds of the rate found in women (BHF 2003). It is not clear why this difference exists although genetic factors may be significant. Other groups with raised mortality include Irish-, Scottish- and Polish-born immigrants.

Genetic predisposition

CHD frequently occurs in families, and the presence of CHD in a first degree relative before the age of 50 years in men and 55 years in women is a strong independent risk factor. Genetic susceptibility may be linked to traits that are known to exist in families or to processes as yet not understood. Interaction between genes and the relationship between genes and environmental factors may play a part. The Human Genome Project is likely to hold the key to identifying the genetic factors underlying CHD (Bentley 2000). Recombinant DNA technology has already identified 'candidate genes' implicated in CHD risk. These include the insulin receptor gene, the ACE gene, those involved in coagulation factors, growth factors and vessel wall proteins. Interactions between genetic and environmental factors appear to have an effect on lipid metabolism, plasma homocysteine levels and the pharmacological response to many commonly prescribed medications (Ellsworth et al 1999). Genetic research into cardiovascular disease needs to become integrated with preventative medicine and public health initiatives. It may become routine for individuals to be offered a blood test to establish their risk of developing CHD. While facilitating decisions around who should be targeted for treatment this may also pose ethical dilemmas around who should be tested and the consequences for employment and insurance cover etc. for individuals once the results are known. Confirmation of increased risk of premature death from CHD can be both empowering and debilitating and individuals will need to be supported through the screening process and beyond.

Social class

It is acknowledged that inequalities in social environments lead to variations in health and life expectancy with those in the lower social classes fairing worse (DoH 1995a, 1999a). Level of income affects an individual's ability to make decisions and take actions regarding health which can have both physical and psychological consequences. Defining and measuring social class is fraught with difficulty. Measurements tend to ask for measures of material wealth, housing, education, income and employment status which can be factors determined by choice as well as reflecting disadvantage or privilege. However, measurement of the relationship between social class and CHD in the UK have consistently highlighted an inverse relationship between CHD and social class, with the disease being substantially more common in social classes IV and V (partly skilled and unskilled manual workers). The premature death rate from

CHD for male manual workers, such as builders and cleaners, is 58% higher than for male non-manual workers such as lawyers and doctors (BHF 2003). Part of the excess in these classes is probably due to the aggregation of risk factors for CHD. For example, it has been reported that the age standardized prevalence of smoking is 18% in social class I compared to 42% in social class V (DoH 1999b).

Geographical distribution

International differences

Major geographical variations in the incidence of CHD are apparent. In comparison with the rest of the world, the UK still has one of the highest death rates for CHD. However, in recent years it is in the countries of Eastern and Western Europe, where there has been much recent political and sociological unrest, where death rates from CHD have risen rapidly and are generally higher than in the UK. Among developed countries, only Ireland and Finland have a higher rate than the UK (Figure 1.3). The UK death rate from CHD has not fallen to the same extent as in other countries. For example, the death rate for men aged 35–74 fell by 33% between 1986 and 1996 in the UK, compared to 45% in Denmark and Norway and by 43% in Australia in the same period (BHF 2003).

Regional differences

A north–south divide exists with the incidence of CHD in the UK with death rates being higher in Scotland, Northern Ireland and the North of England than in Wales and the South of England. The premature death rate for men living in Scotland is over 50% higher than in East Anglia.

MODIFIABLE RISK FACTORS

Modifiable risk factors are common and tend to coexist in individuals. Changing lifestyles and complying with treatment regimens is not easy. For those with multiple risk factors, making informed decisions about how to prioritize activities designed to reduce risk is often difficult. Risk factors are

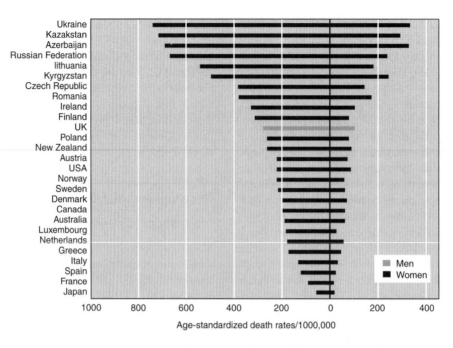

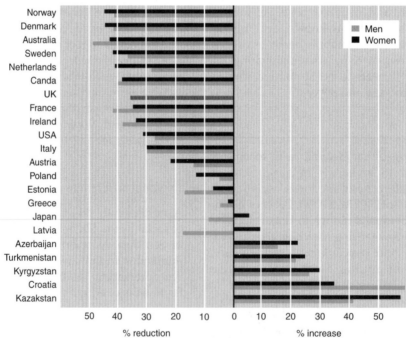

Figure 1.3   Death rates from CHD, men and women aged 35–74, 1996, selected countries (from BHF CHD statistics database 2003, fig. 1.5a).

cumulative with one factor multiplying the risk of another and individuals are more at risk of developing CHD if they have several mild risk factors as opposed to one severe one (Neaton and Wentworth 1992). This next section will highlight those risk factors that can be potentially changed and discuss strategies to support individuals in changing them.

Blood cholesterol

Various blood tests are performed to measure lipid components of the blood and what is being measured and its significance to CHD can be confusing. The various fat components of the blood are summarized in Chapter 8. A high concentration of lipids in the blood is termed hyperlipidaemia.

Total cholesterol

There is a direct link between the risk of CHD and blood cholesterol levels (Law et al 1994) even in populations with low levels. The population of the UK has one of the highest blood cholesterol levels in the world, particularly in women. A raised blood cholesterol level has been defined as being above 5.2 mmol/l with the mean blood cholesterol level for men in England being 5.5 mmol/l and for women 5.6 mmol/l. This compares with a mean of 4.5 mmol/l for the population of Beijing in China (BHF 2003). The prevalence of raised cholesterol increases with age. Reducing population blood cholesterol levels could have a significant effect on CHD mortality and it has been estimated that 10% of deaths could be avoided if the entire population of the UK had a blood cholesterol level of less than 6.5 mmol/l (National Heart Forum 2002). Blood cholesterol levels may also influence the significance of other known risk factors. For example the population of Japan has low cholesterol levels and low CHD mortality, despite high levels of smoking and hypertension.

Familial hypercholesterolaemia affects 2 in every 1000 people in the UK as a result of a mutation of the LDL-receptor gene. It carries a particularly high risk of CHD. Individuals with this condition tend to have a serum cholesterol over 9 mmol/l. They are also likely to have observable signs such as early corneal arcus which is a significant sign in those under 50 years of age.

The role of different lipids and lipoproteins

Lipoproteins are the water-soluble complexes produced from fat-soluble lipids in order to transport fats around the body. They come in different densities which differ in their link with CHD risk. Low levels of high-density lipoprotein (HDL) cholesterol, particularly the HDL2 sub-fraction, and high levels of low-density lipoprotein (LDH) cholesterol are associated with CHD.

HDL cholesterol   The mean HDL-cholesterol level for men in England is 1.3 mmol/l and for women 1.6 mmol/l (BHF 2003). Management guidelines generally recommend treatment for those with HDL cholesterol levels below 1 mmol/l. This is more common in men than in women. One in six men in the general population will have levels lower than this cut off point and the proportion is much higher in men from Pakistani and Bangladeshi communities. A lack of exercise, diabetes, obesity and cigarette smoking are associated with low HDL levels. Pre-menopausal women, those who regularly drink 1–2 units a day of alcohol and those who exercise regularly tend to have higher levels of HDL.

LDL–cholesterol   LDL-cholesterol concentrations are usually estimated indirectly from the relationship between total cholesterol, HDL-cholesterol and triglycerides using the Friedewald formula:

$$LDL = (\text{Total cholesterol} - HDL) \\ - (\text{Triglyceride} \times 0.45)$$

A ratio of HDL to LDL of less than 0.2 increases an individual's risk of developing CHD. Treatment has been recommended for individuals with an LDL-cholesterol of over 3 mmol/l (Wood et al 1998).

Knowing when to initiate cholesterol lowering therapy in patients at risk can be difficult and needs to be related to cholesterol levels and absolute risk, based on the presence or absence of other risk factors. There is evidence to suggest that treatment should be implemented in individuals with average LDL cholesterol and low HDL cholesterol who are at moderate or higher risk for CHD (Gotto 1999).

Lipoprotein A   Lipoprotein A (Lp(a)), although similar to LDL-cholesterol is recognized as a distinct lipoprotein class which may have variable and contrasting effects on different aspects of CHD. It is possibly an independent risk factor for atherosclerotic disease (Bostom et al 1996) and involved in the link between atherosclerosis and thrombosis. The only therapeutic measure that reduces Lp(a) is niacin which is not recommended for routine use.

Triglycerides Triglycerides are the lipids mainly responsible for transporting fatty acids from the liver and intestine to the cells. A high triglyceride level (hypertriglyceridaemia) is associated with increased risk of CHD, probably because this condition is linked with higher levels of LDL-cholesterol and lower levels of HDL cholesterol. There is a significant association between serum triglycerides and hypertension and diabetes and the independent prognostic significance of fasting triglyceride concentration is currently unclear.

Diagnosing hyperlipidaemia

As hyperlipidaemia does not produce symptoms, individuals are not likely to know that they have the condition until they have a blood test to detect it. Individuals may go for screening if they have a family member with hyperlipidaemia or they may be tested opportunistically at health promotion events. Routine screening of population groups is not recommended as it would be costly and there is no evidence to suggest that it would have any health benefit. A knowledge of having hyperlipidaemia does not necessarily lead to appropriate lifestyle adjustments (Irvine and Logan 1994). Individuals may deny the condition, feel that the associated risks do not apply to them or find the necessary lifestyle adjustments too restrictve and difficult to adhere to.

The National Service Framework for CHD (DoH 2000) recommends that total and HDL-cholesterol are measured non-fasting in patients under the age of 75 years who have:

- established arterial disease
- hypertension or diabetes
- a family history of hyperlipidaemia or premature CHD.

It goes on to recommend:

- reassurance and repeat in 5 years if total cholesterol is less than 5 mmol/l
- repeat in one month if total cholesterol 5–7.9 mmol/l and with established arterial disease – treat if still raised
- dietary advice and repeat in three months if total cholesterol 5–7.9 mmol/l without

established arterial disease. Decision to treat based on cardiovascular risk
- repeat in one month and if still raised treat if total cholesterol >8 mmol/l.

Repeat tests should include a fasting lipoprotein profile alongside a full cardiovascular risk assessment, targeted dietary advice and exclusion of secondary causes of hyperlipidaemia which include diabetes, thyroid disorder, renal disease, liver disorder, alcohol and certain drugs.

Blood tests taken at times of acute illness, surgery, trauma and myocardial infarction are likely to produce erroneous results as these conditions can alter serum lipoprotein concentrations. It is best to wait for at least 3 months after the acute coronary event to obtain reliable readings. Prior to that triglyceride levels are likely to be abnormally high and cholesterol levels abnormally low for the individual concerned. Blood cholesterol levels can be reduced by drugs, physical activity and dietary changes, particularly the consumption of saturated fat. The development of HMG-CoA reductase inhibitors, or statins, has been a major advance in lipid-lowering therapy that has revolutionized the treatment of atherosclerosis. Large-scale, randomized controlled primary prevention trials have indicated that statin therapy reduces CHD mortality and morbidity (Shepherd et al 1995, Downs et al 1998). Nurse-run clinics promoting medical and lifestyle aspects of risk factor modification have been shown to be effective in improving lipid management with patients with CHD (Campbell et al 1998) and similar strategies are likely to be of benefit in primary prevention.

Tobacco smoking

The epidemiological evidence that cigarette smoking is associated with an increased incidence of CHD is strong, although weaker than that for lung cancer and other malignancies. Almost 20% of smoking-related deaths are attributable to CHD (Callum 1998) and an individual who smokes 20 cigarettes a day increases their risk of a premature cardiac death fivefold (Freund et al 1993).

The two toxins associated with increased cardiovascular risk are nicotine and carbon monoxide.

Nicotine stimulates catecholamine release and increases myocardial work by increasing the heart rate, blood pressure, and force of myocardial contraction. In addition, there is a thrombogenic action caused by inhibition of fibrinolysis and an increase in platelet aggregation and stickiness. Carbon monoxide attaches itself to the haemoglobin molecule and therefore reduces its oxygen-carrying capacity. It may also cause endothelial dysfunction, increasing permeability to foam cells and predisposing atheroma.

In 1998, 28% of men and 26% of women in Great Britain smoked cigarettes (BHF 2003). The proportion of adult cigarette smokers had been falling sharply since the 1970s, but this decline has now reached a plateau and may even be increasing in younger age groups. There has also been a narrowing of the gap between smoking rates in men and women. Cigarette smoking is more common in manual groups and is generally higher in those living in the North than the South, with the exception of Greater London. Smoking rates vary considerably between ethnic groups in the UK. Rates are particularly high in men from Bangladesh (42% current smokers), Irish (39%) and African Caribbean (42%) communities in the UK (BHF 2003). Government targets aim to reduce overall smoking rates to 24% or less by the year 2010 (DoH 1998) although even if met, this target would only result in preventing 0.5% of deaths from CHD in the UK (National Heart Forum 2002).

When giving advice to those wanting to stop smoking it is worth being aware of the following:

- the overall risk of death from CHD for smokers is twice that for non-smokers
- risk of CHD increases in proportion to the number of cigarettes smoked
- self-reports of the number of cigarettes smoked and the depth of inhalation tend to be inaccurate
- passive smoking is thought to increase cardiovascular risk by about 20%
- inhaling from a pipe carries similar risks to smoking cigarettes
- switching from cigarettes to a pipe tends not to reduce the risk as inhalation patterns remain unchanged
- stopping smoking reduces cardiovascular risk by 50% within 2–3 years and after 10 years the level has reduced to that of non-smokers.

Government recommendations (DoH 2000) advocate that local targets be set up for preventing and reducing smoking prevalence. These local strategies should aim to:

- reduce smoking in public places
- encourage media support and advocacy and work with any national media campaigns
- reduce illegal sales of cigarettes
- support and monitor any bans on advertising
- develop smoking cessation clinics.

Although as many as 70% of smokers want to stop smoking (DoH 1998), this is not easy and services designed to help this process need to provide individualized information and continued support. Government health service circulars (HSC 1998/234 and HSC 1999/087) charge the NHS with integrating brief opportunistic interventions with more intensive support through specialist smoking cessation services, such as specialist clinics, wherever smokers are most likely to benefit. Acute care trusts and primary healthcare teams have a key role to play in smoking cessation as is emphasized by the National Service Framework for CHD (DoH 2000). Many of the new services are being developed and led by nurses. They aim to assess accurately an individual's smoking status and the ways best to help them stop smoking. Intervention options include advice on strategies to stop smoking, support in the use of nicotine replacement therapy (NRT), the use of individual and group therapy sessions and advocating use of the National 'Don't Give Up Giving Up' tobacco helpline service. Smoking cessation clinics have an essential role in providing intensive specialized treatment and expertise. They are developing across the UK in a response to the drive to establish an evidence-based service for smokers who want to quit. These new services have not yet been formally evaluated but would seem to offer an opportunity to support a group at significant risk from CHD.

High blood pressure

Blood pressure levels in the UK are generally high. The incidence of coronary events, stroke and peripheral vascular disease increases with hypertension. The risk of CHD is directly related to both systolic and diastolic blood pressure, although the systolic blood pressure is a more accurate predictor of cardiovascular disease. It is estimated that 14% of deaths from CHD in men and 12% in women are due to a raised blood pressure (defined as a systolic blood pressure of 140 mmHg or over, or a diastolic blood pressure of 90 mmHg or over) (BHF 2003).

There is evidence that hypertension may confer a prothrombotic state as is evident by abnormalities of haemostasis, platelets and endothelial function. Acceleration of atherosclerosis is a feature of hypertension, possibly as a result of changes in arterial compliance and turbulent blood flow facilitating the process of lipid transport into atheromatous lesions. Between 10 and 40% of patients with mild hypertension will develop left ventricular hypertrophy which has consequences for cardiac efficiency. Renal failure is another recognized complication.

Drug treatment and lifestyle changes, in particular losing weight, an increase in physical activity, and a reduction in salt and alcohol intake can effectively lower blood pressure. Hypertension tends to occur more frequently in individuals with other risk factors for CHD and it is likely that an individual receiving treatment for hypertension will also need support to manage other risk factors. The British Hypertension Society guidelines emphasize that the decision to treat needs to be based on the overall cardiovascular risk rather than absolute blood pressure values (Williams et al 2004). These guidelines recommend that drug treatment should be considered for individuals with sustained blood pressures of 140/90 mmHg and over, with optimal blood pressure targets being a systolic blood pressure of less than 120 mmHg and a diastolic blood pressure of less than 80 mmHg. Targets are lower for those with diabetes. The United Kingdom Prospective Diabetes Study (UKPDS 1998) supports reducing blood pressure to under 130/80 in patients with diabetic complications.

It has been reported that patients with an estimated 10-year CHD risk of 15% or greater will have their cardiovascular risk reduced by 25% using antihypertensive treatment and that the incidence of major cardiovascular events will be reduced further with the addition of aspirin (Lip et al 2001). For most individuals with hypertension, a combination of antihypertensive drugs will be required to achieve effective blood pressure control. Low dose

thiazide diuretics or beta-blockers are the drugs of choice for the majority of hypertensive individuals. However, unless there are strong indications for beta-blockade, diuretics or long-acting dihydropyridine calcium antagonists are preferred to beta-blockers in older subjects. Statin therapy has been recommended for hypertensive individuals with a total cholesterol greater than 3.5 mmol/l and established vascular disease, or a 10-year CHD risk greater than 20% (Williams et al 2004). Despite knowledge of the benefits of blood pressure control, it has been estimated that over 70% of men and women with hypertension are not receiving treatment, and of those that are, over two-thirds are not being adequately controlled (BHF 2003). This suggests that current intervention strategies need to be re-examined with a focus on long-term monitoring, individualized tailoring of treatment regimens and support and education to encourage compliance with therapy.

Many individuals do not realize the long-term risks associated with hypertension and may stop taking their medication after a period of time. Blood pressure increases with age, more so after the age of 45, and screening for hypertension tends to start in late middle age and beyond. However, hypertension in young adult men has been significantly related to increased long-term mortality from CHD, suggesting that primary prevention, early detection and control of raised blood pressure are indicated from young adulthood (Miura et al 2001).

OTHER RISK FACTORS

Various other risk factors have been implicated. Some of these are of less certain importance and some are difficult to quantify. Important ones are included below.

Overweight and obesity

Being overweight and obese increases the risk of CHD. Being overweight or obese also denotes an increased likelihood of hypertension, hyperlipidaemia and diabetes mellitus. In industrialized countries the average weight is higher than elsewhere as a result of the amount of food eaten. Food is readily available and what we eat has changed significantly over the last century as our diet has shifted from one which derived energy from carbohydrates in the form of cereals and potatoes, to one which is high in fat from meat and dairy products. The consumption of alcohol has also increased.

There are critical periods in life when weight gain is more likely. In women this period is in puberty, after marriage, after pregnancy and after the menopause. In men it is between 35 and 40 years of age, after marriage and after retirement. Those living in socially deprived areas and smokers who are attempting to stop are also prone to weight gain.

The relationship between an individual and what they eat can be complex with body image and self-esteem being significant factors. Individuals who are overweight are often aware of this without the need for any formal assessment. There are, however, charts developed from insurance company data that give values for 'ideal' weights for particular heights that may be used for confirmation. A more quantitative assessment of obesity is made using the body mass index (BMI) which takes into account the relationship between height and weight:

$$BMI = \frac{Weight\ (kg)}{Height^2\ (m)}$$

In England about 46% of men and 32% of women are overweight with a BMI between 25 and $30\,kg/m^2$. Obesity is taken as a BMI greater than $30\,kg/m^2$. The number of overweight individuals is increasing and this rise is likely to continue as the high level of obesity in children continues into adulthood. The detrimental effect of being overweight is more significant in individuals where the fat is concentrated in the abdomen, known as central obesity. Central obesity can be identified by a high waist to hip ratio (>0.95 in men and >0.85 in women). It is possible for individuals not to register as obese by conventional measurement (BMI) but to have high levels of central obesity. This is particularly the case in Indian, Pakistani and Bangladeshi men in the UK (Joint Health Surveys Unit 2001).

The observed relationship between cardiorespiratory fitness and CHD risk status in adolescents seems to be mediated by fatness, suggesting that primary prevention needs to start in childhood and should concentrate on reversing or preventing undue weight gain (Boreham et al 2001). Weight loss reduces blood pressure in those that are overweight and hypertensive and can also reduce total blood cholesterol. A 10% weight loss in those that are overweight or obese can have significant health benefits. However, preventing weight gain is the best approach in all age groups as once gained, weight is difficult to lose and weight loss difficult to maintain. A healthy diet and adequate levels of physical activity are the best ways to maintain ideal weight.

Low birth weight

Low birth weight and low body mass index at one year have been associated with increased risk for CHD. Also, irrespective of birth weight, both low weight gain and rapid weight gain during infancy are associated with increased CHD risk (Eriksson et al 2001). Improvements in fetal, infant and child growth could lead to significant reductions in the incidence of CHD.

Diet

Almost a third of deaths from CHD in the UK can be attributed to an unhealthy diet. It can be difficult for individuals to make sense of all the diets currently advocated for health, and weight loss. A lifelong balanced diet should be the main objective of any healthy eating advice. The Government's Committee on the Medical Aspects of Food policy (DoH 1994) recommends:

- a reduction in the average contribution of total fat to dietary energy to about 35% (currently estimated to be around 38%)
- a reduction in the average contribution of saturated fatty acids to dietary energy to no more than about 10% (currently estimated to be around 14%)
- a reduction in salt intake to 6 g per day (currently estimated to be around 7 g)
- an increase in the consumption of fruit and vegetables by 50% which equates to at least 5 portions a day
- an increase in starchy foods such as bread, rice, pasta and potatoes
- an increase in the consumption of fish – at least two portions a week, one of those oily.

A high intake of olive oil has been proposed as an explanation for the low incidence of CHD in Mediterranean countries, but it is unclear whether olive oil offers specific benefits beyond its comparatively low content of saturated fat.

Accurate levels of food consumption are difficult to assess, however, progress towards these targets is reported to be slow (BHF 2003). Choice of food can have a social, psychological, economic, religious and cultural context as well as being influenced by availability, health beliefs and values. Whether the lack of a move towards healthier eating is due to lack of knowledge or a lack of desire or ability to change established habits is unclear. Interestingly, there is little difference in the fat and saturated fat intake of different income level groups, whereas the intake of fresh fruit and vegetables is much higher in higher income households.

The best strategies for promoting healthy eating appear to be those that focus on diet alone or diet plus physical activity, set clear goals based on behavioural change theory rather than just information giving, maintain personal support through long-term contact and provide feedback to participating individuals.

Alcohol

Alcoholics and 'heavy' drinkers (over 4 units a day) have an excess mortality from CHD. This applies particularly to binge-drinkers. A moderate intake of alcohol, particularly one to two glasses of red wine a day, appears to reduce the incidence of coronary events by a fifth when compared to those who do not drink any alcohol (DoH 1995b). A possible mechanism being that alcohol intake raises the level of plasma HDL-cholesterol, inhibits platelets and can reduce stress.

The alcoholic content of drinks varies and in order to make comparisons and give advice, alcohol intake is measured in units. One unit equals one glass of wine or sherry, half a pint of lager or a single whisky or other spirit. Government guidelines currently advise that a regular consumption of between three and four units a day by men and between two and three units a day by women of all ages will not lead to any significant health risk (DoH 1995b). This is consistent with previous advice which advocated an upper weekly limit of

21 units for men and 14 units for women. Giving advice based on daily alcohol intake has benefits as weekly quotas can appear to endorse saving allocated units for heavy binges. The guidelines specifically recommend that consuming in excess of four units in any one day should be avoided.

Over a third of men and a fifth of women in Britain drink more than the recommended daily upper limits. Consumption is higher in younger age groups and while remaining stable in men has increased by around 40% in women over the past decade. This increase is particularly apparent in professional women who are three times as likely to exceed the recommended alcohol levels (BHF 2003).

Physical activity

Regular physical activity lowers blood pressure and improves glucose tolerance and insulin sensitivity. It also gives a sense of well-being. However, regular physical activity is becoming less a feature of lifestyles in the UK as employment is becoming increasingly sedentary and less people walk as part of their daily routine. There is some evidence that vigorous physical exercise has some protective effect against CHD. To be of most benefit the activity needs to be aerobic and regular. Aerobic activity involves using the large muscle groups of the arms, legs and back in a steady rhythmic fashion in order significantly to increase the breathing and heart rate. What is not clear is the optimum duration and intensity of the activity as few studies have simultaneously considered physical activity of different intensities with the risk of CHD. Some reports have suggested that physical activity needs to be vigorous to be effective (Lee et al 1995, Folsom et al 1997), whereas others extend the benefits to more moderate activity (Paffenbarger et al 1993). A more recent study concluded that a 20% reduction in CHD risk could be achieved for total activity levels of more than 4200 kJ per week. This equates to performing activities such as brisk walking, recreational cycling or swimming for 30 minutes a day on most days of the week (Sesso et al 2000). This study also suggested that an active lifestyle may counteract the negative effect of coexisting coronary risk factors. Leisure time physical energy expenditure has been demonstrated to have a beneficial effect on the incidence of fatal or non-fatal

MI and coronary deaths (Wagner et al 2002). Current guidelines recommend 30 minutes of moderate activity on five or more days a week (Joint Health Surveys Unit 1999) which is at present only achieved by about a third of men and a quarter of women. There is evidence that programmes designed to promote physical activity will be more successful if the suggested increase in activity fits into an individual's daily routine (Hillsdon and Thorogood 1996), can be undertaken from home and includes moderate intensity walking as the promoted mode of exercise (Hillsdon et al 1995).

Diabetes

Diabetes significantly increases an individual's risk of developing CHD. It is estimated that about 3% of the adult population have diagnosed diabetes and this number is increasing. The prevalence of diabetes has increased by around two-thirds in men over the past decade (BHF 2003). A significant proportion of those with diabetes will be undiagnosed. The prevalence of diabetes increases with age with almost 10% of those over the age of 75 being diabetic. Men with type 2 diabetes are reported to have a two- to fourfold annual risk of CHD, with an even higher (three- to fivefold) risk in women with type 2 diabetes (BHF 2003). Over 70% of individuals with diabetes will die from macrovascular disease, the majority from cardiovascular disease. Diabetes also increases the effect of other risk factors including raised blood cholesterol, raised blood pressure, obesity and smoking.

Previous diagnostic criteria for diabetes have been broadened in an attempt to include a wider group at increased risk (World Health Organization Expert Committee on Diabetes 1999). The classes are:

- Type 1 diabetes (previously called insulin dependent diabetes mellitus)
- Type 2 diabetes (previously called non-insulin dependent diabetes mellitus)
- Impaired glucose tolerance (fasting plasma glucose under 7 mmol/l; 2 hour post oral glucose tolerance test 7.8–11.1 mmol/l)
- Impaired fasting glucose (fasting plasma glucose between 6.1 and 7 mmol/l).

The classic symptoms of diabetes are polyuria and polydipsea (increased urine output and increased thirst) combined with significant weight loss. For these individuals a diagnosis of diabetes is made through either a random plasma glucose greater than 11.1 mmol/l, a fasting glucose greater than 7.0 mmol/l, or a plasma glucose greater than 11.1 mmol/l two hours following an oral glucose tolerance test. Those that do not have symptoms are likely to be tested opportunistically and a random blood glucose over 5.5 mmol/l indicates the possibility of glucose intolerance.

Diabetes is frequently associated with other risk factors for CHD including being overweight and hypertensive. Weight reduction improves glucose tolerance and is one way the detrimental effects of being diabetic can be reduced.

Haemostatic variables

Raised levels of factors VII and VIII, and fibrinogen, are predictors of CHD mortality. A number of studies (Thompson et al 1991, Muller et al 1985, Tofler et al 1987) have shown that the risk of acute myocardial infarction and sudden cardiac death are more likely to occur at about 0600–1000 hours, a possible explanation being that platelets become more aggregable at these times and are more likely to aggregate at the site of a thrombogenic atherosclerotic lesion and precipitate arterial occlusion.

Hormone levels

The use of hormone replacement therapy (HRT) to reduce cardiovascular risk remains uncertain with recent randomized trials failing to support the promising work of earlier epidemiological studies (Hulley et al 1998, Chin et al 2001).

Vitamin E

Vitamin E consists of a number of compounds that function as lipid-soluble antioxidants. One hypothesis is that vitamin E may slow the progression of atherosclerosis by blocking oxidative modification of LDL cholesterol and thereby decrease its uptake into the arterial lumen. However, several large randomized controlled trials have failed to show any benefit for vitamin E being taken as a dietary supplement. Advice from health professionals needs to reflect the uncertainty over its benefit.

Homocysteine

Homocysteine is derived from the breakdown of the amino acid methionine found in ingested animal protein and levels in the blood are dependent on both genetic and nutritional factors.

Studies have demonstrated the link between homocysteine and CHD with homocysteine levels shown to be an independent risk factor for atherosclerotic vascular disease (Refsum et al 1998). High homocysteine levels induce vascular endothelial dysfunction which predisposes to subsequent atherosclerosis.

It is possible to reduce homocysteine levels by taking vitamin B6, B12 and folate and although it is not known if this reduces the risk of CHD, it seems sensible to advise cardiac patients to eat a diet rich in the B vitamins and folate. However, there needs to be further convincing evidence before measuring blood homocysteine levels becomes routine.

Psychosocial well-being

Defining and measuring psychological well-being is a major problem, however, four different types of psychosocial factor have been linked to increased risk of CHD. These are work stress, lack of social support, depression (including anxiety) and personality (particulary hostility) (Hemingway and Marmot 1999). It is not known how many deaths would be avoided if psychosocial well-being were increased. When asked, individuals will often cite stress or a particular stressful event as contributing to their acute cardiac event and indeed it has been shown that stressful events often precede admission to coronary care (Solomon et al 1969). It is possible that the increased catecholamine activity as a result of sympathetic nerve stimulation may act as a trigger for plaque rupture. Quantifying the effect of stress is difficult and dependent on individual perception. It is also possible that wanting an explanation for a frightening event leads to over-reporting of stress in relation to cardiac events. However, life is full of potential stressors, some more significant than others. One prospective

follow-up study has reported an association between the death of a child and subsequent increased risk of MI in bereaved parents (Li et al 2002).

Apart from influencing mortality figures, psychosocial factors are likely to influence how individuals cope with the day-to-day living with CHD and its management.

Work stress

There is reasonably robust and consistent empirical evidence indicating some causal relationship between work stress and CHD risk (Tennant 2000). It is acknowledged that working in employment which makes very high demands, or in which individuals have very little control over their work, increases the risk of CHD and is more significant than the type or pace of work (Hemingway and Marmot 1999). Women and those under 24 years old are more likely to report having little control over their work (Joint Health Surveys Unit 1996). There is also excessive mortality due to CHD recorded among the unemployed.

Social support

Lack of social support is strongly associated with social class with those in social class V being more than twice as likely to report a severe lack of social support as those in social class I. Inadequate social support or lack of social networks can also have a negative effect on those living with CHD and those recovering from an acute cardiac event.

Depression

There is a special interest in the link between depression and CHD (Creed 1999). The Health Survey for England (Joint Health Surveys Unit 1999) has used the General Health Questionnaire (GHQ12) to assess levels of depression, anxiety, sleep disturbance and happiness in the population. The higher the score, the higher the individual's level of psychological distress. Women tend to have higher scores than men and scores tend to be higher in those over 75 than those in younger age groups.

Personality

Type A behaviour, Type D behaviour, anger and hostility or inadequate coping style have all been shown to influence risk of CHD. Type A characteristics include abrupt gestures, hurried speech, tenseness, impatience and rapid illegible handwriting. Individuals with a classic type A personality strive for success, are very competitive and easily provoked (Friedman and Rosenman 1959). Type D personality, which comprises depression and social inhibition has been found to be closely linked to cardiac risk (Denollet and Brutsaert 1998).

Anger can trigger myocardial ischaemia and may be an independent risk factor for CHD. A high level of anger in response to stress in young men has been found to be associated with an increased risk of subsequent premature cardiovascular disease, particularly myocardial infarction (Chang et al 2002).

Air pollution

Variations in air pollution have been associated with cardiovascular mortality and morbidity. This is thought to occur as a result of increased susceptibility to myocardial ischaemia with increased ambient particle levels leading to a decrease in myocardial oxygen supply and/or an increase in myocardial oxygen demand (Pekkanen et al 2002).

PRIMARY PREVENTION

Primary prevention of CHD refers to its prevention by avoidance of factors known to contribute to its development. The fact that mortality from CHD in the UK fell by over 40% in the decade from 1982 highlights that changes in lifestyle and treatment are of value, since that time span is too short for genetic factors to have had effect.

The second chapter of the National Service Framework for CHD (DoH 2000) focuses on the prevention of CHD and sets a standard that general practitioners and primary health care teams should identify all people at significant risk of CHD but who have not yet developed symptoms and offer them appropriate advice and treatment to reduce their risk.

It is likely that central organization, agreed quality assurance standards, adequate resources and management structures need to be developed in order to make any primary prevention screening programme effective (Rouse and Adab 2001).

The National Service Framework for CHD makes the points that:

- People who have either (a) the symptoms of heart disease, other occlusive arterial disease or peripheral vascular disease or (b) multiple risk factors for heart disease, are three to five times more likely to suffer a major cardiovascular event than those without.
- People's risks can be reduced by up to two-thirds with appropriate treatment and lifestyle changes.
- The progression of established CHD can be slowed and possibly reversed with appropriate intervention.
- The people likely to benefit most from treatment are those at greatest risk.
- Treatment is most cost effective in those at greatest risk.
- Decisions around the allocation of resources for primary prevention need to take into account: the treatment benefit for individuals; the numbers eligible for treatment; cost effectiveness and total resource implications of policies evolving from decisions made.
- The first priority is to identify, advise and treat those with clinical evidence of CHD. The second is to do the same for those who are free from symptoms but who have a greater than 30% risk of a cardiac event in the next 10 years.
- New evidence on effectiveness and cost effectiveness of interventions needs to be evaluated and incorporated into policies as appropriate.

For patients with established CHD and individuals at high multifactorial risk of developing CHD, the same lifestyle and risk factor goals are appropriate (Wood 2001).

The National Service Framework recommends the following interventions for those without clinical evidence of CHD but with an event risk greater than 30% over 10 years:

- advice about how to stop smoking including advice on the use of nicotine replacement therapy
- information on other modifiable risk factors and individualized advice about how they can

be reduced (including advice about physical activity, diet, alcohol consumption, weight and diabetes)
- advice and treatment to maintain blood pressure below 140/85 mmHg
- add statins to lower serum cholesterol concentrations either to less than 5 mmol/l (LDH to below 3 mmol/l) *or* by 30% whichever is the greater
- meticulous control of blood pressure and glucose in individuals who also have diabetes.

Further work is needed to determine whether other interventions such as the use of antithrombotic agents (warfarin and/or aspirin) have any benefit in primary prevention (Knottenbelt et al 2002).

As atherosclerosis has been shown to have its origins in childhood with a progression towards clinically significant lesions in young adulthood being strongly influenced by CHD risk factors, true primary prevention must begin in childhood or early adolescence (Zieske et al 2002).

The value of any intervention is best determined by attempting to quantify how it will influence an individual's overall risk of CHD taking into account both the significance of the individual risk factor and its contribution to the overall risk profile for that individual. Evidence from intervention studies that link multiple risk factor intervention with reduced mortality is limited, although this strategy has been shown to benefit high-risk groups such as those with hypertension (Ebrahim and Davey-Smith 2004). Primary prevention strategies often require numerous people to be treated over prolonged periods to prevent illness in a few and so their ratio of cost to benefit may be poor in relation to other clinical activities. This further highlights the need to target those at greatest risk (McNeil et al 2001).

Identifying those at risk

Those with known CHD or with significant risk factors are known to be at high risk of cardiac events and do not need this quantifying to decide on treatment. However, for other groups, their risk for CHD can be derived from population-based epidemiological studies of heart disease that give information about the relationship between risk factors, their interactions and subsequent CHD. Apparently healthy individuals with several mildly abnormal risk factors may be more at risk than those with just one high risk factor and therefore risk factors need to be considered together to determine absolute risk. The Framingham study followed 5000 individuals who were free from heart disease in the 1940s and recorded the prevalence, incidence and prognosis of heart disease as it developed in these individuals over time. Information from the Framingham data has been used to develop mathematical equations of the relationships between quantifiable variables which allow clinicians to calculate an individual's coronary risk (Anderson et al 1990). It is currently the best source of such data, and its use is recommended by the European Society of Cardiology. However, as it is based on a specific population from a North American city and excludes information on the impact of several risk factors including family history and meaningful data from minority groups, its use as a predictive tool for UK individuals has some limitations.

Table 1.4 gives a list of risk assessment tools recommended by the Department of Health (2000) in the National Service Framework for CHD.

Data about risk factors need to be collected systematically to allow the use of the most appropriate calculation tools. The information traditionally available in patient's records is not enough to undertake an accurate risk assessment and more comprehensive methods of data collection need to become routine. One study of general practices in England found that a record of HDL-cholesterol levels was present in less than a quarter of records (McManus et al 2002). This same study also found that both general practitioners and practice nurses

Table 1.4 Risk assessment tools recommended by the Department of Health 2000 (National Service Framework for CHD)

- Coronary risk prediction chart and the associated computer disc (Durrington et al 1999)
- Sheffield risk tables (Wallis et al 2000)
- European coronary risk chart (Wood et al 1998)
- University College London computer program (Hinorani and Vallance 1999)

were able to evaluate the risk of CHD with only moderate accuracy and that there was only moderate agreement between the two professional groups.

Improving the communication between primary and secondary health care is likely to help identify some individuals with significant risk factors for CHD, particularly those experiencing a cardiac event in hospital. Having standardized discharge forms which convey relevant information promptly to the general practitioner may go some way in facilitating this as may the use of faxes and communication by e-mail.

Once individuals at risk have been identified, a record of them, their significant risk factors and treatment regimens may help develop systems of care for treatment and follow up. Effective audit can then be used to monitor the quality of care that is given.

Delivering primary prevention

There need to be well structured and organized systems of care delivery in order to maximize treatment for those at high risk of CHD. Otherwise too many individuals will remain unidentified, inadequately treated and not followed up. There need to be systems in place to (DoH 2000):

- identify those at high risk of CHD using appropriate risk assessment tools
- identify and record modifiable risk factors for those at high risk
- use protocols, guidelines and patient held records to inform practice

- invite identified individuals to special cardiac prevention clinics
- document the delivery of appropriate advice and treatment to this group
- monitor equality of access and uptake of services
- offer regular review.

There is evidence that the process of identifying those at high risk for CHD who would benefit from treatment does not necessarily lead to more people being treated (Ford et al 2001). Primary care providers need to examine the systems they have in place to use risk assessment results appropriately. The shift towards a primary care led NHS, together with other health and policy changes, offer opportunities for nurses to develop their roles in new ways. Introducing nurse-led clinics to support the above process has been shown significantly to increase the numbers of individuals being offered appropriate treatment (Campbell et al 1998).

Offering patients at risk from CHD appropriate treatment does not always lead to this treatment being followed. The decisions around compliance with therapy, particularly drug therapy, are complex. Individuals without symptoms may refuse treatment regardless of the risk reduction offered. There may also be a notable proportion of patients whose level of required risk reduction is considerably greater than what is achievable with treatment (Llewellyn-Thomas et al 2002). Individuals need to be given straightforward individualized advice to help them make informed decisions about compliance with therapy.

References

Anderson KM, Odell PM, Wilson PWF, Kannel WB (1990). Cardiovascular disease risk profiles. *American Heart Journal*, 121: 293–298.

Balarajan R (1991). Ethnic differences in mortality from ischaemic heart disease and cerebrovascular disease in England and Wales. *British Medical Journal*, 302: 560–564.

Beaglehole R (1999). International trends in coronary heart disease mortality and incidence rates. *Journal of Cardiovascular Risk*, 6: 63–68.

Bentley DR (2000). The Human Genome Project – an overview. *Medical Research Reviews*, 20: 189–196.

Bhopal R (2000). What is the risk of coronary heart disease in South Asians? A review of UK research. *Journal of Public Health Medicine*, 22: 375–385.

Bhopal R, Unwin N, White M et al (1999). Heterogeneity of coronary disease risk factors in Indian, Pakistani, Bangladeshi and European origin populations: a cross sectional study. *British Medical Journal*, 319: 215–220.

Boreham C, Twisk J, Murray L et al (2001). Fitness, fatness and coronary heart disease risk in adolescents: the Northern Island Young Hearts Project. *Medicine & Science in Sports & Excercise*, 33: 270–274.

Bostom AG, Cupples LA, Jenner JL et al (1996). Elevated plasma lipoprotein (a) and coronary heart disease in men aged 55 years and younger. A prospective study. *Journal of the American Medical Association*, 276: 544–548.

British Heart Foundation (2003). *Coronary Heart Disease Statistics Database*. BHF, London.

Callum C (1998). *The UK Smoking Epidemic: Deaths in 1995.* Health Education Authority, London.

Campbell NC, Thain J, Deans HG et al (1998). Secondary prevention clinics for coronary heart disease: randomised trial of effect on health. *British Medical Journal*, 316: 1434–1437.

Chang PP, Ford DE, Meoni LA et al (2002). Anger in young men and subsequent premature cardiovascular disease: the precursors study. *Archives of Internal Medicine*, 162: 901–906.

Chin BS, Futaba K, Jethwa A, Lip GY (2001). The impact of coronary heart disease in determining use of hormone replacement therapy in a general practice population (Comment). *International Journal of Clinical Practice*, 55: 515–518.

Clarke KW, Gray D, Keating NA et al (1994). Do women with acute myocardial infarction receive the same treatment as men? *British Medical Journal*, 309: 563–566.

Creed F (1999). The importance of depression following myocardial infarction. *Heart*, 82: 406–408.

Davies MJ (1987). Pathology of ischaemic heart disease. In *Ischaemic Heart Disease* (KM Fox, ed.), MTP Press, Lancaster, pp. 33–68.

Denollet J, Brutsaert DL (1998). Personality, disease severity and the risk of long term cardiac events in patients with a decreased ejection fraction after myocardial infarction. *Circulation*, 97: 167–173.

Department of Health (1994). *Nutritional Aspects of Cardiovascular Disease. Report of the Cardiovascular Review Group on the Committee on Medical Aspects (CoMA) of Food Policy.* HMSO, London.

Department of Health (1995a). *Variations in Health: what can the Department of Health and the NHS do? Report of the Variations Sub-group of the Chief Medical Officer's Health of the Nation Working Group.* HMSO, London.

Department of Health (1995b.) *Sensible Drinking. The Report of an Inter-Department Working Group.* The Stationary Office, London.

Department of Health (1998). *Smoking Kills: A White Paper on Tobacco.* HMSO, London.

Department of Health (1999a). *Saving Lives: Our Healthier Nation.* Department of Health, London.

Department of Health (1999b). *Health Survey for England: Cardiovascular Disease 1998.* Stationery Office, London.

Department of Health (2000). *The National Service Framework for Coronary Heart Disease.* Department of Health, London.

Downs JR, Clearfield M, Weis et al (1998). The AFCAPS/TexCAPS Research Group. Primary prevention of acute coronary events with lovastatin in men and women with average cholesterol levels: results of AFCAPS/TexCAPS. *Journal of the American Medical Association*, 279: 1615–1622.

Durringtom P, Prais H, Bhatnagar D et al (1999). Indications for cholesterol-lowering medication: comparison of risk–assessment methods. *Lancet*, 353: 278–281.

Ebrahim S, Davey-Smith G (2004). Multiple risk factor interventions for primary prevention of coronary heart disease (Cochrane Review). In: The Cochrane Library, Issue 1. John Wiley, Chichester.

Ellsworth DL, Sholinsky P, Jaquish C, Fabsitz RR, Manolio TA (1999). Coronary heart disease. At the interface of molecular genetics and preventive medicine. *American Journal of Preventive Medicine*, 16: 122–133.

Eriksson JG, Forsen T, Tuomilehto J et al (2001). Early growth and coronary heart disease in later life: longitudinal study. *British Medical Journal* 323: 572–573.

Folsom AR, Arnett DK, Hutchinson RG et al (1997). Physical activity and incidence of coronary heart disease in middle-aged women and men. *Medicine & Science in Sports & Exercise*, 2: 901–909.

Ford DR, Walker J, Game FL et al (2001). Effect of computerised coronary heart disease risk assessment on the use of lipid lowering therapy in general practice patients. *Coronary Health Care*, 5: 4–8.

Freund KM, Belanger AJ, D'Agostino RB et al (1993). The health risks of smoking. The Framingham Study: 34 years of follow up. *Annals of Epidemiology*, 3: 417–424.

Friedman M, Rosenman RH (1959). Association of specific overt behavior pattern with blood and cardiovascular findings. *Journal of the American Medical Association*, 169: 1286–1296.

Gotto AM Jr (1999). Lipid management in patients at moderate risk for coronary heart disease: insights from the Air Force/Texas Coronary Atherosclerosis Prevention Study (AFCAPS/TexCAPS). *American Journal of Medicine*, 107(2A): 36S–39S.

Heart Protection Study Group (2002). MRC/BHF heart protection study of cholesterol lowering with simvastatin in 20 536 high risk individuals: a randomised placebo-controlled trial. *Lancet*, 360: 7–22.

Hemingway H, Marmot M (1999). Psychosocial factors in the aetiology and prognosis of coronary heart disease: review of prospective cohort studies. *British Medical Journal*, 318: 1460–1467.

Hillsdon M, Thorogood M, Anstiss et al (1995). Randomised controlled trials of physical activity promotion in free living populations: A review. *Journal of Epidemiology and Community Health*, 49: 445–453.

Hillsdon M, Thorogood M (1996). A systematic review of exercise promotion strategies. *British Journal of Sports Medicine*, 30: 84–89.

Hinorani AD, Vallance P (1999). A simple computer program for guiding management of cardiovascular risk factors and prescribing. *British Medical Journal*, 318: 101–105.

Hulley SB, Grady D, Bush T et al (1998). Randomised trial of estrogen plus progestin for secondary prevention of coronary heart disease in post-menopausal women. *Journal of the American Medical Association*, 280: 605–613.

Irvine MJ, Logan AG (1994). Is knowing your cholesterol number harmful? *Journal of Clinical Epidemiology*, 47: 131–145.

Joint Health Surveys Unit (1996). *Health Surveys for England 1994.* The Stationery Office, London.

Joint Health Surveys Unit (1999). *Health Surveys for England 1998.* The Stationery Office, London.

Joint Health Surveys Unit (2001). *Health Surveys for England. The Health of Minority Ethnic Groups 1999.* The Stationery Office, London.

Kannel WB, Larson M (1993). Long term epidemiological prediction of coronary disease. *Cardiology*, 82: 137–152.

Kannel WB (2002). Coronary heart disease risk factors in the elderly. *American Journal of Cardiology*, 11: 101–107.

Knottenbelt C, Brennan PJ, Meade TW. Medical Research Council's general practice research framework (2002). *Archives of Internal Medicine*, 162: 881–886.

Law MR, Wald NJ, Wu T et al (1994). Systematic under-estimation of association between serum cholesterol and ischaemic heart disease in observational studies: data from the BUPA study. *British Medical Journal*, 308: 363–366.

Lee IM, Hsieh CC, Paffenbarger RS et al (1995). Exercise intensity and longevity in men: the Harvard Alumni Health Study. *Journal of the American Medical Association*, 273: 1179–1184.

Llewellyn-Thomas HA, Paterson JM, Carter JM et al (2002). Primary prevention drug therapy: can it meet patients' requirements for reduced risk? *Medical Decision Making*, 22: 326–329.

Li J, Hansen D, Mortensen PB et al (2002). Myocardial infarction in parents who have lost a child: a nationwide prospective cohort study in Denmark. *Circulation*, 106: 1634–1639.

Lip GY, Edmunds E, Beevers DG (2001). Should patients with hypertension receive antithrombotic therapy? *Journal of Internal Medicine*, 249: 205–214.

Liu JLY, Manìadakis N, Gray A, Raynor M (2002). The economic burden of coronary heart disease in the UK. *Heart*, 88: 597–603.

Lukkarinen H, Hentinen M (1997). Assessment of quality of life with the Nottingham Health Profile among patients with coronary heart disease. *Journal of Advanced Nursing*, 26: 73–84.

McEwen J (1993). The Nottingham Health Profile: a measure of perceived health. In *Quality of Life: Key Issues in the 1990s* (Walker SR, Rosser, eds), Kluwer Academic, London, pp. 111–130.

McKeigue P, Sevak L (1994). *Coronary Heart Disease in South Asian Communities*. Health Education Authority, London.

McManus RJ, Mant J, Meulenijks CF (2002). Comparison of estimates and calculations of risk of coronary heart disease by doctors and nurses using different calculation tools in general practice. Cross sectional study. *British Medical Journal*, 324: 459–464.

McNeil JJ, Peeters A, Liew D, Lim S, Vos T (2001). A model for predicting the future incidence of coronary heart disease within percentiles of coronary heart disease risk. *Journal of Cardiovascular Risk*, 8: 31–37.

Miura K, Daviglus ML, Dyer AR, et al (2001). Comment. *Archives of Internal Medicine*, 162: 610–611.

Muller JE, Stone PH, Turi ZG et al (1985). Circadian variation in the frequency of onset of acute myocardial infarction. *New England Journal of Medicine*, 313: 1315–1322.

National Heart Forum (2002). *Coronary Heart Disease: Estimating the Impact of Changes in Risk Factors*. The Stationery Office, London.

Neaton JD, Wentworth D (1992). Serum cholesterol, blood pressure, cigarette smoking and death from coronary heart disease. Overall findings and differences by age for 316 099 white men. Multiple Risk Factor Intervention Trial Research Group (1992). *Archives of Internal Medicine*, 152: 56–64.

Paffenbarger RS, Hyde RT, Wing et al (1993). The association of changes in physical activity level and other lifestyle characteristics with mortality among men. *New England Journal of Medicine*, 328: 538–545.

Pekkanen J, Peters A, Hoek G et al (2002). Particulate air pollution and risk of ST segment depression during repeated submaximal exercise tests among subjects with coronary heart disease: the exposure and risk assessment for fine and ultra fine particles in ambient air (ULTRA) study. *Circulation*, 106: 933–938.

Pinto RJ (1998). Risk factors for coronary heart disease in Asian Indians: clinical implications for prevention of coronary heart disease. *Indian Journal of Medical Sciences*, 52: 49–54.

Refsum H, Ueland PM, Nygard O et al (1998). Homocysteine and cardiovascular disease. *Annual Review of Medicine*, 49: 31–62.

Rouse A, Adab P (2001). Is population coronary heart disease screening justified? A discussion of the National Service Framework for Coronary Heart Disease (standard 4). *British Journal of General Practice*, 51: 834–837.

Salomaa V, Rosamond W, Mahonen M (1999). Decreasing mortality from acute myocardial infarction: effect of incidence and prognosis. *Journal of Cardiovascular Risk*, 6: 69–75.

Sesso H, Paffenbarger R, Lee IM (2000). Physical activity and coronary heart disease in men: the Harvard Alumni health study. *Circulation*, 102: 975–980.

Shepherd J, Cobbe SM, Ford I et al (1995). The West of Scotland Coronary Prevention Study Group: prevention of coronary heart disease with pravastatin in men with hypercholesterolemia. *New England Journal of Medicine*, 333: 1301–1307.

Solomon HA, Edwards AL, Killip T (1969). Prodromata in acute myocardial infarction. *Circulation*, 40: 463–471.

Tennant C (2000). Work stress and coronary heart disease. *Journal of Cardiovascular Risk*, 7: 273–276.

Thompson DR (1990). *Counselling the Coronary Patient and Partner*. Scutari, London.

Thompson DR, Sutton TW, Jowett NI et al (1991). Circadian variation in the frequency of onset of chest pain in acute myocardial infarction. *British Heart Journal*, 65: 177–178.

Tofler GH, Brezinski D, Schafer A et al (1987). Concurrent morning increase in platelet aggregability and the risk of myocardial infarction and sudden cardiac death. *New England Journal of Medicine*, 316: 1514–1518.

Tunstall-Pedoe H, Kuulasmaa K, Amouyeln P et al (1994). Myocardial infarctions and coronary deaths in the World Health Organization (MONICA) project. Registration procedures, event rates, and case fatality rates in 38 populations from 21 countries in four continents. *Circulation*, 90: 583–612.

Tunstall-Pedoe H, Kuulasmaa K, Mahonen M et al (1999). Contribution of trends in survival and coronary event rates to changes in coronary heart disease mortality: 10 year results from 37 WHO MONICA project populations. *Lancet*, 53: 1547–1557.

UKPDS (1998). The United Kingdom Prospective Diabetes Study Group 38. Tight blood pressure control and risk of macrovascular complications in type 2 diabetes. *British Medical Journal*, 317: 703–713.

Wagner A, Simon C, Evans A et al (2002). Physical activity and coronary event incidence in Northern Ireland and France: The Prospective Epidemiological Study of Myocardial Infarction (PRIME). *Circulation*, 105: 2247–2252.

Wallis EJ, Ramsay LE, ul Haq I et al (2000). Coronary and cardiovascular risk estimation for primary prevention: population validation of a new Sheffield table in the 1995 Scottish health survey population. *British Medical Journal*, 320: 671–676.

Williams B, Poulter NR, Brown MJ et al (2004). British Hypertension Society guidelines for hypertension management 2004 (BHS-IV): Summary. *British Medical Journal*, 328: 634–640.

Wood D, de Backer G, Faergeman O et al (1998). For the Second Joint Task Force of European and other societies on coronary prevention. Prevention of coronary heart disease in clinical practice. *European Heart Journal*, 19: 1434–1503.

Wood D (2001). Joint European Societies Task Force. Established and emerging cardiovascular risk factors. *American Heart Journal*, 141: S49–57.

World Health Organisation Expert Committee on Diabetes Mellitus (1999). *Diagnosis and Classification of Diabetes Mellitus and its Complications*. WHO, Geneva.

Zieske AW, Malcom GT, Strong JP (2002). Natural history and risk factor of atherosclerosis in children and youth: the PDAY study. *Pediatric Pathology and Molecular Medicine*, 21: 213–237.

Further reading

Hatchett R, Thompson DR (eds) (2002). *Cardiac Nursing: A Comprehensive Guide*. Harcourt, London.

Jowett NI, Thompson DR (2003). *Comprehensive Coronary Care*, 3rd edn. Baillière Tindall, London.

Stewart S, Moser DK, Thompson DR (eds) (2004). *Caring for the Heart Failure Patient*. Martin Dunitz, London.

Chapter **2**

Cardiac structure and function

The heart is a double pump which maintains both pulmonary and systemic circulations. The basic function is:

- to transport oxygen and other nutrients to the body cells
- to remove carbon dioxide and metabolic waste products from the tissues and the lungs
- to convey substances such as water, electrolytes and hormones from one part of the body to another
- to support the immune system
- thermoregulation.

CARDIAC STRUCTURE

The heart is a hollow, fibromuscular cone-shaped organ about the size of the person's fist and weighing between 230 and 340 g. It is located in the mediastinum, one third lying to the right of the sternum and the rest to the left. The top of the heart is usually termed the base and lies in an oblique position behind the sternum. The lowest point of the heart is referred to as the apex and this lies to the left in the fifth intercostal space behind the mid-clavicular line (Figure 2.1).

The heart consists of two specialized pumps (one left and one right), each of which contains two valves. Each side of the heart contains two chambers, an atrium and a ventricle. The atria and ventricles are separated by a band of fibrous connective tissue which provides a framework for the heart valves. The thin-walled atria serve to 'prime' the thick-walled ventricles. Blood enters and leaves each heart chamber through one way valves, which

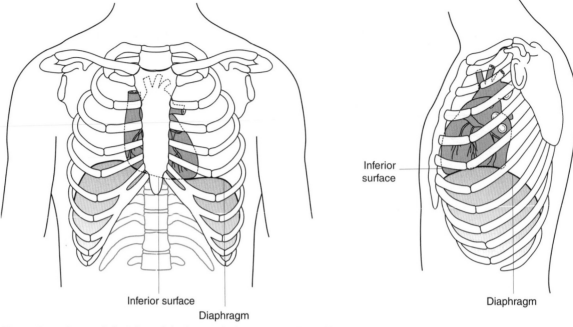

Figure 2.1 Anatomic location of the heart within the thoracic cavity.

open and close in a coordinated manner so that one closes before the other opens thus ensuring one directional blood flow through the heart. The right and left sides of the heart are separated by the inter-atrial septum and the interventricular septum.

The flow of blood through the heart

Deoxygenated blood from the body returns to the right side of the heart through the superior and inferior venae cavae and into the right atrium. From the right atrium the blood passes through the tricuspid valve into the right ventricle. Contraction of the right ventricle, simultaneous with that of the left ventricle, forces blood through the pulmonary valve into the pulmonary artery and to the lungs. Oxygenation occurs in the lungs, after which the blood returns to the left atrium via the pulmonary veins. From the left atrium, blood passes through the mitral (bicuspid) valve into the left ventricle. The oxygenated blood is then ejected from the left ventricle through the aortic valve and to the aorta and the body via the systemic circulation.

Cardiac cycle

This is the cyclical contraction (systole) and relaxation (diastole) of the two atria and the two ventricles. Each cycle is initiated by spontaneous generation of an action potential in the sinus node.

Diastole

During diastole each chamber fills with blood. Blood enters the relaxed atria and flows passively into the relaxed ventricles. Diastole usually lasts 0.4 s.

Systole

During systole the blood is expelled. Both atria and ventricles contract almost simultaneously. The duration of atrial systole is about 0.1 s and that of ventricular systole 0.3 s. Thus, the combined duration of systole is about 0.4 s.

Heart rate

The normal heart rate is about 70 beats/min in the resting adult, and the duration of the cardiac cycle is about 0.8 s.

Volume

The volume of the heart is some 700 ml at the end of diastole, whereas the actual volume of muscle is about 300 ml; therefore, the cavities may contain about 400 ml of blood (end-diastolic volume), an amount that is much greater than the quantity expelled by both ventricles each time they contract (about 140 ml).

Provided that the heart receives excitation along the normal pathways and the heart rate remains constant, each successive cardiac cycle follows the same pattern of systole and diastole.

Valves of the heart

In order to understand the cardiac cycle it is important to appreciate the role of the heart valves in coordinating blood flow.

The atrioventricular valves are the tricuspid and the mitral (bicuspid) valves which allow passage of blood from the atria to the ventricles. The tricuspid valve is situated between the right atrium and the right ventricle and has three cusps or leaflets (flaps): septal, anterior and posterior. The mitral valve has two cusps and controls the inlet from the left atrium to the left ventricle. The cusps of the valves are tethered to the ventricular walls by fan-shaped chordae tendineae of varying lengths and thicknesses.

When the valves are open, their cusps hang loosely into the ventricles and blood passes through them. The valves are passive and the cusps close during systole when the build up of pressure in the ventricles causes the blood to push up against them and push them together. This prevents the blood flowing back into the atria in a retrograde manner. The chordae tendineae prevent the ventricular pressure pushing the cusps back into the atrium.

The semilunar valves are the pulmonary and aortic valves. Both are three cusped valves which help control the exit of blood from the ventricles. The pulmonary valve lies between the right ventricle and the pulmonary artery and is the gate to the pulmonary outflow tract. The aortic valve helps regulate the flow of blood from the left ventricle into the aorta. The aortic valve is stronger than the pulmonary valve as it has to cope with the higher pressures in the left side of the heart. At the origin of each of the aortic valve cusps is a slight dilatation or sinus known collectively as the sinuses of Valsalva. The right coronary artery

arises from the right aortic sinus and the left coronary artery from the left aortic sinus.

The semilunar valves close passively at the end of systole because ventricular contraction causes the pressure in the ventricles to rise above that behind the valves in the aorta and the pulmonary trunk. This forces the cusps backwards and the valves open allowing blood to be pumped out into the pulmonary and systemic circuits. When the pressure in the ventricles falls below that of the major vessels, blood will begin to flow backwards until the cusps fill with blood and close the valve.

Chambers of the heart

The atria

The atria are thin-walled muscular chambers that form the most anterior aspect of the heart.

The right atrium forms the lower right lateral border on the chest radiograph. It is a thin-walled chamber that receives the venous return to the heart from the superior and inferior venae cavae. It also receives blood from the cardiac sinus and the anterior cardiac veins. The right AV orifice and the tricuspid valve perforate the right atrial floor. The interatrial septum features a fibrous oval depression known as the fossa ovalis which marks the site of the fetal foramen ovale.

The left atrium is the most posterior heart chamber and lies to the midline behind the right ventricle. It is the only chamber not normally seen in the chest X-ray. The left atrium receives blood from the pulmonary veins. The pressure in the left atrium tends to be higher than that in the right as the left atrium is slightly smaller and less distensible.

Atrial function

The atria serve as reservoirs for blood returning to the heart from the pulmonary and systemic circulations. They are able to adapt to the volume of blood they receive by distending when they are full and reducing in size when venous return is reduced.

In atrial systole, contraction of the right atrium usually very slightly precedes that of the left. The muscular contraction forces blood from the atria through the AV valves into the ventricles during the last phase of passive ventricular filling. This causes small increases in the pressures in both the atria and the ventricles because the AV valves are still open. As there are no valves between the right atrium and venae cavae, some blood is expelled backwards during atrial systole causing a rise in venous pressure. At the end of atrial systole the blood continues to move through the valves because of its inertia. The delay of electrical transmission at the AV node allows the atria to contract completely before ventricular contraction starts.

The ventricles

The ventricles are divided by the intraventricular septum which ensures that two separate circulations are maintained. Both ventricles have a spiral arrangement of muscles to ensure that blood is propelled into the respective outflow tracts (the aorta and pulmonary artery) during systole.

The right ventricle is located directly beneath the sternum and extends from the tricuspid valve to the apex. It is much smaller than the left ventricle and has thinner walls reflecting its role as pump into the low resistance pulmonary circuit.

The left ventricle forms the lower lateral cardiac border and lies posteriorly and left of the right ventricle. It lies approximately in the fifth intercostal space within the mid-clavicular line. As it normally ejects blood against a higher resistance than the right ventricle, the walls of the left ventricle are more muscular than those of the right ventricle.

Ventricular function

Ventricular function begins soon after the start of ventricular excitation. The pressure of blood in the ventricles begins to rise while that in the relaxing atria is falling. The cusps of the AV valves close and then bulge backwards momentarily into the atria. This momentary backward bulging of the AV valve cusps produces slight transient increases of pressure in the atria. After the closure of the AV valves the blood pressure rises in both ventricles. Because both the AV and the semilunar valves are closed, the volume of intraventricular blood remains constant. During this isovolumetric (isometric) phase of ventricular contraction the ventricles alter their shape, becoming plumper. When the rising ventricular pressures exceed the pressures

in the aorta and pulmonary artery the semilunar valves open, the isometric phase ends and the ejection (isotonic) phase of contraction begins. At the end of this phase the ventricular muscle relaxes, and when the pressures fall below those in the aorta and pulmonary artery the semilunar valves open.

Throughout ventricular systole the ventricular volume falls. Simultaneously, blood has been entering the atria. Because the AV valves are closed the intra-atrial pressure gradually rises. After the closure of the semilunar valves, the pressure in the ventricles falls rapidly and is soon below that in the atria. At this point the AV valves open and blood flows passively from the atria to the ventricles, at first very fast, later more slowly.

Tissues of the heart

The main mass of the heart consists of muscular tissue (the myocardium). Blood and lymphatic vessels, nerves and specialized conduction cells are found in the myocardial tissues.

The epicardium

The epicardium is a single layer of mesothelial cells over a layer of connective tissue containing small blood vessels, elastic fibres and nerves. In places it is separated from the myocardium by a layer of adipose tissue which carries the coronary blood vessels.

The myocardium

The myocardium is thickest towards the apex and thins towards the base, a reflection of the differing amounts of work undertaken by different parts of the heart. The myocardium is composed of specialized involuntary cardiac muscle. Myocardial cells are grouped into bundles within connective tissues and these bundles carry the small blood vessels, lymphatic vessels and autonomic nerve fibres. There is a large density of capillaries in the myocardium to meet the high oxygen demands of the cardiac muscle. The muscles of the myocardium are both transverse and longitudinal and are in close contact with each other so that once contraction is initiated it spreads throughout the entire network of muscle cells.

The endocardium

The endocardium is the inner lining of the heart and is much thinner than the epicardium. It consists of a lining of endothelial cells, a middle layer of dense elastic connective tissue and an outer layer of loose connective tissue containing small blood vessels and specialized conducting tissue. The endocardium is thought to be the source of several chemical mediators that are involved in vasoregulation, including nitric oxide (NO_2) which is a powerful vasodilator and endothelin which is a vasoconstrictor. The heart valves are formed from folds of endocardium thickened by a core of fibrous tissue.

Cardiac cells

The heart is composed of two major types of cardiac cells: those specialized for contraction (myocardial cells), and those specialized for impulse formation (automatic cells). Within these two groups there are differences. For instance, myocardial cells in the atria are anatomically and physiologically different from the myocardial cells in the ventricles.

Myocardial cells

Myocardial cells comprise the main bulk of the atria and ventricles. They are complex structures, generally elongated and clustered tightly together in rope-like strands which function to provide a mechanical pumping action for the heart. There are four basic elements in the myocardial cell structure:

1 cell membrane
2 cytoplasm
3 contractile elements
4 sarcoplasmic reticulum.

Each cell contains a central nucleus with numerous myofibrils aligned along the cell's axis, and a large number of mitochondria. The cell is enclosed by its plasma membrane (sarcolemma) through which the cardiac electrical activity exerts its important function.

The myofibrils resemble those of skeletal muscle, with sets of the proteins actin and myosin present

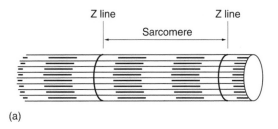

(a)

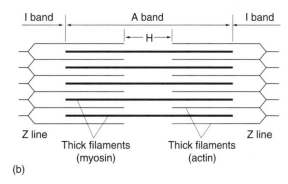

(b)

Figure 2.2 Microscopic structure of myofibrils: (a) myofibrils within a single muscle fibre; (b) myofilaments.

in hexagonally arranged myofilaments (Figure 2.2). Tropomyosin and troponin are also present. In the mitochondria lying close to the myofibrils, the energy of the metabolic substrates (glucose, fatty acids, lactate and pyruvate) is converted to high-energy compounds of creatine phosphate (CP) and ATP. The breakdown of ATP at the myofibrillar bridges releases energy for the contraction of the myofibrils.

Pulmonary circuit

The circulation is a continuous circuit, although it is often conveniently divided into the systemic and pulmonary circuits.

The pulmonary circuit is a low-pressure system with short, wide, thin-walled vessels and a capacity of small volume containing at rest only 500–900 ml of blood.

The pulmonary circulation normally carries all the cardiac output through the lungs at a mean pressure in the adult of 15 mmHg (less than one-sixth of that in the systemic circulation) and hence its resistance to blood flow is one-sixth of the systemic circulation. The total pulmonary blood volume is about 700 ml, with about 60% of this volume in the venous side. The normal pulmonary capillary pressure is about 6–12 mmHg and the normal pulmonary capillary blood volume at rest is about 100 ml (less than half that of the systemic capillaries).

Systemic circuit

The systemic circuit is a high-pressure system which supplies all the tissues of the body, except the lungs, with blood. The aorta functions as a compression chamber or reservoir for blood during the rapid ejection phase from the left ventricle. This is due to the elasticity of the vessel. As the branches arising from the aorta divide, the total cross-sectional area of the arteries, arterioles and capillaries increases and the velocity of blood flow decreases. The arterioles offer the greatest resistance to flow. The capillaries usually have walls consisting of single endothelial cells. Within the capillary bed there is often stasis of flow in some capillaries and an active flow in others. The normal systemic capillary pressure is about 24–35 mmHg and the normal systemic capillary blood volume at rest is about 5% of the total volume (250 ml).

BLOOD SUPPLY TO THE HEART

Coronary arteries

The heart uses vast amounts of energy to function as a pump, which it gets by generating large quantities of adenosine triphosphate (ATP) by oxidative metabolism. Thus, the heart requires a large and continuous supply of oxygen and cannot sustain an oxygen debt for more than a few seconds without becoming severely depressed. Because the myocardial demand for oxygen is so great, the heart requires a rich blood supply.

The heart and the proximal portions of the great vessels receive almost all their blood supply from the two coronary arteries, which arise from the aortic bulb composed of the three aortic sinuses. For functional purposes, the two divisions of the left coronary artery, together with the right coronary artery, are regarded as three coronary arteries supplying the myocardium (Figure 2.3).

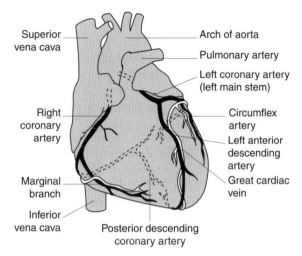

Figure 2.3 The coronary arteries.

The *right coronary artery* arises from the right aortic sinus and supplies the right atrium, right ventricle and posterior aspect of the left ventricle. It runs forward to the atrioventricular (AV) groove, and gives off a small branch to the sinus node. It passes downwards in the groove and rounds the inferior margin of the heart, giving off its marginal branch to supply the right ventricular wall. It then winds around the heart to the posterior aspect and passes down the interventricular groove as the posterior descending branch which supplies the ventricles and interventricular septum. Often a transverse branch continues in the posterior AV groove, supplying branches to the left atrium, before anastomosing with the circumflex branch of the left coronary artery.

The *left coronary artery* is the largest and most important of the main coronary arteries. It arises from the left posterior sinus of the aorta and runs to the left behind the pulmonary trunk and then forward between it and the left auricle to the atrioventricular groove. Here, it divides into its two branches: an *anterior descending branch* and a *circumflex branch*.

The *left anterior descending branch* descends in the anterior interventricular groove to the apex of the heart, where it turns round to ascend a short distance up the posterior interventricular groove, anastomosing with the posterior interventricular branch of the right coronary artery. Diagonal branches

Table 2.1 Regions of the heart supplied by the coronary arteries

Right coronary artery (RCA)
  Right atrium
  Right ventricle
  Inferior left ventricle
  Sinus node
  Atrioventricular node
  Posterior interventricular septum

Left anterior descending (LAD) coronary artery
  Anterior wall of left ventricle
  Anterior interventricular septum
  Apex of left ventricle
  Bundle of His and bundle branches

Left circumflex (LCx) coronary artery
  Left atrium
  Lateral and posterior left ventricle
  Posterior interventricular septum

supply the anterior ventricular wall, and special branches supply the interventricular septum.

The *circumflex* branch passes round the left margin of the heart in the AV groove, supplying branches to the left atrium and the left surface of the heart. In some individuals (15–20%) the circumflex artery gives rise to the posterior descending artery. This is called left dominance. The left marginal branch arises from the circumflex artery, and runs down the left margin of the left ventricle (Table 2.1).

Coronary veins

The veins of the heart drain chiefly into the *coronary sinus* which occupies the posterior part of the AV groove, between the left atrium and left ventricle, and opens into the right atrium. However, some coronary flow from the anterior cardiac veins returns directly to the left atrium and ventricle.

Coronary blood flow

About 4% of the output of the left ventricle passes into the coronary vessels. Therefore the coronary blood flow at rest is about 200 ml. However, as metabolic demands increase, blood flow can increase to more than four to five times resting value. About 70% of the total coronary blood flow

occurs during diastole. This is because during systole the coronary arteries are compressed by contracting myocardium, so that resistance to flow at the time is sharply increased. As the force of contraction of the right ventricle is much less than that of the left, flow in the right coronary artery is less disturbed by systole resulting in relatively more coronary blood flow to the right ventricle than to the left. Also, because the main coronary arteries are on the superficial surface of the heart, and the hindrance to coronary blood flow during systole, the subendocardial region of the left ventricle is more vulnerable to perfusion deficits in relation to oxygen need than the outer two-thirds of the muscle wall.

Coronary blood flow is largely determined by the calibre of the coronary arteries themselves, and is regulated almost entirely by the local metabolic needs of the working heart muscle.

Normally, the heart extracts a high, relatively fixed percentage (65–70%) of oxygen from coronary arterial blood, regardless of physiological conditions. The heart functions exclusively on aerobic metabolism and, unlike skeletal muscle, cannot sustain an oxygen debt. Thus, the most basic regulator of coronary flow is the degree of oxygen need. Since increased oxygen extraction is thus not possible, augmented myocardial oxygen demands must be met by increases in coronary blood flow. This largely depends upon the ability of the coronary arteries to increase their diameter.

Hypoxia is a potent coronary vasodilator and causes a marked increase in flow (up to fivefold). An excess of carbon dioxide and lactic acid causes only slight coronary vasodilatation. Thus, changes in tissue oxygen tensions are probably responsible for most of the variations in coronary blood flow.

Factors that can contribute to increased myocardial oxygen consumption include: increased heart rate; increased myocardial contractility; increased myocardial fibre tension. The latter, systolic wall tension, plays an extremely important role in determining oxygen consumption.

Because pressure work (the mechanical work involved in displacing a pressurized volume of blood) and heart rate are major determinants of myocardial oxygen consumption per minute, the product of heart rate and systolic blood pressure (the 'double product') is often used to predict myocardial oxygen demand. Unfortunately, this index is unreliable because it ignores other major determinants of myocardial oxygen demand: contractile state, ventricular volume and ventricular mass.

Collateral circulation

The coronary arteries are commonly subject to damage; therefore it is important to recognize the significance of the collateral circulation, both the cardiac and extracardiac anastomoses. In the myocardium, there are very rich anastomoses between the right and left coronary arteries, but the vessels involved are small. These anastomoses are genetically determined and it has been shown that a gradual onset of occlusion will allow these vessels to enlarge. However, if there is a sudden occlusion, the necrosis of a segment of cardiac muscle will result.

Collateral circulations are found in about two-thirds of patients with CHD and their incidence increases with age. In the previously healthy young adult who suffers an acute myocardial infarction, significant collateral circulation forms. The arteries anastomosed may increase to a full diameter in a short period of time. After 24 hours the blood flow of the coronary collaterals increases to allow twice as much coronary circulation. After about one month it returns to a normal coronary blood supply. This compensatory mechanism saves many lives.

LYMPHATIC DRAINAGE OF THE HEART

The body also contains a parallel circulation of lymphatic vessels and nodes. The function of the lymphatic system is return to the cardiovascular system the interstitial fluid that enters the body tissues. This is approximately 8 litres a day. There are many fine-walled lymphatic vessels distributed throughout the myocardium. The bundle branches and the atrial surfaces of the AV nodes have a particularly dense lymph vessel supply. Large lymphatic vessels form the subendocardial and subepicardial lymphatic plexuses. The main collecting ducts lie alongside the large blood vessels in the grooves of the heart. There is one large vessel ascending each side of the heart ending in the anterior mediastinal lymph nodes below the arch of the aorta and the bifurcation of the trachea. The lymph finally drains into the thoracic duct.

NERVOUS SUPPLY TO THE HEART

The cardiovascular system is centrally regulated by the autonomic nervous system. This works in conjunction with other mechanisms to minimize fluctuations in cardiac output and mean arterial blood pressure to maintain adequate perfusion of the organs. Intrinsic reflexes respond to stimuli originating in the cardiovascular system and these include:

- baroreceptors which respond to changes in arterial pressure
- cardiopulmonary receptors which respond to changes in blood volume and pressure in the central thoracic compartments
- arterial chemoreceptors which respond to decreased PO_2, increased PCO_2 and increased blood H^+.

Extrinsic reflexes control the cardiovascular response to stimuli originating elsewhere including temperature changes and pain.

All nervous regulation of the heart comes through the sympathetic and parasympathetic branches of the autonomic nervous system. These nerve fibres are intrinsic to the nervous control which can modify cardiac function by changing the heart rate and the strength of myocardial contraction. The control of the autonomic nervous system is via the cardiac centre in the medulla oblongata of the brain.

The sympathetic fibres

The sympathetic fibres originate in the cervical and upper thoracic ganglia and enter cardiac tissue via the superficial and deep cardiac plexuses. Sympathetic fibres supply the sinus node, atrial muscle, AV node, specialized conduction tissue and the ventricular muscle. Stimulation of the sympathetic fibres results in the release of noradrenaline (norepinephrine) which acts specifically on beta-1 adrenergic receptors in cardiac muscle. At rest, cardiac sympathetic nerves exert an accelerating effect on the sinus node. However, this is overridden by the opposite and dominant effect of the parasympathetic vagal tone. Sympathetic stimulation:

- increases the heart rate and the force of contraction

- increases conduction velocity and shortens the refractory period in the AV node.

The parasympathetic fibres

The parasympathetic fibres originate from the vagus nerve. Most of the fibres from the right vagus are thought to terminate at the sinus node and most from the left at the AV node. There is some vagal innervation to the muscle of the atria and ventricle. Vagal stimulation involves the release of acetylcholine which:

- decreases the heart rate and probably the strength of contraction
- increases the refractory period and decreases conduction velocity in the AV node.

ELECTRICAL ACTIVITY

Electrical stimulation is the precursor for myocardial contraction. A regular coordinated cardiac cycle is dependent on a regular coordinated spread of electrical charge throughout the myocardium.

Automaticity

Some specialized cardiac cells are able to initiate an electrical impulse. This property is known as automaticity and the cells are known as automatic cells or pacemaker cells.

Automatic cells

Automatic cells fire off at different rates in different parts of the heart muscle. The electrical control of the heart normally originates from the cells with the fastest intrinsic rate. This is usually the sinoatrial (SA) node which discharges spontaneously at a rate of about 80 per minute. The intrinsic rate of discharge is lower in automatic cells of the AV node (60 per minute) and lower still in the cells of the ventricles (40 per minute). This means that if the sinus node cells fail to fire, escape rhythms originating from cells elsewhere prevent rhythm failure. If other automatic cells develop faster rates of discharge than the sinus node, they will take over the pacemaker function of the heart.

Conductivity

Both myocardial cells and automatic cells can transmit or conduct impulses, but the specialized conduction tissues are used preferentially and they facilitate a more rapid and coordinated movement of electrical charge through the heart. Each cell generally makes an electrically conductive physical connection (a nexus) with two or more neighbours. Adjacent cells are held together by a complex system of interdigitating projections – intercalated discs. Electrical resistance through these is about 1/400 the resistance through the outside membrane of the myocardial fibre, allowing virtually free diffusion of ions. Thus, impulses can travel from one myocardial cell to another without any significant impedance. The myocardial cells are so tightly bound that stimulation of any single cell causes the impulse to spread to all adjacent cells, eventually spreading throughout the entire latticework of the myocardium – the all-or-nothing principle. Thus, cardiac muscle is said to be a syncytium. In fact, the heart is composed of two separate syncytia, atrial and ventricular, which are separated by the fibrous ring, but the electrical activity can be conducted from the atrial syncytium to the ventricular syncytium by way of the AV junction.

Action potential in myocardial cells

An action potential is the temporary change in the electrical charge of a cell which comes about as a result of the activity of ion channels in the cell membrane allowing changes in the inward and outward flow of electrically charged ions. The rate of change in electrical charge and the magnitude of the charges varies between myocardial cells and the specialized automatic cells of the conduction system.

Ions can have a positive or a negative electrical charge and their relative concentrations will affect the overall electrical charge of the environment they are in. Ions that have a positive charge are called cations and those with a negative charge anions.

Ions will be attracted towards environments with the opposite electrical charge (negatively charged ions will be attracted towards positive ions). Ions will also obey the principles of osmosis and diffusion and naturally move down concentration gradients. Movement of ions across cell membranes also depends on the ability of the ions to move across the membrane, i.e. the permeability of the membrane to that particular ion. Movement of ions against a concentration gradient requires energy.

The ions primarily involved in the generation of a cardiac action potential are sodium (Na^+), potassium (K^+) and calcium (Ca^{2+}). Others, e.g. chloride (Cl^-), however, are also needed. Inside the cell the predominant positively charged cation is K^+ and the predominant negatively charged anions are the proteins, sulphate and organic phosphate. Outside the cell, the predominant cations are Na^+ and Ca^{2+} and the predominant anion is Cl^-.

At rest

In the normal resting state the membrane potential of cardiac muscle is negatively charged at about $-90\,mV$, and about $-95\,mV$ in the specialized conduction system. Whereas the cell membrane is impermeable to the large group of negatively charged anions in the intracellular fluid, its permeability to the positively charged Na^+ and K^+ varies. In the resting state, the cell membrane is approximately 30 times more permeable to K^+ than to Na^+. Therefore K^+ moves out of the cell according to its concentration gradient, but it is also attracted by the negatively charged intracellular environment.

Although extracellular Na^+ is strongly attracted to the negatively charged intracellular space by both its concentration and electrical gradients, very little N^+ movement occurs because of the low membrane permeability during the resting phase.

The relative concentration of N^+ and K^+ and the electrical difference across the cell membrane in the resting phase are maintained by the energy consuming 'sodium pump'. This pump transfers K^+ into the cell and extrudes N^+ in a ratio of about $2–5\,K^+$ to $1\,N^+$. This imbalance in ion transfer helps maintain both the resting membrane potential of $-90\,mV$ and the concentration of Na^+ and K^+ within the cell.

In order for an action potential to be initiated, the interior of the cell membrane has to become more positively charged and this occurs when the cell membrane is at a threshold potential of about $-65\,mV$. This change in charge results from transmission from an adjacent cell through the intercalated discs.

There are three distinct stages of cellular activity in the generation of an action potential:

1 *Polarization.* In the resting state, where the cell has a membrane potential of $-90\,mV$, the cell is said to be in a state of polarization.

2 *Depolarization.* When electrical activation of the cell occurs, changes in the cell membrane permeability result in marked shifts in ion concentrations. Thus, after excitation the polarity of the charge on the membrane is reversed and the membrane potential changes rapidly from its normally very negative value to a slightly positive value of $+30\,mV$. This positive portion is called the *reverse potential*. This state of depolarization reflects the marked influx of positively charged Na^+ (accompanied by a moderate but more sustained influx of Ca^{2+}) into the intracellular environment.

3 *Repolarization.* When the resting state is restored, due to K^+ gradually returning to the cell as Na^+ is pumped out again, the cell is said to be in a state of repolarization. However, simultaneous fluxes of Ca^{2+} between the cell and extracellular fluid and within the cells plays an important role.

Phases of the action potential

The action potential, as recorded from a ventricular myocardial cell, has five distinct phases (Figure 2.4):

0 *(depolarization)*: which is represented by the initial abrupt upstroke, or spike, of the action potential curve. During this phase, membrane permeability to Na^+ is markedly increased. The rapid influx of Na^+ is thought to occur through fast channels specific for Na^+.

There are three phases of repolarization or recovery:

1 *(rapid phase of repolarization)*: the initial downstroke after depolarization. This is the brief change towards the repolarization process, during which the membrane potential returns to $0\,mV$. This phase reflects a brief influx of negatively charged Cl^-.

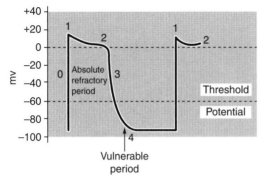

Figure 2.4   Phases of the action potential of a single myocardial cell: phase 0, terminal phase of depolarization; phase 1, early and rapid repolarization; phase 2, slow repolarization (the plateau); phase 3, terminal phase of relatively rapid repolarization; phase 4, resting potential.

2   (*plateau*): reflects a balance between the slow secondary inward Na⁺ and Ca²⁺ current and outward K⁺ repolarizing currents. After the initial spike the membrane remains depolarized (0.15 s for atrial muscle to 0.3 s for ventricular muscle), exhibiting a plateau, followed by the abrupt descent which represents repolarization. This phase reflects a moderate and sustained influx of Ca²⁺ which accompanies the more marked, but less sustained, influx of N⁺. This influx is balanced by a decreased efflux of K⁺. Thus, the net effect is a relative balance of positive charges and gives rise to the plateau.

3   (*rapid descent after the plateau*): membrane permeability to K⁺ increases markedly, thus returning the membrane potential to its resting level of −90 mV and thus ending the action potential.

4   (*interval between the end of repolarization and the subsequent action potential*).

Once the depolarization process has started it is inevitably transmitted along the length of the cell to the adjacent cells. In this manner a single electrical stimulus can depolarize the whole heart (Figure 2.5).

The velocity of conduction of the action potential in both atrial and ventricular muscle fibres is about 0.4 metres per second (m/s).

The myocardium is normally refractory to re-stimulation during the action potential. The normal

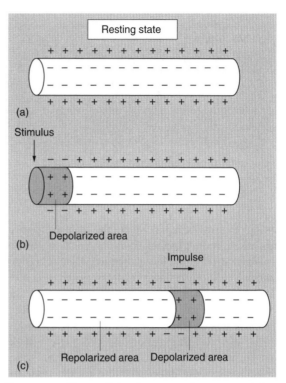

Figure 2.5   Myocardial cell transmembrane potential: (a) at rest; (b) during depolarization; (c) during repolarization.

refractory period of the ventricle is 0.25–0.3 s, which is about the duration of the action potential. In addition, there is a relative refractory period of about 0.05 s during which the muscle is more difficult than normal to excite. The normal refractory period of the atrium is about 0.15 s and is therefore much shorter than that for the ventricles. The relative refractory period is an additional 0.03 s. Therefore, the rhythmical rate of contraction of the atria can be much faster than that of the ventricles.

Action potential in automatic cells

The automatic cells are specialized heart cells whose function is to regulate the contraction of the myocardial cells by providing the initial electrical stimulation. These cells possess three specific properties: automaticity; excitability; conductivity.

Their contractile elements are sparse, and the cells do not contribute significantly to the cardiac contraction. In the automatic cell, the resting membrane potential is slightly less than −90 mV

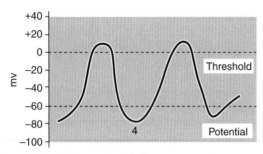

Figure 2.6 Action potential of spontaneously discharging pacemaker cell.

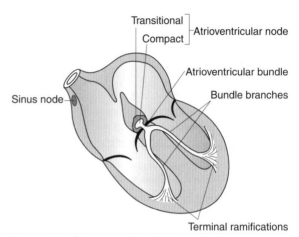

Figure 2.7 Representation of the conducting system of the heart.

(as in the myocardial cell), the depolarization upstroke is more gradual, there is no plateau during repolarization and the descent to phase 4 is more gradual. Although these cells are polarized, their state of polarization never remains constant and they are able to initiate phase 4 depolarization spontaneously (Figure 2.6).

The electrical charge on the cell surface leaks away until the threshold is reached, when spontaneous complete depolarization occurs over the whole cell surface simultaneously and spreads to adjacent cells whether they are myocardial cells or automatic cells. If it spreads to a myocardial cell, then that cell will contract. If it spreads to another automatic cell, then that cell will be depolarized before it can discharge itself. Whichever cell reaches threshold level first will go on to complete depolarization and discharge all the remaining automatic and myocardial cells.

The automatic cell with the most rapid leakage rate will maintain its position as the principal pacemaking cell. Normally the principal pacemaker is located within the sinus node.

Conducting system of the heart

The automatic cells are found in the cardiac conduction system. This conducting system consists of the:

- sinus node
- atrioventricular (AV) junction (the AV node and AV bundle)
- ventricular conducting tissue (the right and left bundle branches and the peripheral ramifications of the bundle branches) (Figure 2.7).

Sinus node

The sinus node is the normal site of initiation of the inherent regular rhythm. It is situated at the junction of the superior vena cava with the right atrium. The node is spindle shaped, about 25 mm long and 3 mm wide. The blood supply is varied. The nodal artery is often found extending throughout the length of the sinus node and arises from the right coronary artery (60% of cases) or the left coronary artery (40% of cases). There are numerous nerve endings in the node, the parasympathetic fibres being derived from the right vagus.

Internodal tracts It is possible that specialized pathways exist in the atrium linking the sinus and atrioventricular nodes. However, there is no histological evidence of such pathways, the conduction occurring preferentially along the thick muscle bundles of the right atrium.

Atrioventricular junction

The AV node lies between the opening of the coronary sinus and the posterior border of the membranous interventricular septum. The node is divided into a transitional zone and a compact portion. Its important function is to cause a delay of about 0.04 s in atrioventricular transmission. Two important advantages result from this delay:

1 postponement of ventricular excitation until the atria have had time to eject their contents into the ventricles

2 limitation of the maximum number of signals which can be accommodated for in transmission by the AV node.

The AV node receives its blood supply from a specific artery which is a branch of the right coronary artery (90% of cases) or the left circumflex artery (10% of cases). There is a rich nerve supply, with parasympathetic fibres being derived from the left vagus.

The AV bundle extends from the AV node, along the posterior margin of the membranous portion of the interventricular septum, to the crest of the muscular septum. Here it bifurcates into the right and left bundle branches. The AV bundle is oval or triangular in cross-section. It and the proximal few millimetres of both bundle branches are supplied by the terminal branch of the AV nodal artery from behind, and from the septal branches of the left anterior descending artery.

Ventricular conducting tissue

The right and left bundle branches extend subendocardially along both septal surfaces. The right bundle branch is a cord-like structure which passes down the side of the right ventricular septum towards the apex. The left bundle branch is an extensive sheet of fibres which passes down the smooth side of the left ventricular septum. The initial part of the left bundle branch is a continuous fan which breaks up into three interconnecting divisions: anterior, middle and posterior. Both bundle branches are supplied by septal arteries from the left anterior descending artery.

Excitation–contraction coupling

This means the mechanism by which the action potential causes the myofibrils to contract. The electrical excitation of a cardiac cell membrane is due to the generation of a local circuit current by the membrane action potential. Due to positive feedback, this current is responsible for the propagation of the action potential. The intercalated discs help by providing a low electrical resistance between the cells.

The sarcoplasmic reticulum is a series of fine branching tubules (T-tubules) forming channels or invaginations from the surface membrane of the cell down to the contractile elements, which allows changes occurring at the cell membrane to be rapidly transmitted to the contractile elements to provide the link between the electrical and mechanical activity of the heart.

Myofibrils occupy most of each muscle fibre which are transversely striated. These striations are divided into bands. The deeply coloured A bands alternate with the I bands. In the centre of each A band is a Z line, and the region between each Z line is known as a sarcomere. In the I bands there are thin myofilaments composed mainly of actin. These are attached to a part of the Z line (Z discs) and extend into the H bands where they interdigitate with a system of thicker filaments composed mainly of myosin.

When the muscle changes in length, the thick and thin myofilaments slide over each other. Thus, when an action potential passes over the cardiac muscle membrane, the action potential also spreads to the interior of the myocardial cell along the membranes of the T-tubules. This in turn results in the release of calcium from the cisternae of the sarcoplasmic reticulum and the T-tubules into the sarcoplasm. Calcium then diffuses into the myofibrils where it catalyses the chemical reaction that activates the sliding of the actin and myosin filaments along each other. The sarcomere shortens and the myofibrils contract. At the end of contraction, the calcium in the sarcoplasm is rapidly pumped back into the sarcoplasmic reticulum and the T-tubules. It can be seen that the strength of myocardial contraction is partly dependent upon the concentration of calcium.

Sequence of excitation

Normally, the activating impulse from the sinus node spreads in all directions. It travels at a rate of about 1 m/s and reaches the most distant portion of the atrium in about 0.08 s, and approaches the AV node. Here, a delay of about 0.04 s in AV transmission occurs while atrial systole is completed. After leaving the AV node, the wave of excitement passes rapidly along the specialized muscle fibres of the AV bundle, bundle branches and peripheral ramifications of these branches causing contraction of the ventricular musculature.

REGULATION OF NORMAL MYOCARDIAL FUNCTION

At rest the normal heart pumps about 5 litres of blood each minute. However, during severe exercise it may be required to pump up to six times this amount. On average, the adult resting stroke volume (SV) (the quantity of blood ejected during systole) is about 70 ml. If the heart rate (HR) is 80 beats/min then the cardiac output (CO) is about 5.6 litres/min. Thus:

$$CO \text{ (litres/min)} = HR \text{ (beats/min)} \times SV \text{ (ml/beat)}$$

Heart rate and stroke volume are the primary determinants of cardiac output. To alter cardiac output to meet changing bodily demands for tissue perfusion, the heart rate or stroke volume (or both) must be altered. These mechanisms normally operate together to increase the cardiac output as required. If either the heart rate or stroke volume increases while the other remains unchanged, the cardiac output will increase. Compensatory adjustments in heart rate and stroke volume are essential to cardiac functioning.

Although cardiac output is a traditional measure of cardiac function, it differs markedly with body size. Thus, a more accurate measure is the cardiac index, which is the cardiac output per minute per m^{-2} of body surface area. Usually it is about 3.2 litres/min.

The primary factors which determine myocardial functioning and cardiac output are:

1 preload (filling of the heart during diastole)
2 afterload (resistance against which the heart must pump)
3 contractility of the heart
4 heart rate.

Preload (Frank–Starling mechanism)

The classical exposition of myocardial pumping performance was provided by Starling in the Linacre Lecture of 1915, published in 1918 (Starling, 1918). Much of Starling's law of the heart was based on the work of Frank in 1895 and hence it is often referred to as the Frank-Starling law of the heart. This law states that, within its physiological limits, the heart will pump whatever amount of blood enters the right atrium (i.e. the rate of venous return).

Preload is the tension exerted on a muscle as it begins to contract. Cardiac output is the quantity of blood pumped by the left ventricle into the aorta each minute, and the venous return is the quantity of blood flowing from the veins into the right atrium each minute. The venous return may vary and this intrinsic ability of the heart to adapt to changing loads of inflowing blood is called the Frank-Starling law of the heart. Within certain limits cardiac muscle fibres contract more forcibly the more they are stretched before contraction begins. This stretching of fibres is achieved by increasing venous return to the heart, which results in greater filling. Thus, the more forceful contraction which ensues empties the heart more efficiently. Once the venous return increases beyond the physiological limits of the heart's ability to adapt, the myocardium begins to fail.

Preload, then, is a function of the volume of blood presented to the left ventricle and also the compliance (the ability of the left ventricle to stretch). It may be described as left ventricular end-diastolic pressure (LVEDP). Preload is best measured haemodynamically as the pulmonary artery wedge pressure.

Afterload

Afterload is the force opposing ventricular ejection and is a function of both arterial pressure and left ventricular size. An increase in afterload usually means an increase in the work of the heart. Examples of increased afterload would include aortic impedance (e.g. aortic stenosis), vasoconstriction (increased systemic vascular resistance) and increased blood volume or viscosity.

Contractility (inotropism)

Contractility or inotropism is an intrinsic property of the heart. The rate (chronotropic force) and force (inotropic force) of contraction can be increased by sympathetic nervous stimulation. The sympathetic nerves of the heart and circulating adrenaline, noradrenaline or dopamine improve the speed and strength of contraction (positive inotropic effect), whereas myocardial hypoxia, ischaemia or beta-blockers can decrease cardiac contractility (negative inotropic effect). The contractile state can be measured by the ejection fraction (EF). This is the ratio of the stroke volume ejected from the left ventricle per beat to the volume of blood in the left ventricle at the end of diastole (left ventricular end-diastolic volume). It is expressed as a percentage, normal being at least greater than 50%.

Heart rate (chronotropism)

Heart rate or chronotropism is an important factor in cardiac performance. It is slowed by the vagus nerve by releasing acetylcholine (negative chronotropism) and increased by stimulation of the sympathetic nerves of the heart releasing adrenaline and noradrenaline (positive chronotropism). Both parasympathetic and sympathetic fibres innervate the sinus node and AV node. In addition, there are sympathetic fibres that terminate in myocardial tissue.

Blood pressure

Blood pressure is defined as the force that the blood exerts upon the vessel walls. Systolic blood pressure is the pressure when the ventricles contract and blood is forced into an already full aorta. This produces a pressure of about 120 mmHg. When the heart is relaxed during diastole, the arterial pressure falls to about 80 mmHg.

Blood pressure is maintained through the interaction of many variables including:

- *Cardiac output*: cardiac output is dependent on the heart rate and the stroke volume. An increase in cardiac output will lead to an increase in both systolic and diastolic blood pressure.

- *Blood volume*: blood pressure falls when there is a fall in the absolute volume of blood as in haemorrhage or a fall in the circulating blood volume available to the tissues as in anaphylactic or septic shock.

- *Peripheral resistance*: normally the artery walls are in a state of mild constriction controlled by the sympathetic vasoconstrictor nerves. In order to maintain an adequate blood supply to the tissues

at all times, selective vasoconstriction and vasodilatation occur in response to metabolic need.

- *Elasticity of the arterial walls*: the arteries need a degree of elasticity in order to propel the blood forward. Recoil of the artery walls maintains pressure in the arteries during diastole. Elasticity is lost with ageing as a result of atheromatous deposits. This means that the arterial walls can not accommodate the effect of the ventricles forcing blood out into the circulation during systole and so the systolic blood pressure rises.

- *Venous return*: muscular contraction, particularly of the leg muscles puts pressure on the veins and forces the blood forward. Changes in intrathoracic pressure during respiration also augment the force of the left ventricle in moving blood back towards the heart. The blood moves in one direction as a result of one-way valves and returns to the right side of the heart via the superior and inferior venae cavae. The volume of blood re-entering the heart has a direct influence on the volume pumped out under the Frank-Starling relationship.

DISEASE OF THE CORONARY ARTERIES

It is generally accepted that a tubular conduit develops restriction to ordinary flow if the lumen is narrowed by 75% or more.

The causes of coronary artery narrowing are many, although coronary atherosclerosis is the leading one accounting for more than 90% of all cases of CHD. Other causes include thrombus, spasm, embolism, dissection or aneurysm. Coronary lesions manifest themselves as heart disease when:

- the chronic stenosis exceeds 75% of the vessel lumen and compromises flow, especially with increased flow demand; or
- the atheromatous plaque fissures and ulcerates acutely, develops superimposed thrombosis, and causes an abrupt diminution or even total loss of blood supply.

Atherosclerosis

Atherosclerosis is a complex disease characterized by focal proliferation of smooth-muscle cells and accumulation of lipid lesions within the intima of large and medium arteries. Atherosclerotic changes are found in almost all patients presenting with acute myocardial infarction (MI). Atherosclerosis is a dynamic process with phases of stability and instability.

Pathogenesis of atherosclerosis

Atherosclerosis was once thought to be a normal part of ageing but it has now been demonstrated that there is a causal link with specific dietary and blood lipids. The progression of atherosclerosis is now thought to be a dynamic inflammatory process that is readily modifiable (Weissberg 2000). Many processes have been implicated in the pathogenesis of atherosclerosis including:

- inflammation
- endothelial injury
- local adherence of platelets
- lipoprotein oxidation
- lipoprotein aggregation
- action of macrophages
- foam cell formation
- smooth muscle alterations.

There has been much debate over which process, if any, could be regarded as the key event in early atherosclerosis to start the chain of events leading to lesion formation in an otherwise normal artery. Several theories have been postulated to explain the pathogenesis of atherosclerosis including the following.

Changes in the endothelium Endothelial breakdown (denudation), injury and activation have all been put forward as being precursors of atherosclerosis (Ross 1993). Endothelial damage has been assumed to be central in the initiation and progression of atherosclerotic plaques. Certainly, endothelial damage has been linked to smooth-muscle cell migration and proliferation, the most essential component of early atheroma, via the release of platelet-derived growth factor. When the injury is minor and brief, the endothelium will heal and regress leaving a slightly thickened intima. However, long-lasting or repeated injuries may lead to lipid accumulation and further smooth-muscle cell proliferation. Agents injurious to the endothelium are probably numerous, but include raised low-density lipoprotein (LDL) levels, haemodynamic forces and various chemicals, such as tobacco. This hypothesis has been questioned because it is now clear that many developing atheroma are covered by an intact endothelial layer throughout most stages of the lesion progression with only the most complicated and ulcerated lesions losing their endothelial layer.

Lipid infiltration hypotheses This postulates that there is increased permeability of the endothelium to atherogenic lipoproteins. This can occur as a result of smoking, abnormal blood lipid profiles and hypertension.

Response to retention of lipoproteins This hypothesis considers that it is not the enhanced endothelial permeability to lipoprotein influx that is the key pathological event, but the trapping and retention of lipoproteins within the arterial wall (Williams and Tabas 1995). It is thought that once trapped the lipoproteins become modified through the action of enzymes and oxidants, accumulate and then stimulate an inflammatory response (Williams and Tabas 1995).

Turbulent blood flow Arterial segments at branch points or during hypertension are subjected to turbulent blood flow and show a predisposition to lesion development. Because of the response to injury hypothesis, the connection between blood flow and atherogenesis has led to many studies on the effects of shear stress on the endothelium.

Lipoprotein oxidation Lipoprotein oxidation has been proposed to be central to atherogenesis, a theory which is supported by the fact that compounds with antioxidant actions (such as vitamin E) can reduce atherosclerosis in experimental situations, although the clinical benefits remain unclear. Oxidized modification of LDL by oxidants derived from macrophages and endothelial and smooth-muscle cells can lead to the generation of highly atherogenic oxidized LDL within the vascular wall. Oxidized LDL attracts circulating monocytes which penetrate the endothelium, lodge underneath it and mature into macrophages. It is thought that these macrophages accumulate large quantities of oxidized LDL which eventually become the cholesterol rich foam cells forming the fatty streak.

Inflammation and infection Atherosclerosis bears many similarities to inflammatory/autoimmune diseases like rheumatoid arthritis and multiple sclerosis. It is possible that there are antigens linked to atherosclerosis and a vaccination against atherosclerosis has been postulated (Hansson 2002). Significant association has been reported between infection (*C. pneumoniae, Helicobacter pylori*, cytomegalovirus, herpes simplex virus) and the extent of atherosclerosis (Espinola-Klein et al 2002).

Atherosclerotic plaques

Atheromatous lesions may range from the flat, lipid-rich lesions (fatty streaks) which may be precursors of advanced raised lesions, to the raised fibrous plaques which project upward from the surface. All raised plaques contain varying proportions of lipid, smooth-muscle cells and a connective tissue matrix rich in collagen and glycosaminoglycans.

Fatty streaks, which are localized accumulations of lipid within the arterial intima, may begin in early childhood. Monocytes carried by the blood stream penetrate the arterial wall and become foam cells within the intima by absorbing LDL-cholesterol. These lesions are benign in themselves as they cause minimal disruption to blood flow. They are however thought to be the precursors of more advanced atheromatous lesions.

By middle age some of the fatty streaks will have developed into atherosclerotic or fibrous plaques. These are focal lesions where the arterial wall is grossly abnormal. These plaques may be several centimetres across and are found most often in the aorta, the coronary and internal carotid arteries and the circle of Willis. As the plaque develops, there is an increase in the numbers of very smooth muscle cells and the deposition of fibrous connective tissues to form a tough fibrous cap. This fibrous cap projects into the vascular lumen, restricting the flow of blood. When the stenosis reaches about 50% of the lumen diameter, blood flow becomes restricted enough to produce ischaemia when myocardial demand increases. This leads to stable or exertional angina.

Advanced plaques often have large areas of endothelial damage or erosion which serve as sites for thrombus formation on their surface. These type one lesions tend to have smooth regular edges and the fibrous cap remains intact. It is the loss of endothelium that stimulates platelet adhesion and thrombus (blood clot) formation. Pools of extracellular lipid and cell debris collect beneath the fibrous cap. In type two lesions, which are more common, the fibrous cap ruptures or tears away. Type two lesions have irregular edges and may show up on angiography. Fibrous cap rupture may be exacerbated by mechanical factors such as arterial spasm. Plaques susceptible to rupture are those with a large lipid pool, low numbers of vascular smooth muscle cells in the fibrous cap, high numbers of macrophages and a thin fibrous cap. There is evidence that it is the smaller lesions (causing less than 50% lumen occlusion) that are responsible for acute events (Falk et al 1995). As a result of the cap rupture, blood enters the lesion or plaque and platelet-rich thrombi (blood clots) are formed both within and on the surface of the lesion.

Thrombosis

Plaque rupture triggers the formation of platelet-rich thrombus, an essential event in the pathophysiology of acute coronary syndromes which are initiated by abrupt myocardial ischaemia as a result of platelet thrombus formation on ruptured or eroded atherosclerotic plaques. The platelets in the circulation become exposed to thrombogenic stimuli within the plaque or in the exposed subendothelial layers. These include lipid laden macrophages, collagen, adhesive protein (von Willebrand factor vWF) and platelet glycoprotein 1 b (GP1b). Adhesion of platelets to subendothelial vWF is followed by platelet activation. Platelet activation results in the platelets changing shape and becoming more proagulant.

Platelet aggregation is the last stage in the formation of a platelet-rich thrombus. The final common pathway to platelet aggregation is activation of the platelet glycoprotein IIb/IIIa receptor which enables adhesive proteins to bridge the platelets together to form a thrombus. These thrombi may be large enough to cause partial or complete occlusion of the artery resulting in ischaemia or necrosis of the muscle being supplied. The thrombi or the material leaking from the ruptured lesion may be carried upstream and block smaller arteries also resulting in small areas of myocardial necrosis or microinfarcts. The endothelium over the lesion may be unstable. This can lead to repeated thrombus formation. Spontaneous breakdown of the thrombus (thrombolysis) followed by the development of a further thrombus results in short, time-limited episodes of vessel occlusion, transient symptoms and ECG changes. The thrombus may also produce vasoconstrictor agents such as serotonin which can induce vasospasm. The damage to the muscle by repeated thrombus formation from an unstable plaque may be negligible or may result in small areas of necrosis detectable by troponin estimation.

The risk of an acute coronary syndrome depends on the number of plaques which are vulnerable to rupture. Many plaques responsible for acute coronary syndromes are not visible on angiography. In the future cardiovascular magnetic resonance imaging (MRI) may be able to determine plaque vulnerability and the risk of acute coronary syndrome by assessing the size of the lipid pool within the lesion and the integrity of the fibrous cap.

Non-fatal chronic thrombi may gradually be replaced by connective tissue and reabsorbed into the lesion to form a stable plaque.

Coronary artery spasm

The heart can be rendered ischaemic by mechanisms other than fixed atherosclerotic lesions of the coronary arteries. Angiographic studies performed with patients having clinical or provoked attacks have provided direct evidence that vasospasm can cause partial or complete coronary obstruction. Coronary vasospasm is an abnormal increase in coronary vasomotor tone involving one or more epicardial coronary arteries with or without atherosclerotic lesions. In about 10% of acute coronary patients, transient coronary artery spasm may serve to alter adversely the balance between myocardial supply and demand. Acute infarction often occurs in patients with the 'variant' form of angina described by Prinzmetal et al (1959). Because the coronary arteries lie on the epicardial surface of the ventricle, the effect of

arterial spasm is to produce subepicardial ischaemia. This manifests as ST elevation on the ECG. Coronary artery spasm may be responsible for the diurnal distribution of episodes of transient acute ischaemia in patients with variant angina and myocardial infarction. The former tends to exhibit peaks of ischaemic episodes between 0400 and 0600 hours, and the latter between 0600 and 0800 hours (Muller et al 1985, Thompson et al 1991). What precisely induces vasospasm is unknown in most cases.

MYOCARDIAL ISCHAEMIA

The development of myocardial ischaemia is a dynamic process in which increased myocardial oxygen demand or decreased coronary blood flow are the main but not the sole determinants. Ischaemic chest pain typically occurs during periods of increased oxygen demand such as exercise, during tachycardia or other cardiovascular stresses. The increased demand requires an increase in myocardial blood flow which an obstructed coronary vessel cannot accommodate. Critical restriction to ordinary flow occurs when the diameter of the vessel lumen is reduced by more than 50% (equivalent to 75% stenosis if the vessel is circular), usually resulting in angina pectoris.

Oxygen demand

Oxygen demand depends mainly upon heart rate, myocardial contractility and systolic wall tension.

Heart rate

An increase in heart rate increases myocardial oxygen consumption by increasing the frequency of cardiac contractions per unit of time. In addition, this increase in heart rate leads to an increase in contractility. When the heart rate increases, systolic timing does not alter very much and the increased heart rate shortens diastole. Since coronary perfusion takes place in diastole there is less filling time for the coronary arteries to meet the increased demands placed upon it by the increased heart rate. Angina may therefore result.

Myocardial contractility

Factors that increase myocardial contractility, such as inotropic drugs and thyrotoxicosis, also increase the rate of myocardial oxygen consumption.

Systolic wall tension

Tension in the myocardial wall is an important determinant of cardiac energy utilization and myocardial oxygen consumption. According to the Laplace relationship, systolic wall tension is directly proportional to the ventricular systolic pressure and the ventricular radius and inversely proportional to the ventricular wall thickness. Thus, oxygen consumption will be increased by factors such as high blood pressure.

Oxygen supply

In general, the delivery of oxygen to the myocardium varies with coronary blood flow, which is in turn determined by perfusion pressure. Myocardial oxygen supply may be compromised by abnormalities of the vessel wall, in blood flow, or in the blood itself.

Abnormalities of the coronary vessel wall

Coronary blood supply may be impaired by fixed (atheroma) or reversible (spasm) lesions. Both atheroma and spasm are usually always present in patients with angina, although their precise contribution to impairing myocardial perfusion at any given time will vary.

Abnormalities in blood flow

Aortic valve disease will reduce perfusion of the coronary arteries and impair oxygen supply. Hyperviscosity syndromes may result in myocardial ischaemia by slowing blood flow.

Abnormalities in the blood

Anaemia will prevent adequate oxygen carriage and may provoke angina.

Metabolic consequences of myocardial ischaemia

Normal cardiac function is dependent upon an adequate supply of high-energy phosphate compounds, in particular ATP. Under aerobic conditions ATP is produced in the mitochondria by the process of oxidative phosphorylation.

Although traditionally, myocardial ischaemia has been defined as a state of the heart when there exists an imbalance between oxygen supply and demand, such a definition excludes the removal of metabolites, particularly heat and carbon monoxide, as important a function of myocardial blood flow as the supply of oxygen and substrate. A more precise definition is that myocardial ischaemia is characterized by an imbalance of ATP consumption and blood flow. Ischaemia occurs either when ATP consumption increases above the rate of ATP production that can be sustained by a given blood flow, or when blood flow is reduced so that the existing rate of ATP consumption cannot be maintained.

Because oxidative metabolism supplies the high-energy phosphate compounds necessary to sustain cardiac activity, the utilization of oxygen by the myocardium can be used as a measure of energy expenditure. The myocardium uses 8–10 ml of oxygen per 100 g of muscle per minute in resting subjects.

When hypoxia occurs, oxidative phosphorylation is inhibited and intracellular stores of ATP decline dramatically. Although the myocyte is capable of producing limited amounts of ATP under hypoxic conditions, the reduced perfusion that characterizes ischaemia leads to the accumulation of metabolites that have inhibitory effects on anaerobic energy production. Thus, the availability of oxygen in the cell determines whether metabolic processes can occur aerobically or anaerobically.

The primary metabolic disturbance in the hypoxic or ischaemic myocardium is that aerobic synthesis of high-energy phosphate compounds is blocked by the lack of oxygen; consequently, a shift to anaerobic metabolism occurs. However, anaerobic metabolism of glucose, for instance, provides a yield of two high-energy phosphate bonds per molecule, whereas oxidative metabolism yields 38. Instead of extracting lactic acid from the arterial blood, the hypoxic heart produces lactic acid as the end-product of anaerobic metabolism. If blood flow to hypoxic myocardial cells decreases below a critical level, as occurs in ischaemia, lactic acid and other metabolites accumulate and the intracellular pH falls. As a result, anaerobic metabolism is inhibited and, ultimately, the production of high-energy phosphate compounds halts.

Localized ischaemia may be intermittent and have reversible effects, but it causes decreased myocardial function. Following the total occlusion of a coronary artery, there is sufficient oxygen in the tissue, and high-energy phosphates (ATP and CP) within the myocardium, to supply energy for about two and seven heart beats, respectively. Myocardial contraction declines rapidly and developed tension ceases within about 90 s, leading to characteristic haemodynamic alteration. The ventricular stroke volume is diminished, which results in decreased cardiac output, while rising left ventricular filling pressures cause decreased compliance in the left ventricle. The electrocardiogram (ECG) is altered after about 30 s and pain is experienced at about 60 s.

Acidosis that occurs, together with the rapid accumulation of potassium in the extracellular space following the onset of ischaemia, probably account for electrophysiological changes in the conduction velocity, rate of depolarization, resting membrane potential and duration of the action potential. These changes coincide with the occurrence of ventricular arrhythmias.

MANIFESTATIONS OF CORONARY HEART DISEASE

The manifestations of coronary heart disease (CHD) are dependent on the extent and suddenness of the obstruction to coronary blood flow, the length of time the myocardium has a reduced blood supply and the myocardial oxygen demand at the time. Clinically, CHD can be categorized into stable and unstable coronary syndromes and sudden death. Stable coronary syndrome refers to stable angina. Unstable coronary syndromes include unstable angina and acute myocardial infarction, now increasingly being grouped under the diagnostic label of acute coronary syndrome (ACS).

Stable angina

Angina pectoris is a transient, reversible episode of inadequate coronary circulation. It is a symptom and not a disease.

The word angina is derived from the Greek word *anchien* (meaning to choke). It was originally mentioned by Heberden in a lecture before the Royal College of Physicians of London in 1768. His observations were published four years later: 'They who are afflicted with it, are seized while they are walking, (more especially if it be uphill and soon after eating) with a painful and most disagreeable sensation in the breast, which seems as if it would extinguish life, if it were to increase or to continue; but the moment they stand still, all this uneasiness vanishes' (Heberden 1772).

The amount of effort that precipitates the pain is variable. Atypical angina pain bears no known relation to effort. Characteristically, it is:

- a discomfort located in the chest or adjacent areas
- being caused by myocardial hypoxia secondary to inadequate coronary blood flow
- not being associated with myocardial necrosis.

The characteristic feature of angina is pain that is precipitated by exercise (effort) or emotion, or both, and is relieved by rest. Typically, the duration of an anginal attack is 2–5 min. The term *stable angina* refers to angina which is worse in cold weather or after a heavy meal and is relieved by rest.

Acute coronary syndromes

Unstable angina, non-ST segment elevation myocardial infarction (NSTEMI) and ST segment elevation myocardial infarction (STEMI) represent a continuum along the same disease process characterized by plaque rupture followed by intermittent or sudden reduction in coronary blood flow.

Unstable angina

In unstable angina, occlusion tends to be transient and episodic resulting in prolonged and increasing episodes of angina occurring at rest with no obvious precipitating factors. The coronary vessels often show type II plaques undergoing fissuring associated with non-occlusive luminal thrombi. Progression to myocardial infarction at 30 days is 20%.

Myocardial infarction

Myocardial infarction refers to the necrosis of a portion of myocardium as a result of a reduction, interruption or cessation in blood flow. Interruption of myocardial blood flow and the resulting ischaemia leads to cessation of myocardial systolic function. Generally, myocardial cells are irreversibly injured by 30–40 min of total ischaemia. The essential feature is myocardial necrosis. Regional infarction tends to involve the area of myocardium supplied by one branch of a major coronary artery. Diffuse infarction is thought to involve the subendocardial area and occur as a result of a fall in overall myocardial perfusion either due to widespread atheromatous damage or severe myocardial hypertrophy and elevated ventricular diastolic pressure.

The concept that plaque fissuring and thrombosis underlies most episodes of acute myocardial infarction is supported by angiography which, when carried out within an hour of onset of infarction, shows an occluded artery in 90% of cases. This figure declines with time because of spontaneous dissolution of the thrombus by natural thrombolytic mechanisms.

Around the zone of dead infarcted tissue is a 'zone of injury' (Figure 2.8). This tissue cannot contract but may be salvaged if an adequate blood supply can be quickly established. Superimposed on the zone of injury, and separating it from undamaged tissue, is the ischaemic zone. This tissue can usually be salvaged if treatment is prompt.

During the first 6 hours after the onset of symptoms (evolving phase), hydrogen ions accumulate in the myocardium, calcium ions are displaced from the contractile proteins in the endoplasmic reticulum and the myocardium becomes acidotic. The membrane action potential is altered as potassium ions migrate outside the cell and sodium ions enter it, predisposing to oedema and swelling. There is increased risk of arrhythmias.

The infarcted area is at first red owing to extravasation of the red cells (infarct means 'stuffed-in' with red cells). The area later appears pale as the necrotic muscle swells and squeezes out the extravasated blood. Finally, the infarcted area is replaced by fibrous scar tissue over the course of 4–6 weeks.

Location of infarction   Traditionally, infarctions were classed by the area of damage, although there has now been a move to use ECG criteria, specifically ST elevation, as this helps inform treatment decisions. Infarcts can be classed according to the region of myocardial muscle damaged or the area of the heart where the infarcted area is situated. In a *subendocardial* infarction necrotic tissue is on the endocardial surface. An *intramural* infarction involves damage to the interior of the myocardium; and an *epicardial* infarction involves just the epicardial surface. A *transmural* infarction involves the full thickness of the ventricular wall, the endocardium and the epicardium.

Infarction may be located in the *anterior* region of the left ventricle if the left anterior descending artery is occluded (where it may involve the septum and papillary muscles); in the *posterior* region of the left ventricle if the left circumflex artery is occluded; or in the *inferior* (diaphragmatic) region if the right coronary artery is occluded. Because of the frequency of involvement of the left ventricle, classification according to location is usually in reference to this chamber. Each classification is further divided to designate the particular section of the wall involved: *lateral* or *septal*. The former involves the far side of the wall of the chamber and the latter involves the interventricular area of the anterior, posterior or inferior wall.

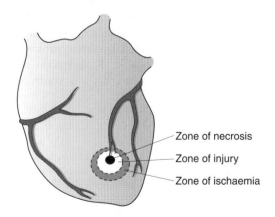

Figure 2.8   Zones of necrosis, injury and ischaemia.

Sudden cardiac death

The terms sudden cardiac death and myocardial infarction have often, mistakenly, been regarded as synonymous. Sudden cardiac death means a death from natural causes in which the individual dies within one hour of the first symptoms. Almost three-quarters of sudden deaths will be in individuals with CHD, about half of whom will be unaware that they have any cardiac disease. Sudden cardiac death may have a thromboembolic or an electrical trigger. The cause is often indeterminable at post-mortem as changes that would have become apparent do not manifest themselves in the short period from onset to death. When contrasted to the arterial lesions of acute myocardial infarction, there is a lower incidence of total occlusion in sudden cardiac death with only a third of cases having an occlusive thrombus indicative of a developing infarction.

About a quarter of sudden cardiac deaths are thought to be due to the onset of ventricular fibrillation (VF), but the mechanism of induction of VF is unclear, although it may, in part, be due to intramyocardial emboli or ionic events which accompany a short period of myocardial ischaemia.

Since the immediate cause of death is potentially reversible, education of the public in emergency cardiopulmonary resuscitation, and the provision of support services, including rapid defibrillation, can result in a considerable saving of lives (Stiell et al 1999).

Ventricular remodelling

Remodelling refers to the changes in the structure of the myocardial cells following infarction. It involves the necrotic tissue being replaced by scar tissue and is significant to left ventricular function and prognosis. Remodelling takes about 4–6 weeks, although it begins within 24 hours of coronary occlusion. It involves:

- the infarcted area becoming progressively thinner and expanding (develops within hours)
- lengthening and hypertrophy of the remaining non-infarcted myocardium to increase the shape and volume of the ventricle (continues over months or years leading to progressive dilatation).

Initially remodelling is a beneficial compensatory mechanism as it leads to reduced filling pressures and increased stroke volumes. In large infarcts (those with an ejection fraction less than 40%), and those with persistent occlusion of the infarct-related artery, dilatation may lead to ventricular failure and death. This emphasizes the importance of preventing infarct expansion and remodelling through:

- early and complete reperfusion of the infarct-related artery
- reducing the workload of the heart and limiting ventricular expansion through the use of ACE inhibitors.

Myocardial stunning

Myocardial stunning refers to a period of reduced contractility following a transient period of ischaemia. This can occur following thrombolysis, angioplasty or cardiac surgery and explains why ventricular function may improve days or even weeks after successful reperfusion therapy.

Myocardial hybernation

Myocardial hybernation occurs when there is adequate blood flow to the myocardium to prevent necrosis, but not enough to allow the myocytes to initiate contraction. This occurs in peri-infarction tissue. Unless the situation becomes prolonged, the myocytes remain viable. Reperfusion strategies aim to prevent permanent loss of contraction in peri-infarct tisssue.

References

Espinola-Klein C, Rupprecht HJ, Blankenburg S et al (2002). Impact of infectious burden on extent and long-term prognosis of atherosclerosis. *Circulation*, 105: 15–21.

Falk E, Shah PK, Fuster V (1995). Coronary plaque disruption. *Circulation*, 92: 657–671.

Hansson G (2002). Vaccination against atherosclerosis: science or fiction? Editorial. *Circulation*, 106: 1599–1601.

Heberden W (1772). Some account of a disorder of the breast. *Medical Transactions of the Royal College of Physicians of London*, 2: 59–73.

Muller JE, Stone PH, Turi ZG, et al (1985). Circadian variation in the frequency of onset of acute myocardial infarction. *New England Journal of Medicine*, 313: 1315–1322.

Prinzmetal M, Kennamer R, Merliss R, Wada T, Bor N (1959). Angina pectoris, I. A variant form of angina pectoris. *American Journal of Medicine*, 27: 375–388.

Ross R (1993). The pathogenesis of atherosclerosis: a perspective for the 1990s. *Nature*, 362: 801–809.

Starling EH (1918). *The Linacre Lecture on the Law of the Heart*. Longmans, Green, London.

Stiell IG, Wells GA, Field BJ et al (1999) Improved out-of-hospital cardiac arrest survival through the inexpensive optimization of an existing defibrillation program: OPALS study phase II. Ontario Pre-hospital Advanced Life Support. *Journal of the American Medical Association*, 281: 1175–1181.

Thompson DR, Sutton TW, Jowett NI et al (1991). Circadian variation in the frequency of onset of chest pain in acute myocardial infarction. *British Heart Journal*, 65: 177–178.

Weissberg PL (2000). Atherogenesis: current understanding of the causes of atheroma. *Heart*, 83: 247–252.

Williams K, Tabas I (1995). The response to injury hypothesis of early atherosclerosis. *Arteriosclerosis, Thrombosis and Vascular Biology*, 15: 551–561.

Chapter 3

Coronary care

INTRODUCTION

The concept of coronary care comprises:

1 Pre-hospital care with community involvement and early management
2 Coronary care in hospital
3 Post-hospital care with progressive rehabilitation and secondary prevention.

THE NATIONAL PERSPECTIVE

The National Service Framework for Coronary Heart Disease was published in March 2000 (DoH 2000a) and has been the catalyst for many developments in coronary care since that date. The framework aims to:

- set national standards and define service models for coronary heart disease
- establish strategies to support implementation
- develop performance milestones against which progress within predetermined time scales can be measured
- form part of a range of measures designed to raise quality and equity in service introduced in 'The New NHS: modern, dependable' (DoH 1997) and 'A First Class Service' (DoH 1998).

The document is in line with the wider Government agenda of ensuring a modern, standardized, equitable, evidence-based quality health service (DoH 1997, 1999a, 2000b).

The National Service Framework sets out a 10-year programme aimed at setting standards to reach a target of reducing heart disease and cerebral vascular accident by 40% by the year 2010 (Mayor 2000). Substantial resources (£50 million) were targeted for coronary heart disease which have helped move the framework into clinical practice. The framework sets out 12 standards for the prevention, diagnosis and treatment of coronary heart disease including an 8-minute response time for the availability of a defibrillator and someone trained in its use to reach people with symptoms suggestive of a heart attack.

The National Service Framework encompasses the clinical governance agenda in that it encorporates and aims to encourage the use of evidence-based practice, particularly the use of evidence-based guidelines. It has been the impetus for many cases where nurses are taking the lead in developing services, such as rapid access chest pain clinics, expanding cardiac rehabilitation programmes, to encompass a wider range of CHD patients and heart failure nurses.

The National Institute for Clinical Excellence (NICE) is the body charged with bringing together all the evidence relating to available treatment options for specific conditions, appraising the evidence and producing clinical guidelines to inform practice. The Commission for Health Improvement (CHI) charged with responsibility for monitoring standards and evaluating the response to government targets has, of 2004, been superseded by a new body, the Healthcare Commission.

The use of guidelines and the evidence underpinning the care of coronary patients is discussed elsewhere in this book.

The NHS Modernisation Agency, established in 2001 to support the NHS and partner organizations in modernizing services and improving patient experiences and outcomes, includes a specific area of work called the CHD collaborative which supports achievement of the National Service Framework for CHD standards at local level.

Pre-hospital care

The National Service Framework (NSF) for CHD has encouraged the development of systems to deliver the time-dependent elements of cardiac care as soon as appropriately competent individuals are available, such as defibrillation carried out by pay first responders and pre-hospital thrombolysis.

Response to symptoms

An individual with acute cardiac symptoms needs to get professional help as quickly as possible. Only then will skilled help be available within the 'window of opportunity' for time-dependent treatments, including defibrillation and reperfusion. Patients with ischaemia are most likely to develop ventricular fibrillation (VF) in the first hour or so after symptom onset. They are more likely to survive this if they are in the presence of emergency services personnel who are able to perform defibrillation (Norris 1998, United Kingdom Heart Attack Study Collaborative Group (1999)).

In order for appropriate treatment to be given promptly, an individual with cardiac symptoms needs to recognize that there is a problem, appreciate the seriousness of the problem and then take action to summon professional help. Often patients call for help too late. This is something that needs to be addressed in public health education strategies.

Targeting the most appropriate patients

Rapid diagnosis and early risk stratification of patients presenting with acute chest pain are important, not only to identify patients likely to benefit from early intervention, but also, once an acute cardiac event has been excluded, to ensure that those with other cardiac or non-cardiac symptoms receive appropriate treatment.

Paramedic ambulance crews are often the first health care professionals to assess patients with chest pain and their ability to identify correctly patients with acute coronary syndromes has huge implications for subsequent management and outcomes. There is increasing evidence that appropriately trained paramedics, equipped with facilities to obtain a 12-lead electrocardiogram and working with set protocols, are able accurately to diagnose myocardial infarction and decide on which patients should be admitted to CCU (Banerjee and Rhoden 1998). This study illustrated how the paramedics' diagnoses resulted in appropriate patients bypassing the Accident and Emergency (A&E) Department and going directly to coronary care.

Fast response

Intensive coronary care will not influence community mortality rates in people who do not get to hospital or get to hospital late. It is now established that most deaths (in the order of 60%) associated with acute myocardial infarction occur in the first hour after onset and that death is usually due to VF. Thus, the recognition and immediate implementation of resuscitation measures and rapid and smooth transport to hospital is essential. Likewise, restoration of myocardial blood (reperfusion) supply needs to be prompt to ensure most benefit. The ambulance service have an established role in providing a rapid response to those calling for help with chest pain. Emergency calls are now triaged to ensure that life-threatening emergencies are given top priority with a standard set that by April 2001 three-quarters of such calls would meet the standard of a response in 8 minutes (DoH 2000a).

When patients initially call their GP, the best action is for an ambulance to be called before the GP travels to see the patient.

Appropriate treatment

Whoever first attends the patient, the priorities are the same: rapid response of vital signs, any immediate life-saving measures and then ensuring the patient gets as quickly as possible to a place where reperfusion, stabilization, reducing the risk of complications and ongoing monitoring are available.

The National Service Framework for CHD (DoH 2000a) advocates that patients with MI should receive certain interventions prior to hospital arrival. This means that all patients with suspected MI should initially be managed in an environment where these interventions are possible. These interventions are:

- cardiopulmonary resuscitation in the event of cardiac arrest
- high concentration oxygen
- pain relief (such as 2.5–5 mg of diamorphine intravenously; 5–10 mg morphine intravenously; with an antiemetic)
- aspirin (at least 300 mg orally)
- immediate transfer to hospital.

Coronary care in hospital

Patients with cardiac problems will be cared for in a variety of settings depending on how and where they present, and the structure and availability of specialist resources.

Patients who are stable

Rapid access chest pain clinics Rapid access chest pain clinics are being developed as a consequence of the National Service Framework for CHD (DoH 2000a) which states (Standard 8) that 'people with symptoms of angina or suspected angina should receive appropriate investigation and treatment to relieve their pain and reduce their risk of coronary events'. The NSF required at least 50 Rapid Access Chest Pain Clinics to be opened by April 2001, a figure that was well exceeded. They have developed to ensure that people who develop new symptoms that their GP considers might be the result of angina can be assessed by a specialist within two weeks of referral. They are designed to provide 'one stop' services so that patients undergo a basic clinical assessment and investigation (blood tests, ECG, exercise test) to confirm or exclude coronary disease and facilitate risk stratification. They aim to reduce waiting times and to reduce deaths and non-fatal cardiac events among people waiting for assessment and investigation. They also aim to enhance the quality of the service by developing high-quality information systems for audit and performance information. Rapid Access Chest Pain Clinics are an exciting opportunity for developing nursing roles and linking in with cardiac rehabilitation and primary prevention services. Although a relatively new concept, the clinics are being well evaluated and have been shown to provide the GP with a firm diagnosis in over 90% of cases (Newby et al 1998).

Patients with symptoms suggestive of acute coronary syndrome should not be referred to a Rapid Access Chest Pain Clinic but enter the emergency care system. Those with established

CHD should not be referred to the clinic but rather be re-referred to the Cardiology Outpatients Department.

Patients who are unstable

Triage strategies Reducing the time from when the patient arrives at the hospital or first experiences symptoms to the time that they are in a position to receive optimum treatment is likely to save lives. Cutting down the number of people the patient has to see and the effective use of multidisciplinary systems that facilitate rapid assessment of all patients presenting with chest pain will help, as will accelerated clinical pathways, admission protocols and admitting department triage systems. Identifying those patients who need coronary care and those who do not are important processes in appropriate patient management. The value of a high quality handover from ambulance or other emergency staff should not be underestimated. Initial evaluation, including a history and physical examination and 12-lead ECG is conclusive in only a minority of patients (Karlson et al 1991) and so the use of cardiac markers is becoming standard to stratify further the risk for such patients, following protocols for marker testing over 6–12 hours. Creatine kinase MB (CK-MB), cardiac troponin (I or T) and in some cases myoglobin are the most commonly used cardiac markers.

Nurses are often the first hospital staff to assess patients presenting with chest pain and their management decisions have been shown to match those of medical staff (Quinn 1995). An example of a triage document is given in Figure 3.1.

For such strategies to be effective, appropriate patients need to be selected and their movement through the process coordinated. While this is likely in areas with cardiac nurses, it is less so for the patient who experiences chest pain in a general ward area or in another speciality. Patients can go from having stable angina to unstable angina, acute myocardial infarction or even sudden death within days of first presentation and ongoing assessment is important. Having a specialist cardiac nurse available to support other clinical areas in identifying and securing appropriate treatment is one way these patients could be better managed.

Accident and emergency departments

The majority of patients with suspected cardiac chest pain are seen first in the A&E department (Birkhead et al 1999) even if the hospital has a direct admission coronary care unit. The efficacy of this will depend on:

- the pressure of work and the time delay before the patient is appropriately assessed
- the cardiac assessment skills of those first seeing the patient
- the availability and ability of staff in A&E department to initiate and monitor thrombolytic therapy and other first line treatments without delay
- what happens to the patient after any initial treatment (ease and speed of transfer to a suitable environment for ongoing care)
- the work of the coronary care unit (specialist CCU staff may feel de-skilled).

Some hospitals have specialist nurses who are able to assess cardiac patients and administer thrombolysis in the A&E department following agreed protocols. There is also scope for this role to have a wider function, incorporating assessment, decision making and initiating therapies for a range of patients presenting with acute coronary syndromes. This is likely to be an effective way to expedite initial management for the most unstable and at risk group of CHD patients (Kucia et al 2001). However, there are potential drawbacks to this service including the de-skilling of A&E department staff and inequalities in care as a result of the service not being available over the 24-hour period (Quinn and Morse 2003). Not all patients will meet the criteria for treatment under the predetermined protocol and it has been argued that this limits and potentially delays some treatments, as anything other than the straightforward will still have to be seen by a physician (Rhodes 1998).

The development of new nursing roles is discussed further later in this chapter.

Chest pain units

About 500 000 patients attend emergency departments in the UK each year (DoH 2001) and between

ACUTE TRIAGE ASSESSMENT

Admitted at: Time................ Date...............   999   GP referral   TIME SYMPTOM ONSET......

CARDIAC ARREST → → → → → → YES → → CCU

↓ NO

CARDIAC PAIN/SYMPTOMS			
1. Band-like pain across centre of chest	Y/N	↓	
2. Gradual onset of pain.	Y/N		
3. Pain came on at rest.	Y/N	↓	
4. Pain radiating to arms or neck or back	Y/N		
5. Episode associated with SOB	Y/N	↓	
Sweating	Y/N		
Nausea/vomiting	Y/N	*SOUNDS ACUTE*	
6. Symptoms associated with activity	Y/N	*CARDIAC* → →	*YES* → → *CCU*
7. Increasing in frequency over last few days	Y/N	↓	
8. Like previous ischaemic chest pain/		*NO*	
symptoms?	Y/N N/A		
9. Relieved by GTN?	Y/N N/A	↓	
10. Any other significant details including:			
– patient interpretation of symptoms			
– significant risk factors		↓	
– previous cardiac history suggesting			
MI/unstable angina?			
Details:	Y/N N/A	↓	
↓ NO		↓	
12-LEAD ECG SHOWS ACUTE MI		↓	
Brief details:		*ECG*	
		SUGGESTIVE OF MI? →	*YES* → → *CCU*
1. Significant ST elevation?	Y/N	↓	*&*
2. LBBB	Y/N	*NO*	*thrombolytic assessment*
↓ NO		↓	
ACUTE 12-LEAD ECG		↓	
Associated with presence or <u>risk</u> of significant	Y/N		
symptoms.		↓	
ECG shows (describe & tick):			
*significant ischaemia		↓	
*complete heart block		*NEEDS MONITORING/*	
*irregular heart rate		*TREATMENT ON CCU* →	*YES* → → *CCU*
*bradycardia			
*tachycardia		↓	
Is currently experiencing (underline)			
Pain, dyspnoea, dizziness, palpitations,		↓	
hypotension (BP=)		*NO* → →	*NO*→ →*TRANSFER*
Other details:			

↓ NO   ↓ NO

DECISION FOR <u>EARLY</u> TRANSFER TO MEDICAL WARD/EMU made at time............by. sig.......... Grade.......

ACTION taken: stay on CCU   transfer EMU   Transfer ward   discharge home   Time:

TRANSFERRED on (date).......... at (time)............... To: Home   EMU   Wd 11   Wd 2   Wd 6   Other..........

INITIAL DIAGNOSIS: MI   UNSTABLE ANGINA   STABLE ANGINA   ARRHYTHMIA   HEART FAILURE   NON-CARDIAC

FINAL DIAGNOSIS: MI   UNSTABLE ANGINA   STABLE ANGINA   ARRHYTHMIA   HEART FAILURE   NON-CARDIAC

BP = blood pressure, CCU = coronary care unit, ECG = electocardiogram, EMU = emergency medical unit, GTN = glyceryl trinitrate, LBBB = left bundle branch block, MI = myocardial infarction, SOB = shortness of breath.

Figure 3.1   Example of a triage document (Leicester General Hospital).

20 and 30% of all medical admissions are for acute chest pain (Capewell and McMurray 2000). This number is likely to increase as the public and GPs respond to education campaigns that advise calling an ambulance for chest pain suggestive of an MI (Clancy 2002). There is a need to develop strategies to prevent wards becoming swamped with patients who do not need to be there. However, as the pressure to avoid inappropriate admissions rises, so potentially will the number of inappropriate discharges. One UK study has demonstrated that about 6% of patients discharged from an emergency department had prognostically significant myocardial damage (Collinson et al 2000b). Chest pain units allow patients admitted with suspected cardiac pain to be assessed by experienced staff in order to avoid unnecessary hospital admission and ensure appropriate management of those that need to be admitted (Farkouh et al 1998). They also aim to shorten patient stay and save money. They are separate from the A&E department, thus avoiding any conflict of interest with other types of patients. They usually take patients who have already been assessed as low to medium risk and monitor them closely for 6–12 hours, undertaking further tests including serial ECGs, ST segment monitoring and biochemical assays. Like other relatively new initiatives in coronary care, their role has yet to be formally evaluated in the UK is only beginning (Goodacre et al 2004), although in the USA they have been well evaluated. Reported benefits include (Gibler 1997):

- identification and subsequent admission of high risk patients who might otherwise have been discharged
- improved care for patients with ST segment elevation MI with decreased time to thrombolysis or acute mechanical intervention.

Coronary care units

Coronary care units were essentially designed to serve three purposes (Jowett and Thompson 1989):

1 the provision of a separate area within the hospital for the care and surveillance of patients with acute myocardial infarction or other cardiac disorders, such as unstable angina, heart failure, cardiac arrhythmias and cardiogenic shock

2 the provision of care by nurses and physicians with specialist training

3 the provision of personnel and equipment immediately available for resuscitation.

The management of patients with an acute cardiac event requires rapid assessment, stabilization, re-establishment of adequate cardiac blood flow, relief of pain, treatment of complications including resuscitation and patient support and education. Roughly half of all acute coronary patients admitted to a coronary care unit have a complicated clinical course, and these complications often occur soon after admission. In general, patients with larger myocardial infarctions have more complications and a poorer prognosis. However, much depends upon how much myocardium is viable. Intervention to salvage ischaemic myocardium has become a major target in the modern management of the coronary patient, and pharmacological and mechanical therapies directed at improving oxygen supply and reducing myocardial work have assumed increasing prominence. Thrombolysis is the single most important advance in coronary care since defibrillation. It is now routine hospital practice unless specific contraindications exist.

HISTORY AND PRESENT STATUS OF CORONARY CARE

Vesalius had written about cardiac resuscitation in the sixteenth century, and there had been sporadic reports of success in restarting the arrested heart. However, it was Hooker et al (1933), using animal experiments, who proposed a specific method of cardiac resuscitation involving rhythmic manual massage of the heart through a thoracotomy followed by defibrillation. Fourteen years elapsed before Beck et al (1947) successfully applied Hooker's technique to a 14-year-old boy in the operating theatre who had developed VF following chest surgery. Later, Beck et al (1956) and Reagan et al (1956), working independently, used this method for the first time outside the operating theatre in acute coronary patients. At about the same time, Zoll et al (1956) reported that VF could be terminated by defibrillation (using an alternating current, AC, device) delivered externally through the intact chest wall. A few years later, Lown et al (1962) first described a direct current (DC) defibrillator.

Incorporating the technique of Zoll and his colleagues, Kouwenhoven et al (1960) demonstrated that the heart could effectively be massaged without thoracotomy by rhythmic external compression of the chest wall. Combined with mouth-to-mouth resuscitation, this would maintain an oxygenated blood supply to vital organs until external defibrillation could be applied. These advances formed the basis of cardiopulmonary resuscitation as we know it today. Soon after, Julian (1961) suggested that all medical, nursing and auxiliary staff should be trained in these new techniques of resuscitation.

Based on these concepts, the coronary care unit was developed whose goal was to provide a group of patients assembled under the surveillance of skilled personnel with electrocardiographic and resuscitation facilities in a specialized setting. The first coronary care units were established, more or less independently, in the early 1960s in Kansas, Toronto, Philadelphia, Sydney and London (Day 1972). Brown et al (1963) ingeniously converted an old electroencephalograph into a four-channel electrocardiograph, thereby greatly adding to an understanding of arrhythmias.

Despite such advances, many patients were needlessly dying because usually no one was available at all times who could interpret the electrocardiogram (ECG) pattern. Thus, nurses were trained in ECG recognition and interpretation, and defibrillation.

Centralized viewing of the ECG, and the installment of alarm systems, revolutionized coronary care. A major impact was the responsibility that nurses assumed in providing 24-hour monitoring. Other responsibilities that the coronary care nurse assumed, which were delegated by physicians, included the initiation of intravenous drug therapy, the assistance in routine haemodynamic monitoring and the obtaining of arterial and venous blood samples. They were to be especially skilled in cardiopulmonary resuscitation.

Thus, it was soon apparent that the major factors in determining the success of the coronary care system were the competence and training of the nurse.

Although the original concept of the coronary care unit nurse was in the immediate detection and prompt resuscitation of patients with VF following acute myocardial infarction, the emphasis was later extended to the possible prevention of lethal arrhythmias by the administration of new anti-arrhythmic drugs.

The management of patients with suspected MI has changed dramatically since Herrick's description of the syndrome in 1912. In the early 20th century, patients with MI were nursed in bed for long periods with minimal therapeutic intervention apart from narcotic analgesia. The feasibility of treating acute MI patients with thrombolytic therapy to disperse thrombus and limit infarct size was first described by Fletcher et al in 1958. Intravenous streptokinase was administered over a 30-hour period to 28 patients within 6–72 hours of symptom onset. In the next two decades over 30 trials compared intravenous streptokinase with placebo but were not thought to have demonstrated signi-ficant clinical benefit. Interestingly, subsequent meta-analysis of these trials (Lau et al 1992) demonstrated a favourable outcome in the treatment groups, leading to the conclusion that intravenous streptokinase could have been saving lives 20 years previously. Thrombolytic therapy did not become routine treatment for MI until the 1980s.

The latter years of the 20th century saw significant advances in early defibrillation, infarct limitation and secondary prevention. However, until the advent of thrombolytic therapy there was an argument for managing older patients with uncomplicated MI at home (Hill et al 1978).

With rapidly increasing technology and advances in therapeutics and pharmacology, together with the expertise of nursing and medical staff, the role of coronary care units continued to expand.

Current status of the coronary care unit

The coronary care unit now has an important role in the management of a wider range of acute coronary syndromes and other medical disorders, including heart failure, cardiogenic shock and serious cardiac arrhythmias. Thus, perhaps the term 'coronary care unit' is a misnomer, and 'cardiac care unit' a more accurate term.

Use of the coronary care unit

Contemporary coronary care usually commences in the pre-hospital setting and continues in the emergency department for the majority of patients. On-going management is best placed on the coronary care unit. There is evidence that MI patients managed on a medical ward fare less well than those on a coronary care unit (Lawrence-Mathew et al 1994). Coronary care units are relatively well resourced, and the challenge lies in ensuring that the most appropriate patients are able to benefit from these resources. This is more likely if there is:

- accurate initial assessment, including risk stratification, of potential patients to ensure that those not requiring a coronary care bed are triaged to a less intensive environment
- ongoing assessment of patients and developed decision-making processes to ensure that patients who no longer require coronary care are identified
- nursing empowerment and skill to make discharge decisions
- development of appropriately used step-down beds
- the capacity to move patients promptly to other areas when they no longer require coronary care
- care of low-risk patients on telemetry systems on cardiac wards
- systems in place to identify patients elsewhere who would benefit from coronary care and being able to transfer these patients promptly to the coronary care environment
- appropriate staff skill mix.

At any one time there is likely to be a proportion of patients in a coronary care unit who do not need to be there. The wide range of presenting symptoms in patients, a lack of specialized assessment skills in those to whom the patient presents and limited diagnostic equipment make it difficult accurately to identify and exclude acute cardiac disorders. As many as 30% of admissions to a coronary care unit may be non-cardiac and other cardiac patients who are admitted may not require such intensive care. The focus of coronary care remains the rapid reperfusion of MI patients with ST elevation. These patients are often stable within 6 hours and the challenge is often finding a bed for them in a less intensive environment. It is not unknown for MI patients to be discharged directly from the coronary care unit as there are no beds on cardiac wards. Conversely, many cardiac patients who would benefit from the coronary care environment, such as those with unstable angina or non-ST segment elevation MI are admitted via accident and emergency departments and admission wards and never reach a coronary care unit. There is evidence that nearly two thirds of this group of patients are cared for outside a coronary care unit environment (Collinson et al 2000a).

Coronary care unit resources

Environment   Coronary care units are traditionally comparatively well resourced, although there is probably now more pressure to justify new purchases and capital outlay. Nurses are having to become more *au fait* with making purchasing decisions, developing business plans and bidding for limited funds.

Coronary care units need to evoke a calm and reassuring atmosphere and yet be places where high technology can be used appropriately to help monitor and manage care. They need to allow the entry of as much natural light as possible and have air conditioning. There needs to be some control over 'through traffic', such as an entrance buzzer, in order to minimize disturbance and to be able to advise visitors when it is inappropriate to visit. Procedures such as temporary pacing or cardioversion are best carried out away from the main bed areas. Space around the bed needs to be wide enough to enable resuscitation to take place safely and for portable equipment such as X-ray and echocardiogram machines to fit around the bed space.

Most units have a combination of side rooms and small bay areas. Side rooms allow privacy and limit disturbance for other patients, although it can mean that patients feel isolated, unsafe and are unwilling to ask for help. Not being able to see a clock can increase feelings of disorientation and lack of control. Patients are more difficult to observe in side wards and having a number of side wards may have implications for staffing levels. Patients who are stable often benefit from talking to others in a similar position, an opportunity which is lost if all the beds are separate. Bed areas need to have piped oxygen and suction and cardiac monitoring facilities which relay recorded information to a central consul. Beds need to be easily movable and enable the patient to rest in a variety of sitting positions. Patients who are unstable will need a bedside commode and to wash by their bed, but thereafter may be able to walk to the toilet or washroom. These facilities should be single sexed and have emergency buzzers and slide opening doors.

Relatives of coronary care patients frequently want to talk in private about care and may also need somewhere to sit quietly if they are distressed. Patients also benefit from having somewhere away from the main bed area to discuss their treatment options and receive health care advice.

Trying to accommodate these activities in the ward nursing office is not ideal and has implications for confidentiality and day to day unit management. Staff rest rooms adjacent to the unit mean that staff can leave the clinical area for a break but can still be called upon in an emergency. A seminar room equipped with education resources and audio-visual aids, that is available to the multidisciplinary team is useful for meetings and education sessions.

Staffing   Admission rates to coronary care units have increased exponentially since the advent of thrombolytic therapy for patients with acute myocardial infarction (Hobbs 1995). The period of most intense patient care tends to occur in the period immediately after admission. Due to limiting infarct size, patients arguably require less intervention for complications following myocardial infarction. Staffing levels have tended not to reflect increased throughput and there is wide variation between units. The British Cardiac Society recommends that there should be one cardiologist for every 50 000 of the district population, with a minimum of two cardiologists in acute hospitals. Patients are usually investigated and medically treated by trainee physicians and their supervising consultants. However 24-hour care, which involves ongoing assessment, coordinating care, monitoring the effects of treatment and anticipating and responding to changes in the patient's condition is

provided by the nursing team who are the key to successful patient management.

The British Cardiac Society (2002) recognizes the importance of adequate nurse staffing and recommends a ratio of 1 nurse to 2 patients in CCU. There are no recognized work load indices for coronary care units to quantify ideal staffing levels. It is the *potential* needs of patients rather than their actual needs which need to be considered. A coronary patient can be stable and require minimal care one moment and the next need the skills of a full resuscitation team. A unit can have empty beds and have patients ready for transfer and then admit two or three acutely unwell patients over a short period of time. Also, it is the skills of the nurses which are important, not the numbers.

There are various methods for estimating the size and skill mix of nursing teams, all of which have strengths and weaknesses. The methods can be grouped into:

- professional judgement
- nurses per occupied bed
- acuity-quality methods
- time-task/activity approaches
- regression-based systems.

Triangulating two or more methods may give more confidence that appropriate staffing levels have been determined.

Nursing shift systems   Flexible methods of working, including job share, term-time working, more part-time workers, supernumerary student status and the move away from permanent night staff have all contributed to making the process of ensuring appropriate nursing numbers and skill mix an ever more complex problem. The relatively new working time regulations (Department of Trade and Industry 1998) further complicate the picture. Many coronary care units have explored different shift systems in an attempt to solve local staffing problems. There has been a significant increase in the number of nurses working 12-hour shifts. Good quality research in the field of shift work and its influence on efficiency and effectiveness of care delivery is limited, with researchers tending to focus on different aspects of shift work with conflicting findings emerging (Fitzpatrick et al 1999). With such limited evidence on which to base decisions, practice has tended to change through a process of trial and error. Many units now offer a mixture of shifts which, while suiting the individuals concerned may not be best for patient care or for staff development.

Step-down units

The provision of intermediate or step down beds can bridge the gap between the more intensive coronary care and management in a general ward. They are a useful response to the ever increasing demand for coronary care beds in the face of limited resources and there is growing interest in developing ways of identifying those patients for whom CCU is not necessary (Quinn et al 2000).

Patients can be transferred within the first 24 hours if they are stable, free from ischaemic pain, heart failure, hypotension or compromising arrhythmias. As with deciding who should be admitted *on* to a coronary care unit, the decision as to who should be moved *off* is more effective if there are guidelines and protocols to work with. The transfer decision needs to be reviewed on each ward round and documented so that the health care team and the patient are all aware of the plan. Hopefully this avoids the situation where a patient, who is obviously ready to move, has to wait until the next consultant visit for this to be put into action. experienced coronary care nurses are likely to be able to make appropriate transfer decisions, although the key to this probably lies in the development of specific and sensitive decision algorithms (Quinn et al 2000). Step-down units are usually staffed by coronary care nurses and this allows therapeutic nurse–patient relationships to continue. It also gives the opportunity for specialized staff to carry on with patient support and advice in a less busy environment at a time when the patient is more ready to receive it. Group rehabilitation sessions on the ward are one option and encourage patients to listen to and learn from others in a similar position. Discharge planning can begin as soon as the patient goes on to the step-down unit to encourage a coordinated and timely approach.

It is all too easy to see the step-down beds as an extension of the coronary care unit and if mismanaged, this can lead to unsafe work loads and a disruption of the step-down environment for other patients.

Standards for coronary care

Ideally, any patient admitted to any hospital across the country should expect to receive the same standard of evidence-based high quality coronary care. The British Cardiac Society sets specific standards in its Clinical Governance Peer Review Scheme. These include:

- all main facilities for cardiac patients within the same area of the hospital
- adequate space with separate rooms for ECG, stress testing, ambulatory monitoring, reception, consultant office, junior staff office, secretarial office
- arrangements for rapid assessment of patients with suspected angina, e.g. rapid access chest pain clinics supported by clear referral criteria and protocols for investigation
- smoking cessation clinic
- time from GP referral to specialist 2 weeks for new onset chest pain
- time from GP referral to consultant 4 weeks for other cardiac problems
- coronary care unit under administrative control of a cardiologist
- 4 coronary care beds per 100 000 population
- facilities for temporary pacing, Swan-Ganz catheters/direct arterial pressure monitoring and adequate radiation protection
- bed occupancy less than 85%.

The nurse in coronary care

Since the introduction of the coronary care system, the nurse's role has not remained static, but has continued to develop, accompanying the changing needs of patients and the rapid advances in medicine and technology. Nurses have always been central to the development and success of coronary care units (Quinn and Thompson 1999). Developments in the nursing role have centred on the evolution of the nursing function and professional and legal responsibility and autonomy. Nursing often has to redefine its function in terms of patient needs and be prepared to move outside the sphere of traditional nursing.

Traditionally, according to Benner (1984) there are seven domains of nursing practice, all of which apply to coronary care nursing:

1 the helping role
2 the teaching–coaching function
3 the diagnostic and patient monitoring function
4 the effective management of rapidly changing situations
5 administering and monitoring therapeutic interventions and regimens
6 monitoring and ensuring the quality of health care practices
7 organizational and work-role competencies.

Initially, doctors were delegating medical responsibilities to nurses who, impressed by this, automatically assumed them. In many instances this had the deleterious effect of reducing the quality and quantity of *nursing* activity. Much of the coronary care nurse's time has been spent supporting the aims and aspirations of medical colleagues, often resulting in stereotyped and unthinking behaviour.

Nursing traditionally aims to help individuals maintain as near to normal lifestyles as possible and to help them in those activities which they would normally be able to perform themselves (Henderson 1966, McFarlane 1980). Doing this effectively relies on a good nursing assessment of what the patient is like normally and how they have been affected by their condition and admission to hospital. Nursing is now an increasingly complex activity, partly because medical knowledge and technology have advanced so rapidly and become more complex, and partly because a body of knowledge and skills peculiar to nursing has assumed greater importance.

Nursing responsibilities for patients admitted with CHD include:

1 identifying and prioritizing the ongoing nursing needs of the patient
2 devising and implementing appropriate nursing care for each patient
3 making observations of the patient's response to treatment
4 anticipating care needs

5 being involved in and contributing to decisions about patient treatment
6 coordinating procedures, tests and personnel for the patient – ensuring continuity of care
7 being involved in decisions about transfer and discharge
8 initiating preventive measures to protect the patient from complications
9 supporting and educating the patient and family
10 translating relevant research findings into actual nursing practice
11 instituting change in order to improve patient care.

The nurse is thus responsible for controlling and manipulating the patient's environment so as to promote well-being and comfort while carrying out the established objectives of care.

In the coronary care unit the nurse has more opportunity than any other member of the health care team to observe the patient continuously and to influence patient care. For a short while the patient may be dependent on the nurse for many activities of living. Neglecting basic care in favour of the technical and specialized is an easy trap to fall into. The focus on rapid diagnosis, rapid intervention and prompt transfer or discharge may mean that actions such as listening to a patient's concerns, providing a bowl for a wash or explaining what is happening to a worried relative can get neglected.

In order to operate effectively, the nurse needs to possess a depth of knowledge and a range of skills and expertise. Nurses need to assess and interpret the needs of the patient and family, make judgements and decisions, set priorities and take responsibility for the delivery of care and its outcome. In addition it is necessary to be aware of a range of medical treatment strategies in order to help inform junior medical staff, anticipate treatment and discuss management options with patients and their families. It is important that technical competencies and interpersonal skills go hand in hand.

NURSE EDUCATION

As professional workers, nurses have a responsibility to themselves as well as to patients and others to maintain their professional knowledge and competence (Nursing and Midwifery Council 2002). It is important to continue to be educated about nursing, health care and political issues. This includes frequent and systematic updating of knowledge and skills by reading relevant literature and staying informed about political and professional issues as well as those related to clinical practice. Staff development is intrinsic to this process, and should be seen as an obligatory, not an optional, part of professionalism.

When coronary care units were first established, nursing education programmes in coronary care were initially virtually non-existent. The few that did exist were unstructured, with nurses determining their own needs and seeking ways to meet them. Early programmes tended to focus on pathophysiology, technology, pharmacology and therapeutics at the expense of psychological, social, moral, ethical, cultural and spiritual aspects of care.

Nursing has been identified as being different from other professions in that it places great emphasis on formal, post-basic education. In an attempt to meet some of the educational and clinical needs of the specialist nurses the Joint Board of Clinical Nursing Studies (JBCNS), set up in 1970, provided post-basic courses for registered nurses. The JBCNS was superseded by the National Boards for Nursing, Midwifery and Health Visiting which were responsible for post-basic nursing courses until 2002. These courses evolved over the years, becoming increasingly more academic, arguably at the expense of developing good clinical skills to prepare nurses for clinical decision making. Nurses completing them were increasingly demonstrating a perceived (and actual) lack of clinical skills and confidence. Technical competence has been identified as a learning priority in intensive and coronary care nurses (Little 1999). The restructuring of post-basic education since the demise of the National Boards is an opportunity to re-examine course outcomes and methods of assessment. There is also scope to examine shared learning opportunities with other professionals and other strategies to enhance the process of life-long learning. Options include flexible learning and increased use of information technology.

A real problem for the coronary care nurse today is balancing specialist education with the statutory and mandatory training that is becoming an annual requirement to meet the standards of bodies such as the Clinical Negligence Scheme for Trusts (CNST). There is a potential danger that a so-called specialist nurse will be *au fait* with corporate knowledge at the expense of the knowledge required to care for patients. An appraisal of what knowledge or competencies are needed for specific roles and to minimize risk to the patient, the nurse and the organization seems a sensible way forward.

NURSING EXPERTISE

Towards the end of the last decade, the United Kingdom Central Council for nursing and midwifery (UKCC) re-examined the concepts of advanced and specialist practice and concluded that there was a need for a clear, robust framework to minimize confusion. The terms are still used interchangeably even within the same hospital. There is some debate as to whether the development of nursing expertise requires education and training or whether it evolves through experience. Other points for debate focus on how expertise is quantified and how it is assessed.

Extensive clinical experience has been shown to outweigh educational attainment when nurse's expertise is judged by their peers (Thompson et al 2001). Development of expertise is likely to require periods of observing and reflecting on the work of more experienced role models and is also dependent on the support of others (Manley 2000).

Benner (1984) considers that nurses develop in a series of stages:

1 *Novice*: has little understanding of the contextual meaning of facts learnt from textbooks. Behaviour is governed by rules and tends to be inflexible and not always appropriate. Takes in little in a novel situation.
2 *Advanced beginner*: has coped with enough real situations to begin to note the priorities and relevance of aspects of the various situations. Needs support and help in setting priorities, as she tends to operate on guidelines.
3 *Competent*: begins to see own actions in terms of long-range goals or plans of which is consistently aware. Analytically contemplates the problem.

4 *Proficient*: perceives situations based on experience and recent events. Tends not to have to 'think out' the situation; understands it as a whole, holistic understanding. Can recognize when the expected normal picture does not materialize.

5 *Expert*: no longer relies on an analytical principle, but has an intuitive grasp of each situation and can concentrate on what is important rather than spending wasteful time on alternative diagnoses and situations.

Benner believes that expertise develops through a process of comparing clinical situations with each other in order to develop a deep understanding. Expertise is now recognized as a benchmark within career frameworks (DoH 1999b,c) and expert practice is also a core sub-role of advanced nurse practice.

The Scope of Professional Practice (UKCC 1992) recommended that nurses advance their practice through additional training and later it was recommended that all advanced practitioners study at Master's level and there are now specific courses to facilitate this (Dunn and Morgan 1998). However, since March 1997 there are no standards for advanced practice and the term specialist practice has come to embody nursing care that exercises higher levels of judgement, discretion and decision making in clinical care and incorporates clinical practice, care and programme development, clinical practice development and leadership (UKCC 2001). To use the title specialist practitioner an individual must have a clinical recordable qualification following a course of at least 4 months relevant to the area of practice and evidence that they have consolidated their experience. The individual's employer also needs to go on record that they are confident that the individual has the relevant skill and knowledge for the role.

Many of the skills needed to undertake the role of a so-called expert coronary care nurse fall into a technical domain which can be broken down into discrete competencies. It has been argued that these competencies can be carried out by any health care worker who has been appropriately trained and if this is the case, there is an argument against having so many qualified staff on a coronary care unit.

To counter this, it has been proposed that expert nurses are able to give additional care and therapy while they are completing tasks (Kitson 1987).

OPPORTUNITIES FOR NURSING

NHS Trusts need to recognize the value of and, indeed, require nurses with knowledge and skills beyond initial registration. This is to provide services that are appropriate for the level of patient need (Williams et al 2001). The concept of the extended role was used for nurses who took on functions that were once the remit of other professions. This term was officially 'laid to rest' some years ago as it was recognized that it may well have been limiting practice (Quinn and Thompson 1995). The term role expansion reflects a deeper development of a nursing role that continues to recognize the therapeutic potential of the core nursing function (Ersser 2000). The document 'Making a Difference – strengthening the nursing, midwifery and health visiting contribution to health and health care' (DoH 1999b) attempted to clarify new career structures to help develop professional leadership, extend the clinical career ladder for those who might otherwise have entered management and foster opportunities for sideways movement between practice, education and research. The NHS Plan (DoH 2000b) further supported the development of nursing roles.

The concept of specialist nursing posts is not new. Clinical nursing roles have developed in response to changes in the government agenda, health care delivery systems and professional roles. The New Deal and changes to junior doctors' hours (National Health Service Management Executive 1991) proved to be a significant driver for change and many nurses now work in different ways to those of 10 years ago. Cardiac nurses have traditionally worked as part of a multidisciplinary team and have taken on many expanded roles. Many have been actively involved for some time in roles that involve teaching and guiding their medical colleagues through the realities of clinical life (Quinn and Thompson 1995). Nurses now lead services, have recognized patient case loads and make complex clinical decisions. In coronary care nursing, nurses lead cardiac rehabilitation programmes, smoking cessation clinics and chest pain, heart failure and hypertension clinics. The National Service Framework (DoH 2000a) has provided further opportunity for nurse-led services including rapid access chest pain clinics and nurse-led thrombolysis. Ideally nurse-led roles need to be cost effective, fit in with the health care system and be practical (Thompson et al 2001). The roles are still new and there is comparatively little evidence as to their effectiveness. While there is some evidence that nurses are able to function in roles that require them to emulate physicians, for example making thrombolysis decisions (Quinn et al 1998, Somauroo et al 1999), it is questionable that this is the best way to evaluate *nursing* roles. Nurses may well bring extra dimensions to the roles that are difficult to quantify by traditional research methods.

Health Service Circular 1998/161 sets out plans to develop nurse consultants posts whereby, in theory, expert nurses could develop their role as clinical leaders while retaining day-to-day contact with patients. Four interrelated functions essential for the nurse consultant role were identified. These were:

- an expert practice function (minimum 50% of time in practice)
- a professional leadership and consultancy function
- an education, training and development function
- a practice and service development function.

These posts were to be new posts, not automatic rewards for experienced clinical nurse specialists and not to be dependent on specific qualifications. As there has been no formal funding, posts have tended to develop around areas financially supported from other sources and are not always based on local need. Formal evaluation of these relatively new roles in coronary care is awaited.

The impact of a pay structure (Agenda for Change) which aims to reward generic competencies across professional groups may allow nurses to develop their roles in new ways (DoH 1999c).

RELATIONS WITH OTHER HEALTH PROFESSIONALS

The concept of coronary care is based on a team approach, with the nurse and physician sharing the responsibility for patient care. Individual professions need to appreciate the collaborative role of all members of the coronary care team, especially the relationship between the nurse and physician.

Frequently, in the coronary care unit, as with other specialized areas, the roles of the nurse and physician overlap, particularly concerning issues relating to medical and technical aspects of care where difficulties may arise regarding role clarification.

The doctor must also appreciate that the nurse needs to take into account their own professional code of conduct as well as their legal obligations, and that individual professional accountability is an integral part of nursing practice.

Nevertheless, problems will continue to occur. For instance, if certain technologies are available, why not use them regardless of the patient's age or condition? If not, who makes such a decision? What is the nurse's role in such a situation, particularly when they regard themselves as patient advocate? Clearly such issues are complex and not easily resolved. But, by mutual respect and intelligent, constructive debate with other professionals, such problems are not insurmountable. The discrepancies in authority between the multidisciplinary roles are beginning to be met by the formalization of treatment plans, guidelines and critical/integrated pathways.

In intensive care areas, including coronary care, there is often a high workload, with many responsibilities and emotional demands, and although many people relish this atmosphere, others may find it overpowering. Ashworth (1986) made reference to the classification of staff (and patients) as 'drains' or 'radiators'. The former group leave one emotionally and physically drained and exhausted after an encounter, whereas the latter radiate warmth and other good qualities, leaving one feeling better than before. Coronary care units need to develop a functional maturity where each staff member is a 'radiator' of professional competence and support.

NURSING STRESS

Working in an environment with critically ill (or potentially critically ill) patients and an unpredictable workload is a possible source of working stress for the coronary care nurse. The relationship between the nurse and the patient, particularly if they are seriously ill or dying, is also potentially a major source of nursing stress. The threat of losing a life often goes against nursing perceptions of success, and feelings of failure or inadequacy may ensue. Nurses in coronary care are assuming an increasing responsibility for patient care management and are also expected to be familiar with an array of technical equipment. A further problem for many nurses is the patient who displays negative emotions when trying to cope with their condition, or who is considered demanding, attention seeking, continually asking questions and seeking reassurance and support.

Workload stress is a particular source of stress experienced by nurses (Healy and McKay 2000). A large study of over 4000 Royal College of Nursing members (Seccombe and Smith 1996) revealed increasing levels of workload stress with almost 60% of the sample claiming to have worked in excess of their contracted hours in their latest working week. The emphasis on shorter patient stay, day-case facilities for certain procedures (such as cardioversions), and the success of certain treatments, means that there is potential for a faster patient through put and a more dependent patient case load. Staffing establishments have not tended to reflect this, so the same number of nurses are having to work harder. Increased paper work and having to respond to government targets in terms of audit and data collection, which are seen to detract from patient care, may be a developing source of stress in coronary care nurses.

Ehrenfeld and Cheifetz (1990) identify three main sources of stress as:

1   inadequate or poor communication with doctors or other staff
2   dealing with a dying patient and his/her family
3   overload and/or inadequate resources.

Sawatzky (1996) identified patient care factors as the highest stressor identified by a group of critical care nurses, although lack of control over situations was also ranked highly.

The patient's family may be a source of stress for nursing staff. There is a danger that the nurse may feel emotionally drained and have difficulty in balancing the time she gives to the needs of the patient and those of the family.

Interpersonal relationships with colleagues are a potential source of stress for the nurse. The close, but often blurred, role of the doctor and the nurse particularly has the potential for producing uncertainty and conflict. Personality clashes between nurses are not uncommon and may be exacerbated in the coronary care unit.

Supervisory behaviour and leadership styles can have a mitigating or buffering effect on nurses' stress. Leaders who are perceived to be closely monitoring nurses in their performance of duties so as to prevent mistakes, have been shown to generate higher levels of emotional exhaustion among their staff (Stordeur et al 2001). This behaviour was perceived as lack of trust and the nurses felt unsupported.

The environment itself may be stress-producing. For example, the relative isolation of the coronary care unit and its unique layout, technology, high percentage of qualified staff, high staff–patient ratio and other factors, such as internal rotation of staff shifts, may add to the problem. Many nurses find that the coronary care unit is typified by periods of relative inactivity interspersed with episodes of crisis. Unlike most other critical care areas, coronary care patients are usually conscious and look generally well, with no apparent signs of injury or distress. Thus, the extensive personal communications among staff reported on intensive care units, and cited as a source of escape from the work situation, are likely to be curbed on the coronary care unit where the nurses are aware that they are being observed by their patients.

High stress levels are likely to be reflected in high staff turnover. Unrealistic expectations may contribute to feelings of inadequacy and dissatisfaction, and a lack of peer support and counselling may contribute to staff being unable to face up to the demands of their job.

Burnout

According to Freundenberger (1974), burnout means 'to fail, wear out or become exhausted by making excessive demands on energy, strength or resources'. Much of the literature on nurses and burnout is from the 1980s, although it could be argued that recent advances in technology and increasing care demands make it more likely in the coronary care nurse of today. A more recent study highlighted that burnout was more of a risk for those nurses who demonstrated a low level of hardiness (Collins 1996). Interpersonal conflict, management of the unit, the nature of direct patient care and inadequate knowledge and skills are further contributory factors. The precursor for burnout and its manifestations may be recognized by others prior to being noted by the person affected. Changes observed may be grouped as follows:

- physical, e.g. fatigue, headache and changes in appetite
- cognitive, e.g. poor concentration, decreased creativity and poor judgement
- psychological, e.g. feelings of dehumanization, suspicion and helplessness
- behavioural, e.g. decreased performance, increased illness and physical distancing from patients.

Dewe (1987) identifies six coping strategies that nurses reported using to cope with burnout:

1 problem-oriented behaviour
2 trying to unwind and put things into perspective
3 expressing feelings and frustrations
4 keeping the problem to oneself
5 accepting the job as it is
6 trying not to let the stress get at one.

Ehrenfeld and Cheifetz (1990) list four disparate ways which nurses might use to deal with stress:

1 active coping strategies aimed at solution of the problem
2 diverting responsibility to others for finding a solution to the stressful problem
3 passivity or avoidance of dealing with the problem
4 activity not directed at solution of the stress problem.

Although most nurses are able to recognize when they are stressed and feel able to relieve this in some way, it is likely that coronary care nurses would benefit from supportive structures within their working environment. Factors such as promoting positive aspects of the job; staff appraisal and feedback; peer support; adequate teaching, clinical supervision; adequate meal breaks; and safe staffing levels are likely to minimize nursing stress. Effective communication between all groups of staff working in the coronary care unit would seem to be vital.

References

Ashworth P (1986). Doctors, nurses and others in ICU – 'drains' or 'radiators'. *Intensive Care Nursing*, 1: 165–167.

Banerjee S, Rhoden WE (1998). Fast-tracking of myocardial infarction by paramedics. *Journal of the Royal College of Physicians of London*, 32: 36–38.

Beck CS, Pritchard WH, Feil HS (1947). Ventricular fibrillation of long duration abolished by electric shock. *Journal of the American Medical Association*, 135: 985–986.

Beck CS, Weckesser EC, Barry FM (1956). Fatal heart attack and successful defibrillation. *Journal of the American Medical Association*, 161: 434–436.

Benner P (1984). *From Novice to Expert: Excellence and Power in Clinical Nursing Practice*. Addison-Wesley, Menlo Park (CA).

Birkhead J, Goldacre M, Mason A et al (1999). *Health Outcome Indicators: Myocardial Infarction*. Report of a working group to the Department of Health. National Centre for Health Outcomes Development, Oxford.

British Cardiac Society (2002). Fifth report on the provision of services for patients with heart disease. *Heart*, 88 (suppl 3): 1–56.

Brown KW, MacMillan RL, Forbath N (1963). Coronary unit. An intensive care centre for acute myocardial infarction. *Lancet*, 2: 349–352.

Capewell S, McMurray J (2000). Chest pain – please admit: is there an alternative? *British Medical Journal*, 320: 951–952.

Clancy M (2002). Chest pain units. *British Medical Journal*, 325: 116–117.

Collins MA (1996). The relation of work stress, hardiness, and burnout among full time hospice workers. *Journal for Nurses in Staff Development*, 12: 811–815.

Collinson J, Flather MD, Fox KA et al (2000a). Clinical outcomes, risk stratification and practice patterns of unstable angina, and myocardial infarction without ST elevation: Prospective registry of Acute Ischaemic Syndromes in the UK (PRAIS UK). *European Heart Journal*, 21: 1450–1457.

Collinson PO, Premachandran S, Hashemik K et al (2000b). Prospective audit of the incidence of prognostically important myocardial damage in patients discharged from an emergency department. *British Medical Journal*, 320: 1702–1703.

Day HW (1972). History of the coronary care unit. *American Journal of Cardiology*, 30: 405–407.

Department of Health (1997). *The New NHS, Modern, Dependable*. Department of Health, London.

Department of Health (1998). *A First Class Service*. The Stationery Office, London.

Department of Health (1999a). *Saving Lives: Our Healthier Nation*. The Stationery Office, London.

Department of Health (1999b) *Making a Difference: Strengthening the Nursing and Midwifery and Health Visiting Contribution to Health and Health Care*. Department of Health, London.

Department of Health (1999c). *Agenda for Change: Modernising the NHS Pay System*. HSC 1999/227. Department of Health, London.

Department of Health (2000a). *The National Service Framework for Coronary Heart Disease*. Department of Health, London.

Department of Health (2000b). *The NHS Plan. A Plan for Investment, a Plan for Action*. HMSO, London.

Department of Health (2001). *Restoring Emergency Care. First Steps to a New Approach*. Department of Health, London.

Department of Trade and Industry (1998). *Working Time Regulations*. Statutory Instrument 1998 No 1833. The Stationery Office, London.

Dewe PJ (1987). Identifying strategies nurses use to cope with work stress. *Journal of Advanced Nursing*, 12: 489–497.

Dunn L, Morgan E (1998). Creating a framework for clinical practice to advance in the West Midlands region. *Journal of Clinical Nursing*, 7: 239–243.

Ehrenfeld M, Cheifetz FR (1990). Cardiac nurses: coping with stress. *Journal of Advanced Nursing*, 15: 1002–1008.

Ersser S (2000). Editorial. *Journal of Clinical Nursing*, 9: 665–657.

Farkouh ME, Smars PA, Reeder GS et al (1998). A clinical trial of a chest pain observation unit for patients with unstable angina. Chest Pain Evaluation in the Emergency Room (CHEER) Investigators. *New England Journal of Medicine*, 339: 1882–1888.

Fitzpatrick J, White A, Roberts J (1999). Shift work and its impact upon nurse performance: current knowledge and research issues. *Journal of Advanced Nursing*, 29: 18–27.

Fletcher AP, Aikjaersig N, Smyrniots FE et al (1958). The treatment of patients suffering from early myocardial infarction with massive and prolonged streptokinase therapy. *Transcripts of the Association of American Physicians*, 71: 287–296.

Freundenberger HJ (1974). Staff burn-out. *Journal of Social Issues*, 30: 159–165.

Gibler WB (1997). Chest Pain Units: Do they make sense now? *Annals of Internal Medicine*, 29: 168–171.

Goodacre S, Nicholl J, Dixon S et al (2004). Randomized controlled trial and economic evaluation of a chest pain observation unit compared with routine care. *British Medical Journal*, 328: 254–257.

Health Service Circular 1998/161. *Nurse Consultants*. NHS Executive, Leeds.

Health Service Circular 1999/158. *Making a Difference, Strengthening the Nursing, Midwifery and Health Visiting Contribution to Health and Health Care*. NHS Executive, Leeds.

Health Service Circular 1999/217. *Nurse, Midwife and Health Visitor Consultants. Establishing Posts and Making Appointments*. NHS Executive, Leeds.

Healy C, McKay M (2000). Nursing stress: the effects of coping strategies and job satisfaction in a sample of Australian nurses. *Journal of Advanced Nursing*, 31: 681–688.

Henderson V (1966). *The Nature of Nursing*. Macmillan, New York.

Herrick JB (1912). Clinical features of sudden obstruction of coronary arteries. *Journal of the American Medical Association*, 59: 2015–2020.

Hill JD, Hampton JR, Mitchell IRA (1978). A randomized trial of home versus hospital management for patients with suspected MI. *Lancet*, 1: 837–841.

Hobbs R (1995). Rising emergency admissions. *British Medical Journal*, 310: 207–208.

Hooker DR, Kouwenhoven WB and Langworthy AR (1933). Effects of alternating electrical currents on the heart. *American Journal of Physiology*, 103: 444–454.

Jowett NI and Thompson DR (1989). *Comprehensive Coronary Care*. Scutari, London.

Julian DG (1961). Treatment of cardiac arrest in acute myocardial ischaemia and infarction. *Lancet*, 2: 840–844.

Karlson BW, Herlitz J, Wiklund O et al (1991). Early prediction of acute myocardial infarction from clinical history, examination and electrocardiogram in the emergency room. *American Journal of Cardiology*, 68: 171–175.

Kitson A (1987). Raising the standards of clinical practice: the fundamental issue of effective nursing practice. *Journal of Advanced Nursing*, 12: 321–329.

Kouwenhoven WB, Jude JR, Knickerbocker GG (1960). Closed-chest cardicac massage. *Journal of the American Medical Association*, 178: 1064–1067.

Kucia A, Taylor KTN, Horowitz JD (2001). Can a nurse trained in coronary care expedite the emergency department management of patients with acute coronary syndromes? *Heart and Lung*, 30: 186–190.

Lau J, Antman EM, Jimenez-Silva J et al (1992). Cumulative meta-analysis of therapeutic trials for myocardial infarction. *New England Journal of Medicine*, 327: 248–254.

Lawrence-Mathew PJ, Wison AT, Woodmansey PA et al (1994). Unsatisfactory management of patients with myocardial infarction admitted to general medical wards. *Journal of the Royal College of Physicians of London*, 28: 49–51.

Little C (1999). The meaning of learning in critical care nursing: a hermeneutic study. *Journal of Advanced Nursing*, 30: 697–703.

Lown B, Amarasingham R, Neuman J (1962). New method for terminating cardiac arrhythmias. Use of synchronized capacitor discharge. *Journal of the American Medical Association*, 182: 548–555.

Manley K (2000). Paying Peter to pay Paul: reconciling concepts of expertise within competency for a career structure. *Journal of Clinical Nursing*, 9: 357–359.

Mayor S (2000). Heart Disease Framework aims to cut deaths in England. *British Medical Journal*, 320: 665.

McFarlane I (1980). *Essays on Nursing*. King's Fund, London.

National Health Service Management Executive (1991). *Junior Doctors: the New Deal*. NHSME, London.

Newby DE, Fox KA, Flint LL et al (1998). A 'same day' direct-access chest pain clinic: improved management and reduced hospitalisation. *Quarterly Journal of Medicine*, 91: 333–337.

NHS Executive (1996). *Review of Ambulance Performance Standards*. NHS Executive, London.

NHS Executive (1998). *The New NHS: Modern, Dependable*. Department of Health, London.

Norris RM (1998). Fatality outside hospital from acute coronary events in three British Health Districts, 1994–1995. United Kingdom Heart Attack Study Collaborative Group. *British Medical Journal*, 316: 1065–1070.

Nursing and Midwifery Council (2002). Code of Professional Conduct.

Quinn T (1995). Can nurses safely assess suitability for thrombolysis? A pilot study. *Intensive and Critical Care Nursing*, 11: 126–129.

Quinn T, Morse T (2003). The interdisciplinary interface in managing patients with suspected cardiac pain. *Emergency Nurse*, 11: 22–24.

Quinn T, Thompson DR (1995). The changing role of the nurse. *Care of the Critically Ill*, 111: 48–49.

Quinn T, Thompson D (1999). History and development of coronary care. *Intensive and Critical Care Nursing*, 15: 131–141.

Quinn T, MacDermott A, Caunt J (1998). Determining patients suitability for thrombolysis: coronary care nurses' agreement with an expert cardiological 'gold standard' as assessed by clinical and electrocardological vignettes. *Intensive and Critical Care Nursing*, 14: 219–224.

Quinn T, Thompson DR, Boyle R (2000). Determining chest pain patient's suitability for transfer to a general medical ward following admission to a cardiac care unit. *Journal of Advanced Nursing*, 310–317.

Reagan LB, Young KR, Nicholson JW (1956). Ventricular defibrillation in a patient with probable acute coronary occlusion. *Surgry*, 39: 482–486.

Rhodes MA (1998). What is the evidence to support nurse led thrombolysis? *Clinical Effectiveness in Nursing*, 2: 69–77.

Sawatzky J (1996). Stress in critical care nurses: actual and perceived. *Heart and Lung*, 25: 409–417.

Seccombe I, Smith G (1996). *In the Balance: Registered Nurse Supply and Demand*. Report No 315. Institute of Employment Studies, University of Sussex.

Somauroo JD, McCarten P, Appleton B et al (1999). Effectiveness of a 'thrombolysis nurse' in shortening delay to thrombolysis in acute myocardial infaction. *Journal of the Royal College of Physicians*, 33: 46–50.

Stordeur S, D'hoore W, Vandenberghe C (2001). Leadership, organisational stress, and emotional exhaustion amongst hospital nursing staff. *Journal of Advanced Nursing*, 35: 533–542.

Thompson C, McMaughan D, Cullum N et al (2001). The accessibility of research based knowledge for nurses in United Kingdom acute care settings. *Journal of Advanced Nursing*, 36: 11–22.

UKCC (1992). *The Scope of Professional Practice*. UKCC, London.

United Kingdom Heart Attack Study Collaborative Group (1999). Effect of time from onset of coming under care on fatality of patients with acute myocardial infarction: effect of reuscitation and thrombolytic therapy. *Heart*, 80: 114–120.

Williams A, McGee P, Bates L (2001). An examination of senior nursing roles: challenges for the NHS. *Journal of Clinical Nursing*, 10: 195–203.

Zoll PM, Linenthal A, Gibson W, Paul MH, Norman LR (1956). Termination of ventricular fibrillation in man by externally applied electric countershock. *New England Journal of Medicine*, 254: 727–732.

Further reading

Hatchett R, Thompson DR (eds) (2002). *Cardiac Nursing: A Comprehensive Guide*. Harcourt, London.

Jowett NI, Thompson DR (2003). *Comprehensive Coronary Care*, 3rd edn. Baillière Tindall, London.

Chapter 4

Acute care: patient assessment

INTRODUCTION

Deciding what to do for a patient presenting with a possible cardiac problem involves determining what the problem is and then deciding the best way to manage it. It also involves a certain degree of prediction as to the likely consequences of the problem so that care planning can be prioritized. This is a complex process dependent on a wide range of previous experience, knowledge and skills in health professionals. It involves:

- a knowledge of the patient's past medical history, including family history
- a knowledge and assessment of the patient's presenting complaint
- an assessment of how the patient's presenting complaint is affecting the patient
- assimilating information from the above with the results of appropriate diagnostic tests in order to establish a working diagnosis
- deciding on the most appropriate management option for the patient based on best available evidence
- planning how to deliver this treatment most effectively.

Decisions also need to incorporate individual circumstances and patient choice. The plan of care will ultimately be dependent on the resources and treatment options available. This will differ depending on where the patient enters the health care system. Patients are not managed in isolation and the reality is that care has to be prioritized, with the needs of the individual often having to accommodate the needs of a larger case load.

The nurse is frequently the first hospital professional to see the patient and the actions taken by them at this point can act as the catalyst for subsequent patient management. Inaccurate or incomplete initial and ongoing assessment can have serious consequences for patient care. Nurses are with patients over the 24-hour period and have developed an important role as gatekeepers for deciding when patients need medical reviews leading to changes in therapy (Cioffi 2000).

THE DECISION-MAKING PROCESS

Little is really known about the correlation between the information obtained in the assessment process and the decisions reached. It has been argued that nurses make decisions using information processing theory, which relies on earlier knowledge, the observation of cues, the generation of alternative explanations and the generation of a working hypothesis which is then tested against earlier knowledge (Junnola et al 2002). The ability to focus on cues that are relevant is thought to be important (Reischman and Yarandi 2002). Nurses who have worked in area for some time are thought to differ from less experienced staff in both what they know and what they do with this information (Benner et al 1992). They have been shown to need less time to assimilate information than less experienced staff (White et al 1992). In acute situations where there is lots of information to process and emerging information builds up to form a picture of the patient's status then the experienced nurse is thought to be able to 'understand without rationale' (Benner and Tanner 1987) through a process akin to intuition. It is possible th applies to coronary care nurses Although in reality, it is likely t decisions are a mixture of intuitive an lytical processes (Eraut et al 1995, Closs and Cheater 1999).

EVIDENCE-BASED PRACTICE

Evidence-based practice is about intergrating individual clinical expertise and best external evidence (Sackett et al 1996). It has developed through the need to provide health care equitably and effectively in a financially restricted climate (Closs and Cheater 1999). Nursing strategies (DoH 1999, 2000) reiterate the need for an evidence-based culture to become part of *nursing* practice.

Much of the evidence available to nurses caring for coronary patients is medical evidence based on the results of multicentred randomized controlled trials where subjects are randomly allocated to one of two groups, one of which receives standard treatment and the second the intervention being studied. This type of study design is considered the most robust way of assessing the effectiveness of health care interventions (Gray 1997) (Table 4.1).

For a variety of reasons, there is limited evidence from randomized controlled trials available for nurses (Closs and Cheater 1999). Nursing interventions can often not be broken down into discrete measurable variables, and it is difficult for nurses to get the large sample sizes needed to demonstrate that the intervention is effective. Much nursing research is qualitative and carried out on small numbers of patients. While not rated

Table 4.1 Strength of different types of evidence

Type	Strength of evidence
I	Strong evidence from at least one systematic review of multiple well-designed randomized controlled trials
II	Strong evidence from at least one properly designed randomized controlled trial of appropriate size.
III	Evidence from well-designed trials without randomization, single group pre-post, cohort, timed series or matched case-control studies
IV	Evidence from well-designed non-experimental studies from more than one centre or research group
V	Opinions of respected authorities, based on clinical evidence, descriptive studies or reports of expert committees

Gray (1997) p. 61.

ɔ high in the 'hierarchy of evidence', this type of research can give a rich insight into patient experiences. Acute care nurses often fail to incorporate the research that is available into practice, often because they cannot interpret it, feel the nature of where they work is prohibitive or do not have the skills or motivation (McCaughan et al 2002). It is important not to ignore the fact that the proficiency and judgement individuals acquire through experience is an important part of evidence for practice (Sackett et al 1996).

GUIDELINES

Clinical guidelines are systematically developed statements made to assist the practitioner make decisions about appropriate health care (Field and Lohr 1990). Coronary care is increasingly being directed by guidelines which tend to be based on evidence from large clinical trials. However, these tend to focus on aspects of care that are predominately the remit of the medical staff. There is limited information on the use of clinical guidelines in nursing (Thomas et al 1999). Obtaining information for nursing guidelines is difficult as much of the literature is anecdotal and/or comes from a different care environment which may not equate to the UK care setting. Also, nurses do not always have the skills to appraise the quality of nursing research papers that are published.

There are some general questions to ask about clinical guidelines:

- is the objective of the guideline clear?
- is the setting and target population clear?
- is the targeted health condition stated?
- is the process of evidence collection thorough – have efforts been made to collect it all? Has the evidence been appraised? What is the quality of the evidence?
- who developed the guidelines – were all key disciplines involved? Has it been independently reviewed?
- have local circumstances been considered?

Adopting guidelines without thought to the above may result in inappropriate care. Guidelines should not prevent nurses using sound clinical judgement or tailoring care to individual patient's circumstances.

PATIENT ASSESSMENT

Assessment is probably the most important phase of the entire care delivery process. It refers to the collection and interpretation of information, especially facts and, to a lesser extent, perhaps some impressions. Patient assessment is a complicated, detailed and orderly process. The influence of the nurse, often the first person with whom the patient comes into contact on admission to hospital, is paramount. A rapid initial assessment usually gives significant clues to the patient's general condition.

The nature of the assessment will depend on the situation – whether or not it is a crisis or critical care situation. In the coronary care unit, for example, when a coronary patient has just been admitted but appears relatively stable, assessments of all body systems can be made with the aim of supporting those in trouble and maintaining those in health. In the crisis situation, such as a patient suffering a cardiac arrest soon after admission or being a potential candidate for reperfusion, rapid assessment has to be made, concentrating on the system(s) in failure, with the immediate aim of reversal or maintenance.

With experience and knowledge the coronary care nurse should be able to recognize which areas require assessment and which require priority. Nursing assessment should be open-ended and flexible.

Some aspects of nursing assessment will be more relevant than others to certain patients. The spiritual aspects may assume priority for the patient who suspects that they may be dying. Normal priorities and values may change on admission and throughout the recovery period. Once the pertinent information has been gathered it needs to be interpreted in order to identify the patient's problems, checking with the patient (validation) when appropriate. Some problems, such as acute shortness of breath, will be immediately obvious to the observer and will have been identified by the patient. Others will only become apparent after the interpretation of diagnostic tests. It is often the diagnostic labelling of a problem that highlights the significance of a symptom to the patient.

Medical and nursing assessment

It is likely that the patient will be assessed by both a doctor and a nurse in a short period of time after presentation. While both professions will be looking to prioritize management options, it is possible that the way the information is obtained will result in different view points of the same patient. Ideally these perspectives should complement each other and be used to build up a more comprehensive picture of the patient.

There is limited information on how nurses undertake assessments, although it has been suggested that the cognitive strategies involved are similar to those used in medical diagnosis, particularly in relation to the gathering and organization of information, but that the purpose of the information search is different. The medical aim is to establish an explanation of the patient's presenting problem whereas that of the nurse is to provide an accurate picture of the patient's current situation or condition (Crow et al 1995).

Medical assessment follows an established format to elucidate facts and arrive at a conclusion by a process of systematic deduction. In essence, nursing assessment has traditionally been focused on defining problems that the patient, or significant other, has in coping with symptoms, diagnosis and restoring or maintaining health. As cardiac nurses establish nurse-led services and have increasing responsibility for deciding on medical management options for patients (Thompson et al 2002) the style of nursing assessment has shifted to a more medical focus. While this has certain benefits for patients and has allowed new nursing roles to develop, it is important that patient-focused issues are not lost. The coronary care nurse works closely with the physician and some medical information will inevitably be of relevance in establishing a data base. However, the medical assessment *per se* should not become a substitute for a thorough nursing assessment.

Maslow (1970) identified certain human needs which he listed in a hierarchical order as a way of indicating that certain basic needs take priority over others. These needs are equally applicable to the coronary patient. The most basic needs are physiological, aimed at self-preservation. These are the ones that need to be assessed as a priority and are ones that focus the attention of health care professionals in the acute setting. At admission and during the early in-hospital phase, the coronary patient's basic needs of survival and safety are likely to require most attention although, for effective rehabilitation and recovery to be optimal, attention needs to be focused on other needs. Upper level needs are security, belonging, self-esteem and self-fulfilment which, although less significant, still need to be addressed for optimum patient well-being.

If caring for the coronary patient is to be considered to include assisting a person to carry out as near to normal activities as possible, assessment needs to include information about the individual's normal behaviour and how it may have changed as a result of the coronary event and subsequent admission to hospital. The activities of living described by Henderson (1960) and Roper et al (1980) are essentially a reflection of these human needs and, if such an approach is used in coronary care, the patient needs to be assessed in terms of their ability to carry out these activities. The activities of daily living model has formed the basis of patient assessment for over two decades and is still a useful framework for comprehensive patient assessment when the patient's initial survival needs have been addressed. There is a danger that this opportunity to obtain an holistic picture of the patient is lost in today's environment of fast patient throughput and streamlined care pathways.

Data collection

Assessment is compiled through:

1 observation
2 history-taking
3 interviewing
4 physical examination
5 examination of pertinent laboratory findings and diagnostic tests.

A combination of observation, intuition, judgement and previous experience is required for accurate patient assessment. This requires certain skills, not least of which are those of good communication and observation.

Data collection may be subjective, i.e. interviewing and history-taking (symptoms), or objective, i.e. physical examination (signs). This requires a wide range of skills including inspection, palpation and the use of a variety of diagnostic aids such as a thermometer, stethoscope and electrocardiograph.

In the UK, unlike North America, it is still generally uncommon for the nurse, even in areas such as the coronary care unit, to undertake a detailed physical examination of the patient, and it is rare to find a nurse skilled in the techniques of percussion and auscultation. However, there are now increasing opportunities for nurses to develop these skills in order to enhance patient care. Patients may present with multiple disease processes and the ability to undertake a comprehensive patient assessment will help ensure that less obvious problems are not missed.

Certain procedures, such as the establishment of a central venous pressure (CVP) line, need to be initiated by the physician, but the subsequent pressure readings are usually made by the nurse.

The personal attitudes, beliefs, values, biases and moods of the nurse are an important part of the nurse–patient relationship. The nurse may feel competent and place priority on the skills of simple data collecting, but miss more subtle information such as the patient's mood, etc. There is a danger that the technical environment of the coronary care unit may detract from the patient being assessed as a unique individual.

Initial assessment

The priority when first assessing a patient presenting with possible cardiac symptoms is to determine:

- whether the patient is haemodynamically stable or at immediate risk from significantly reduced cardiac output (arrhythmia, heart failure)
- whether the patient is suffering from an acute myocardial infarction that would benefit from time dependent reperfusion therapy
- the need for symptom relief – particularly pain relief.

This involves observing the patient, assessing the nature of the presenting symptoms and details of when these symptoms started; obtaining a *brief* patient history of any significant medical events and treatment (particularly recent surgical intervention),

performing a 12-lead electrocardiogram (ECG) and assessing for signs of inadequate cardiac output. These actions need to be performed promptly and not get delayed by other activities.

On admission and in a crisis, assessment will need to be concentrated on key areas. An experienced nurse needs to be able to perform a brief overall assessment to obtain an overview and establish priorities, and then focus on those areas deemed to be most relevant. Initial attention will be centred on the maintenance of cardiac output and oxygenation, so that if these seem threatened or compromised intervention can be promptly instituted.

The structure of subsequent assessment will depend on the results of the initial assessment. All patients will require a full and detailed assessment and history taking. The skill lies in knowing how to prioritize each part of the assessment process for individual patients.

The initial assessment can, out of necessity, appear hurried and the patient may feel rushed through the process. Patients appear to benefit from recounting the 'story' of their symptoms and their journey into the health care system (Gassner et al 2002). Spending time later going over issues and allowing time for questions is likely to be of benefit to the patient and family. It will also enable assessment of the patient's perception of events which can be useful in planning subsequent care delivery.

An initial assessment, valid enough to shape early priority setting and decision making, can be made without recourse to formal physical examination or diagnostic tests. Identifying the key aspects of a patient's condition can be crucial to the early recognition of a cardiac problem and its complications. Interpretation of symptoms and signs is not always easy, as a patient may have many or none. Also, those that do appear to be of cardiac origin may actually be related to other disorders, and conversely, those resulting from cardiac problems may be attributed wrongly to other body systems.

Certain signs and symptoms will provide evidence of compromised cardiac function, especially acute myocardial infarction. These are:

- new onset of chest pain
- chest pain that occurs during rest, is unrelieved by rest or nitrates, has a duration exceeding 30 min and often lasting for several

hours, and is described as crushing, vice-like, tight or constricting in nature
- shortness of breath at rest, on exertion or when lying flat
- change in cardiac rhythm or rate
- change in blood pressure
- change in level of consciousness
- increased anxiety or restlessness
- sweating or clammy skin.

Important information is obtained from observing the general appearance and behaviour of the patient. Body posture and movement, facial expression, tone of voice and mannerisms, all begin to provide an overall impression as to how they are responding to their symptoms, suspected diagnosis and admission to hospital.

ASSESSMENT OF KEY SYMPTOMS
Chest pain

The nature of cardiac chest pain

Acute central chest pain accounts for 20–30% of emergency medical admissions, whereas chronic chest pain is the commonest reason for referral to cardiac outpatient clinics. The presentation of ischaemic chest pain is very individual and its severity bears little relationship to the underlying pathology.

The pain occurs indirectly as a result of ischaemia to the myocardium due to an inadequate blood supply – usually the result of atherosclerosis and blockage of the relevant coronary artery. The pain is thought to be produced by a combination of reduced coronary arterial pressure distal to the occlusion acting on coronary artery pressor-receptors, myocardial ischaemia stimulating visceral pain receptors, ischaemic neuropathy of the nerves of the heart, and the release of chemicals following tissue breakdown. Insufficient oxygen supply to the myocardium means that complete metabolism of glucose is not possible and lactic acid accumulates as a result of anaerobic metabolism. Lactic acid is known to stimulate the pain fibres found in the coronary arteries. Bradykinin, a polypeptide released from ischaemic myocardial cells, is also known to stimulate pain fibres. Pain

impulses travel to the thoracic sympathetic ganglia and to nerve roots T1–T5 via sympathetic fibres. This means that ischaemic pain is experienced in the region between the lower jaw and the epigastrium and is a widespread rather than a localized sensation. Patients are unable to point to a specific focus for their pain but tend to describe it as radiating.

The nausea and vomiting associated with the pain are apparently related to activation of the vagal reflex. Sweating is a response to sympathetic nerve stimulation. Blood is diverted away from the periphery and the skin appears pale. Occasionally, patients may complain of a violent urge to defecate and a sudden onset of diarrhoea as a result of vagal stimulation.

As many as two-thirds of patients admitted with a suspected heart attack may in fact turn out to have a different medical diagnosis. Ischaemic pain can easily be confused with pain from other sources. The finding that glyceryl trinitrate (GTN) can relieve pain caused by oesophageal reflux can serve to complicate the issue.

The differential diagnosis of the patient with chest pain includes:

- aortic dissection
- pulmonary embolism
- peptic ulcer disease
- pneumothorax
- sternal costochondritis
- renal colic
- herpes zoster
- pancreatitis
- pneumonia
- oesophagitis
- COPD
- cholecystitis/biliary colic
- intercostal myalgia.

Pain may not necessarily be the predominant presenting clinical feature. Atypical features such as a new onset of left ventricular failure (LVF), central nervous system manifestations of a stroke where there is cerebral atherosclerosis and a sudden fall in cardiac output, overwhelming weakness, epigastric discomfort with indigestion-like symptoms, and the sudden onset of mania or psychosis, can all result from an acute myocardial infarction.

The prevalance of 'silent' myocardial infarction is unknown, but it is thought that over a quarter of myocardial infarctions go unrecognized and that half of these (one-eighth of the total) produce no symptoms (Campbell 1988). Patients with diabetes often have atypical symptoms and may not experience chest pain (Airaksinen 2001) and the absence of pain and atypical symptoms have been found to occur more frequently in the elderly (Then et al 2001).

Stable angina involves symptoms that are typically provoked by an activity that increases myocardial oxygen demand. The discomfort is often described as 'band like' and is across the chest with radiation to the arms, shoulders or back. Exercise/exertion and emotional factors are significant. The discomfort is usually relieved within 2–10 minutes by rest. Symptoms are often associated with shortness of breath and tend to be worse in the mornings, coinciding with a peak in blood pressure, after heavy meals and in cold weather.

Unstable angina characteristically presents as recent onset of experiencing angina symptoms (within the past 4–6 weeks). The symptoms of unstable angina are classically described as being like the patient's normal angina but more severe, more frequent and less responsive to nitrate therapy. The discomfort/pain and associated symptoms can also occur in the absence of physical or emotional stress and last longer than 20 minutes.

The Canadian Cardiovascular Society classifies angina into four categories:

- *Class 1*: ordinary physical activity does not cause angina. Angina occurs with strenuous rapid or prolonged exertion.
- *Class 2*: slight limitation of ordinary activity. Angina occurs with walking or climbing stairs rapidly, uphill, after meals, in cold or wind, under emotional stress or only in the few hours after awakening. Angina occurs with walking more than two level blocks and climbing more than one flight of ordinary stairs at a normal pace.
- *Class 3*: marked limitations of ordinary physical activity. Angina occurs with walking one or two level blocks or climbing one flight of stairs at normal conditions.
- *Class 4*: inability to carry out any physical activity without discomfort. Anginal symptoms may be present at rest.

Myocardial infarction has classic symptoms that are hard to miss. An aged or elderly person of either sex complains of central crushing retrosternal chest pain, which comes on at rest, lasts longer than 30 minutes and is not relieved by GTN. The discomfort may radiate or localize to the neck, jaw, back and shoulders. There may be associated nausea and a 'feeling of impending doom'. Autonomic dysfunction may produce profuse sweating and the patient may appear cold and clammy. Difficulties arise because not all patients present classic symptoms. Education strategies to inform the public about how to respond to the symptoms of a heart attack tend to emphasize the associated 'pain'. Yet few patients recognize the sensation as such (Treasure 1998).

One literature review reported that pain radiating to the left or both arms and also to the right shoulder increases the likelihood of that pain being the result of an acute coronary syndrome, whereas pain that is described as pleuritic, sharp or stabbing, or positional pain, or pain reproduced by palpation are all associated with a decreased likelihood of acute myocardial infarction (Panju et al 1998). Pain worsened by respiration or relieved by food, antacids, or sitting forward, is unlikely to be ischaemic. Women may present differently to men. Reviews have highlighted that women with acute myocardial infarction are more likely to have vague or non-classic symptoms (Miller 2002) and that they are more likely to have back and jaw pain, vomiting, indigestion and palpitations (Devon and Zerwic 2002).

Determining whether there is a background of a family history of coronary heart disease (CHD) and significant risk factors are important parts of the assessment process. About half the patients presenting with myocardial infarction will have had a previous heart attack or suffer from angina.

Pain assessment

There are several objectives of pain assessment including:

- to assist in the diagnosis of a likely cause of the pain
- to monitor fluctuations of pain over time
- to evaluate the effectiveness of methods of pain relief

- to work towards relief of patient distress
- to convey human concern and improve and maintain an effective nurse–patient relationship.

Pain assessment is an objective assessment of a subjective experience. The experience of pain is private and personal and individuals differ in the extent to which they admit to it. It is possible that the reporting of pain will depend on its perceived significance, the attitude of those undertaking the assessment (do they appear to believe the pain is real?) and whether it is perceived that anything can be done to relieve the pain.

Nurses have the most contact with patients and yet various studies have highlighted that pain assessment and subsequent pain management are inconsistent (Bondestam et al 1987, Meurier 1998, Meurier et al 1998, O'Connor et al 1995, Thompson et al 1994). Patients need to be aware of the importance of reporting any pain as they may think it is to be expected for them to be in some degree of discomfort if they have a cardiac problem.

Those undertaking pain assessments need to be aware that patients may use words like 'ache' and 'heaviness' to describe their symptoms. The use of metaphors such as 'like an elephant sitting on my chest', 'like needles going through you' or 'like a football inside my chest' is common (Jairath 1999). Patients who do not perceive their discomfort as a *pain* may respond negatively to questions asking about the presence of chest pain.

The reality of having a heart attack may differ from the patient's perceptions gleaned from the media or the accounts of others. Ruston et al (1998) in a qualitative study of patients' experiences of a cardiac event concluded that the myth that a heart attack is a dramatic event needed to be dispelled. This study found that most patients experienced symptoms that were gradual rather than dramatic in onset and that many did not use the word 'pain' to describe their symptoms until they were in the hospital setting.

Usually patients will have experienced pain for a few hours prior to admission and will already be using their own coping mechanisms to try to combat the pain. It is thought that coping responses can be divided into those that involve external factors such as the presence of others, distraction, creating pain in some other area of the body, or by movement such as rocking and swaying, or those that involve internal factors such as trying to focus on something else, daydreaming, and body–mind separation techniques through the use of meditation or relaxation. The newly admitted patient may not have had sufficient time to formulate effective coping mechanisms, as they may be experiencing their first-ever episode of acute pain compounded by the exacerbating effect of fear of diagnosis, death and the unknown.

The gate theory of pain (Melzack and Wall 1965) proposes that pain perception can be greatly influenced by the psychological state of the individual and that cells in the dorsal spinal cord can control the intensity of sensory input from the peripheral nerves by modulating the membrane potentials of the terminals of sensory fibres. People may respond differently to the same pain in differing situations. Chest pain that seems very severe when patients are at home may be reduced when they enter hospital where they believe something can be done to resolve the pain. Anxiety seems to increase the severity of the pain experienced (Sternbach 1968). A patient who believes their chest pain to be due to indigestion may feel the pain to be more intense when told they may have suffered a heart attack.

The perceived significance and expectations of pain are relevant to the pain experienced. Patients may be able to cope with a reasonably severe degree of pain during the day when they have other things to distract them, but find the same degree of pain unbearable at night when they have the opportunity to dwell upon it.

Both the pain experience and an individual's reaction to it will be individual. They will be influenced by the situation, the sociological and cultural experience and perceptions of the patient plus the characteristics of the person assessing the pain. South Asian patients have been found to be more anxious about experiencing chest pain than Europeans (Caturvedi et al 1997). It is common for non-Western societies to have a wider view of pain, linking it to other forms of suffering including emotional distress, interpersonal conflicts and unexpected misfortune (Helman 2000). However, it is dangerous to let stereotypes, particularly ethnic stereotypes influence the assessment process.

According to McCaffery (1990): 'Pain is whatever the experiencing person says it is, existing whenever he says it does'. Patients will use a variety of words to describe the quality of their pain, which may mean different things to individual nurses. Melzack and Torgerson (1971) have categorized these words into three major classes with further subdivisions which later became the basis of the McGill Pain Questionnaire (Melzack 1975). One class describes the sensory qualities of the pain experience in terms of temporal (e.g. 'pounding'), spatial (e.g. 'radiating'), pressure (e.g. 'stabbing'), thermal (e.g. 'hot'), and other qualities. A second class describes the affective qualities of pain in terms of tension (e.g. 'tiring'), fear (e.g. 'terrifying'), and autonomic properties (e.g. 'choking'). The final class describes the evaluative aspects of pain in terms of the subjective overall intensity of the total pain experience (e.g. 'excruciating'). However, pain is still frequently considered in regard to a single attribute: variation in intensity. Although this ignores the qualitative dimensions, it is a useful component of the pain experience. Variation in intensity, moreover, lends itself to numerical or graphic measurement which is particularly useful for the assessment of acute pain such as that commonly presenting in the coronary patient.

The patient is the only person who can accurately give a subjective description of the pain experienced. On admission to a coronary care unit the patient may have been experiencing pain for some time and find it difficult to reappraise the pain. They may have developed coping mechanisms to deal with it and may not appear to the nurse to be in much distress. The patient may feel embarrassed at showing their response to pain (e.g. crying or moaning) in the public setting of the hospital, or alternatively feel that they have to justify the admission by appearing to be in distress with pain.

There is always the possibility that a patient may expect to be in pain because of their condition and thus suffer unnecessarily. The absence of pain behaviour does not necessarily mean the absence of pain. It is possible that because nurses work constantly with patients in pain they may become so accustomed to it that its significance decreases. Nurses working predominantly with patients admitted with presupposed similar problems, e.g. a heart attack, may expect them to experience similar pain. The experience of the nurse may influence the pain assessment. Mason (1981) found that less

experienced nurses inferred higher degrees of patient suffering. If a patient is cared for by several nurses, it is possible that interventions for pain relief will lack consistency.

Assessment of pain includes observing the patient's facial expression (e.g. grimacing), body posture (e.g. guarding), heart rate and blood pressure (e.g. tachycardia), and coping strategies that he may use, and talking with the patient to obtain descriptions of the pain.

Location and radiation   The patient should be asked to identify the affected area, if possible using a figure drawing. Is the pain localized precisely or is it vaguely diffuse? Is it superficial or deep? Does it spread or radiate? Has the location and radiation changed since onset?

Intensity   Using a pain-rating scale is of value in assessing pain intensity. How severe is the pain? Does the pain intensity impair function – if so, how and to what extent?

Quality   The nurse should encourage the patient to be explicit and avoid putting words into their mouth, e.g. 'What does your pain feel like?'

Onset   What was the time of onset?, e.g. 'When did your pain begin?'

Duration   How long has the patient been experiencing this pain?, e.g. 'How long has your pain lasted?'

Variation   Is the pain different at certain time – if so, in what way?

Frequency   How often does the pain occur?

Predisposing factors   What factors precipitate or predispose the pain?, e.g. exertion or exposure to cold.

Aggravating factors   What factors aggravate or exacerbate the pain?, e.g. deep breathing, exertion, stress, caffeine, alcohol, smoking, spicy foods or change in body posture.

Relieving factors   What factors alleviate or relieve the pain?, e.g. GTN, anatacids, rest, massage, warmth or change in body posture.

Associated symptoms   Rarely is one symptom such as chest pain associated with a heart attack.

Therefore, the nurse needs to determine whether the patient has any of the following: shortness of breath, sweating, fever, nausea, vomiting, weakness, cough, pallor, numbness, paraesthesia, palpitations, dizziness or faintness.

Other considerations include:

1 How does the patient consider the pain? Is it bearable? Do they want pain relief?
2 What does the patient attribute the pain to?
3 What has the patient done to try to relieve the pain? Has this helped?
4 Has the patient had similar pain before? What action was taken? Was it effective?
5 Has the patient had experience of other sorts of pain? How does the present pain compare?
6 How does the patient normally cope or respond to pain?

Methods of quantifying pain

Various methods of pain assessment are available, including the visual analogue scale (VAS) (Scott and Huskisson 1976) or 'pain ruler' (Bourbonnais 1981). Such methods are especially useful for the assessment of acute pain, e.g. the ischaemic pain that commonly presents in the acute coronary patient. The VAS is a sensitive and reliable method and can be quick and easy to use by both the person experiencing the pain and the observer (Standing 1997). It can be particularly useful in assessing the effects of pain relief measures. However, some patients find it difficult to conceptualize their symptoms in a linear/numerical manner or may find it hard to understand the instructions of how to use the scale.

Problems with respiration

The rate and character of the patient's respirations should be carefully observed. Normally, the adult should breathe comfortably about 14–20 times per minute. Variations to the normal rate and character include:

- *tachypnoea*: rapid shallow breathing which may indicate pain, anaemia, fever or pulmonary problems
- *bradypnoea*: slow breathing which may occur as a result of opiates, coma, excessive alcohol or increased intracranial pressure

- *hyperventilation*: simultaneous rapid deep breathing which is usually found in extreme anxiety states, diabetic acidosis and after vigorous exercise
- *Cheyne–Stokes respiration*: periodic breathing with increased depth of breathing (*hyperpnoea*) alternating with cessation of breathing (*apnoea*) which is usually found in heart failure
- *dyspnoea*: conscious difficulty or effort in breathing, which is usually found in left ventricular failure and frequently seen in cardiac patients
- *orthopnoea*: difficulty in breathing when lying flat and an early symptom of heart failure.

Changes in respiration may occur in the coronary patient as a result of pain, anxiety, heart failure, anoxia and the effects of certain analgesics.

The nature of dyspnoea

This symptom may be described as difficulty with breathing, shortness of breath or breathlessness. Dyspnoea is a common presenting symptom in coronary patients. It usually results from pulmonary congestion or increased pulmonary venous and capillary pressure. LVF is the classical cardiac cause of acute dyspnoea, with pulmonary oedema causing increased lung rigidity and decreased oxygen transfer. Respiration therefore will require greater effort, which is not helped by oedematous narrowing of the larger airways. Dyspnoea may occur only during exertion or at rest. *Paroxysmal nocturnal dyspnoea* may be viewed as a delayed form of orthopnoea. Dyspnoea can be precipitated by the patient sliding down the bed into the horizontal position. The increase in pulmonary congestion leads to dyspnoea, which is reversed by the patient sitting up or standing.

Respiratory assessment

Respiratory assessment is often neglected and yet it can yield important information on the patient's condition. Normal respiratory work at rest uses about 3% of the total intake of oxygen, but this can increase up to 50% in respiratory distress, resulting in cardiovascular and neurological deterioration. Respiratory work may increase significantly and ventilation and perfusion fall markedly before the signs of hypercapnia and hypoxia become apparent.

Assessment of the respiratory system is best undertaken in a quiet, well lit environment. This is not always easy to achieve in an acute care setting. For a basic assessment the patient should be sitting to allow observation of the chest. Observing for visible cyanosis of the lips, being peripherally cold to the touch and mentally lethargic are signs that the patient is unwell. The airway should be assessed by observing and reporting any abnormal breathing patterns. The rate, rhythm and quality of breathing needs to be noted. Assessment of chest symmetry, skin condition and accessory muscle use, pursed lip breathing and the presence of nasal flaring are also important.

Respiratory rates should be assessed for at least 30 seconds unless there are obvious life-threatening problems. The rate will be increased in lung disease, metabolic acidosis, heart failure, pyrexia, pain and anxiety and will decrease with depression of the respiratory centre occurring as a result of narcotic overload, electrolyte imbalance and cerebral lesions. Increased respiratory effort can be indicative of upper airway obstruction.

The front of the chest should be observed for symmetry of movement. There should be equal expansion of the chest wall on both sides. Paradoxical movement is indicated by abnormal collapse of part of the chest wall during inspiration together with abnormal expansion of the same area during expiration. Paradoxical movement (chest wall moves inward on inspiration) indicates loss of normal chest wall function and a reduced tidal volume. This happen with flail chest which can occur when ribs are broken during cardiac massage. Loss of chest movement on one side of the chest can indicate bronchial obstruction, collapsed lung (pneumothorax, haemothorax or haemopneumothorax) or previous surgical removal of a lung. Delayed chest wall movement is indicative of congestion or consolidation of the underlying lung tissue.

The sternocleidomastiod, scalenus and trapezius muscles in the shoulders and neck need to be observed for accessory use. Patients with chronic obstructive pulmonary disease use these muscles to replace the work of the diaphragm and external intercostal muscles.

Defects of the sternum including funnel and convex chest may limit full expansion of the thorax.

Deformities of the posterior thorax that may limit ventilation include curvatures of the spine such as lordosis, scoliosis, kyphosis and kyphoscoliosis.

Patients who prefer to sit forward with their arms resting on their knees or over the bed table (tripod position) in order to aid lung expansion, may be experiencing early signs of respiratory failure. Patients who become short of breath when sitting upright have a respiratory rate greater than 20 respirations per minute and abnormally shallow respirations may be protectively splinting the chest in response to pain. Abdominal ascites and liver enlargement may also limit downward movement of the diaphragm.

Increased blood flow to the lungs when the patient lies flat may produce shortness of breath when the patient goes to bed. Asking about the number of pillows used to sleep is a useful way of determining if this is a problem.

Inspection of the chest for surgical scars, the lips and fingernails for cyanosis and the digits of the fingers for clubbing are all important parts of the respiratory assessment as are determining whether the patient has productive sputum, a cough or a wheeze.

Pulse oximetry

Pulse oximetry records light readings from blood pulsating in the capillaries. It is a simple non-invasive method of monitoring the percentage of haemoglobin that is saturated with oxygen ($SaO_2\%$). An oximeter probe containing two diodes (one red and one infrared diode) emits light onto a detector opposite (usually on the other side of the finger or ear lobe). The probe is linked to a computerized unit and often a display screen. As oxygenated and deoxygenated blood are different in colour it is possible to determine the ratio of their concentrations when the two are mixed from the relative amounts of red and infrared light absorbed as a light source shines through the capillary bed. The corresponding arterial oxygen saturation is calculated as an average based on results of the previous few seconds worth of recordings

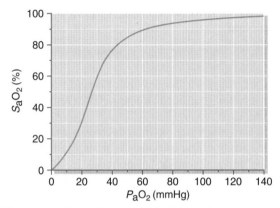

Figure 4.1   The oxyhaemoglobin dissociation curve.

and the results are expressed as a percentage. A saturation of over 95% corresponds to a normal PaO_2 of over 97 mmHg, but a fall in saturation to 90% corresponds to a PaO_2 of 60 mmHg. An oxygen saturation of less than 80% usually equates to severe hypoxia with PaO_2 of less than 45 mmHg. Figure 4.1 shows the relationship between the oxygen saturation (SaO_2) and the PaO_2 of the blood.

Problems with pulse oximetry include:

- motion artefact – the probe needs to be secure and the cable long enough to allow patient movement
- a lop-sided probe – this allows the red and infrared light beams to pass into the detector without passing through the skin thus giving false readings
- excessive ambient light – this produces false readings; direct sunlight or flickering fluorescent light needs to be avoided
- cold extremities/poor circulation can result in non-detection of oxygen saturation
- the probe cannot distinguish abnormal haemoglobin – can get normal readings with carboxyhaemoglobin found in carbon monoxide poisoning
- coloured nail varnish produces inaccuracies
- leaving a probe on when the readings are not being recorded – this causes unnecessary restriction for the patient.

Pulse oximetetry is not without its limitations. For example, it can not give any indication of respiratory failure due to carbon dioxide retention.

Abnormal heart rate and rhythm

Palpitations

Palpitation is an awareness of the heart beat. It is a common symptom regardless of underlying heart disease. Some people complain of a racing heart, and others of thumping or feeling of a missed beat. It should be determined whether they occur on effort or at rest, and whether they begin and end abruptly or gradually. Getting the individual to tap out their palpitations is a good way of determining the rate and regularity of the rhythm. The frequency of the attacks and the accompaniment of breathlessness or pain should be ascertained. Palpitation is an important complaint in those individuals with cardiac rhythm disturbances. The experience of feeling a thumping or pounding in the chest is particularly common and may be anxiety provoking and make people fearful about carrying out daily activities. It may be aggravated by smoking, exercise, stress and excessive intake of alcohol or caffeine. Racing of the heart is usually abnormal if the pulse rate is greater than 130 beats per minute. The experience of missed or dropped beats are more common if the underlying heart rate is slow. Frequent ectopic beats are particularly common in the elderly.

Not all patients with abnormalities of heart rate or rhythm will be aware of this and assessment of the arterial pulse is important even in areas where the patient will be immediately placed on a cardiac monitor. It can indicate qualitative dimensions of the pulse that an ECG tracing will not give.

Assessment of the arterial pulses

Arterial pulses should be examined for rate, rhythm, volume and quality of waveform. The radial artery is commonly used in determining rate and rhythm, although the carotid pulse is better for assessment of volume and waveform, best correlates with the central aortic pressure and reflects cardiac function more accurately than the peripheral vessels. The radial pulse may be difficult to palpate if there is marked vasoconstriction.

An examination of arterial pulses should include palpation of all the major pulses and comparison of the pulse on one side of the body with the corresponding pulse on the other.

Characteristics of the arterial pulse

Rate   The pulse should be counted for 1 min and compared with the apical rate to see if there is a *peripheral pulse deficit*. The rate of the pulse in the normal resting adult averages 70 per minute and is regular, but it varies between 60 and 100 beats/min. Sinus bradycardia (less than 60 beats/min) is frequent following inferior myocardial infarction or in those taking beta-adrenergic receptor blocking agents. Although a slow rate as low as 40 beats/min may be found in the healthy and particularly the athletic, it may be indicative of junctional rhythm or heart block. Sinus tachycardia (more than 100 beats/min) is frequently due to anxiety or pain, although rates in excess of 120 beats/min usually indicate an abnormal tachyarrhythmia.

Rhythm   The normal pulse is regular or may exhibit the gentle slowing and quickening of a sinus arrhythmia. This is usually best appreciated by studying the RR intervals in ECG rhythm strips during respiration. On inspiration, venous return to the heart increases because of the negative intrathoracic pressure. The heart rate therefore increases to cope with the increased load. During expiration, venous return falls and the heart rate slows again. An occasional irregularity in an otherwise regular pulse suggests ectopic beats, and a coupling of beats is due to the alternation of normal and ectopic beats. A totally irregular pulse suggests atrial fibrillation.

Volume   Pulse volume (width or amplitude) depends on the *pulse pressure* (the difference between the systolic and diastolic blood pressure). The pulse is of small volume when the pulse pressure is small and is often found following myocardial infarction. Pulses of large volume are produced by large stroke volumes and are found in anaemia, aortic incompetence and thyrotoxicosis.

Pulse amplitude is categorized into the following levels and compared bilaterally:

     0 = not palpable
    +1 = barely palpable
    +2 = decreased
    +3 = full
    +4 = bounding.

Quality of waveform   Various types of pulse are described:

- *plateau pulse*: low volume, slow rise and slow fall (e.g. aortic stenosis)
- *collapsing pulse*: large volume, rapid rise and rapid fall (e.g. aortic incompetence and heart block)
- *pulsus paradoxus*: volume decreases with inspiration and increases with expiration (e.g. asthma and cardiac tamponade)
- *pulsus alternans*: alternate high-volume and low-volume beats (e.g. LVF).

The patient with suspected cardiac problems needs to be promptly attached to a cardiac monitor and have a 12-lead ECG. This will supplement the information obtained from observation and examination.

Reduced cardiac output

Syncope

Syncope is a transient loss of consciousness due to inadequate cerebral blood flow, resulting in cerebral ischaemia. Vasovagal attacks are the most common cause of syncope and occur following prolonged standing or in response to sudden violent emotion or pain. Syncope on effort may be indicative of aortic stenosis, when the cardiac output through the narrow valve cannot meet the demands of increased activity. Syncope occurring at rest as well as during effort may be due to heart block or arrhythmia. Paroxysmal tachycardias can lead to a marked fall in cardiac output with resulting syncope. Stokes-Adams attacks are associated with complete heart block and sinus arrest. Carotid sinus syncope can occur from stimulation of the carotid sinus either during carotid sinus massage or as a result of restrictive neckware. Micturition syncope occurs in older men as a result of reduced venous return and reduced cardiac output during straining (Valsalva manoeuvre) or because of sudden decompensation of an over-full bladder causing reflex vasodilatation.

Assessment of arterial blood pressure

Arterial blood pressure is an important predictor of morbidity and mortality and is therefore one of the most important clinical observations, yet there is often confusion concerning its measurement and nurses vary in their knowledge of the procedure (Torrance and Serginson 1996). There are many potential sources of error in recording blood pressure, including poor technique and observer bias. Accurate measurements are important as they will affect decisions concerning the patient's management, investigations and outcome.

There are two main methods of determining the blood pressure: direct and indirect. The most accurate method involves the insertion of a tiny pressure transducer unit into an artery for transmission of waveform or digital display on a monitor. For patients who need to be constantly monitored in high dependency situations, the most common technique involves placing a cannula into an artery and attaching a pressure-sensitive device to the external end.

The indirect method of blood pressure measurement is the auscultatory method and is the method used most frequently. This method measures the blood pressure in the brachial artery of the arm and can either be taken by the traditional method of a sphygmomanometer or electronically using a device such as a dynamap.

Equipment   Accuracy in blood pressure measurement depends on correct technique and well-maintained equipment. Equipment errors and poor technique have been found to produce discrepancies in blood pressure readings of more than 15 mmHg (Cambell et al 1990). Mercury sphygmomanometers are more useful than aneroid sphygmomanometers which usually require frequent recalibration and more susceptible to user error (Markandu et al 2000). However, the use of the mercury sphygmomanometer is declining due to the known hazards of the substance. Sphygmomanometers are often poorly maintained and likely to be in poor working order (Carney et al 1995).

Points to check in assessing equipment include:

1 *Manometer*
   ● visibility of meniscus
   ● correct calibration: should be at zero before inflation.

2 *Cuff*
   ● condition, length and width of inflatable bladder
   ● bladder should be at least 80% of the arm circumference in length and 40% of the arm circumference in width – if it is too short the blood pressure will be over-estimated. The arm circumference should be measured at the mid point between the shoulder and the elbow. Once selected, the same cuff needs to be used for all subsequent blood pressure recordings for that patient.

3 *Inflation–deflation device*
   ● control valve – when the valve is closed it should hold the mercury at a constant level
   ● deflation that is too fast or jerky may mean that the systolic pressure is underestimated and the diastolic is overestimated.
   The rubber tubing should be about 80 cm long and have air tight connections that can be separated easily.

4 *Stethoscope*
   ● clean, good condition
   ● well-fitting earpieces.

5 *Maintenance*
   ● service and recalibrate regularly and replace faulty parts.

The Medical Devices Agency (now the Medicines and Healthcare Products Regulatory Agency) has categorized automated non-invasive blood pressure devices into automated, semi-automatic and automatic-cycling devices. These devices measure blood pressure using the oscillometric technique which involves the device pumping up the pressure in the cuff to above the measurement of systolic blood pressure and the cuff deflating in stages. At each stage the amplitude of the blood pressure sound in the brachial artery is recorded. From this amplitude profile, the systolic and diastolic blood pressure are recorded using an algorithm particular to each model. These pieces of equipment can often be set to take readings at preset time intervals and are useful when the nurse is titrating blood pressure response against intravenous drug therapy. They also offer important advantages, such as decreasing observer bias and variability in blood pressure measurement (Rebenson-Piano et al 1989). The patient still needs to be prepared for the cuff inflation and not suffer as a result of reduced direct nurse–patient contact. The British Hypertension Society has produced guidelines for measuring blood pressure by standard sphygmomanometer or semi-automated device (Williams et al 2004).

Ambulatory monitoring allows non-invasive measurement of blood pressure over prolonged periods and gives a more reproducible estimate of the blood pressure. The blood pressure is recorded at intervals, usually every 30 minutes, outside the clinical setting. The individual is asked to keep a diary while they are being monitored so that interpretation has relevance to everyday living. It is particularly useful in patients who experience uncharacteristically high readings when they are having their blood pressure taken by a health care professional. This is known as 'white coat syndrome' and can affect up to a third of the population, particularly the elderly.

New devices for measuring blood pressure use a silicon chip sensor to take a pressure reading. They still require the placement of a cuff around the arm and listening for the Korotkoff sounds through a stethoscope.

Procedure Adequate explanation of the blood pressure recording procedure is necessary to allay any fears of the patient. Ideally, the patient should avoid exertion and not eat or smoke for 30 min beforehand. They should be sitting comfortably in a warm and quiet room.

Several studies have shown a lack of knowledge of the technical aspects of blood pressure measurement. One UK study concluded that only 52% of nurses and 50% of doctors could carry out the procedure correctly (Reeves et al 1998). The patient's arm should be unclothed, supported, slightly extended and externally rotated, otherwise they may perform isometric movements which may give false readings. The arm needs to be supported horizontally on a level with the heart, as the blood pressure rises as the arm is lowered below the level of the heart and increases as the arm is raised. The effect of arm position on blood pressure measurement is particularly important in patients with mild or borderline hypertension (Webster et al 1984). The ideal method of taking a blood pressure recording is to use the sitting position with the arm horizontal and the

antecubital fossa at the level of the fourth or fifth intercostal space.

The person making the recording should also be in a comfortable and relaxed position so that they are unhurried and make careful readings. A cuff with a long and sufficiently wide bladder should be applied to the upper arm, with the tubing placed above so that it does not interfere with auscultation. A cuff that is too small can give a false high reading as the artery is not compressed sufficiently at the appropriate pressure level. A cuff that is too large will produce a falsely low reading as pressure is spread over too large an area and the Korotkoff sounds will be dampened. The centre of the bladder is positioned over the brachial artery, with the lower edge of the bladder 2–3 cm above the point of maximum pulsation of the brachial artery, just above the antecubital fossa. False high readings can be obtained if the bladder is not centred over the brachial artery as more external pressure is needed to compress the artery. If using a mercury sphygmomanometer, the manometer should be vertical and at the recorder's eye level. The brachial artery is palpated with one hand and the cuff inflated for 3–5 s until the pulsation disappears. The cuff is then slowly deflated and a note made of the pressure at which the pulse reappears. This is the approximate level of the systolic pressure, and is useful in patients in whom the auscultatory end-point is difficult to judge accurately.

The stethoscope needs to be placed gently over the brachial artery to the antecubital fossa. A bell end-piece gives better sound reproduction, but a diaphragm is easier to secure with the fingers of one hand. The stethoscope should not be pressed too firmly or touch the cuff, otherwise the diastolic pressure may be grossly underestimated. The cuff is inflated rapidly to about 30 mmHg above the palpated systolic pressure and deflated at a rate of 2 mmHg per second. As the pressure falls, the Korotkoff sounds become audible. The appearance of repetitive clear tapping sounds for at least two consecutive beats (phase I) indicates systolic blood pressure. The point where the repetitive sounds finally disappear (phase V) should be recorded as diastolic blood pressure. Some clinicians prefer to record muffling of sounds (phase IV) as the diastolic pressure. In some patients, for example those who are elderly or have anaemia, the sounds may continue to zero. In such cases, phase IV should be recorded. Sometimes a silent or auscultatory gap occurs when the sounds disappear between the systolic and diastolic pressures. Unless the systolic pressure is palpated first in these cases, the systolic pressure may be underestimated. Whichever is used should be predetermined and recorded in writing. The pressures should be recorded to the nearest 2 mmHg. When all sounds have disappeared, the cuff should be deflated rapidly and completely. One or two minutes should elapse before further measurements are made.

The blood pressure should be measured on at least two separate occasions. If the blood pressure is increased, the mean recording should be noted. Blood pressure recordings in both arms are useful particularly to exclude aortic aneurysms. A difference of 5 mmHg is not uncommon, and the arm with the highest recording should be subsequently used for measurements. Whatever positions are used, they should be specified in the recordings.

The presence of any arrhythmia, anxiety, confinement to bed and whether the patient is receiving any relevant medication should be recorded. A patient resting in bed for two or three days may experience a fall in blood pressure upon standing, and recordings should be made in both lying and standing positions.

Other important mechanical factors that modify the blood pressure values include repeated measurements in a short period of time and rolling up a sleeve which becomes a 'tourniquet' for venous flow.

Changes in blood pressure following acute myocardial infarction

Apart from a circadian pattern in blood pressure, changes occur with increasing age, which particularly affects the systolic pressure, and with physical and mental stress. Blood pressure may be afffected by anxiety, pain, arrhythmias and some medication.

The acute coronary patient may experience initial high blood pressure as a result of pain or stress. Elevated diastolic blood pessure may well fall within the first hour of admission following relief of pain and anxiety. Elevated blood pressure during episodes of angina is a direct result of the decreased blood supply to the heart. Initial hypertension needs to be resolved, to limit the increased workload placed on an already impaired ischaemic left ventricle.

Some patients, often with inferior myocardial infarctions, develop hypotension as a result of activity of the vagal reflex. Hypotension may also occur due to inefficiency of the damaged myocardium to act as a pump, thus reducing cardiac output with the possible development of cardiogenic shock. There is good evidence that a systolic below 100 mmHg in patients with acute myocardial infarction is associated with worse outcome (Morrow et al 2001).

Oedema

Oedema is an abnormal accumulation of fluid in the interstitial tissues and is usually preceded by weight gain from 3 kg to 5 kg of extracellular fluid. It is a relatively late manifestation of heart failure. Oedema will collect preferentially in loose tissues and the distribution of fluid is determined both by gravity and the degree of ambulation. In most patients the legs and feet are affected, but in those confined to bed the fluid accumulates over the sacrum. Greater degrees of oedema will gradually affect the whole of the lower extremities, extending to the torso and eventually the face (anasarca). The oedema characteristically pits when pressure is applied, hence the term *pitting oedema*. The milder grades of oedema are not often noticed by the patient. Oedema is usually, but not invariably, symmetrical in distribution.

Normally, fluid is exuded into the tissues because arterial capillary pressure (30 mmHg) exceeds plasma oncotic pressure (25 mmHg). However, the fluid is forced back into circulation at the venous end of the capillaries because pressure here (12 mmHg) is exceeded by the oncotic pressure (25 mmHg). If the venous pressure rises (as in heart failure), the resorption of fluid is impaired and oedema results.

Assessment of oedema

Oedema is best assessed by pressing the ball of the thumb or the tips of the index and middle fingers down into the skin and maintaining moderate pressure for a few seconds. If there is oedema present the skin has a 'boggy' feel. The external pressure squeezes the oedema fluid away from the pressure point. On removing the thumb or the fingers, the finger impression remains imprinted in the skin for a short while (pitting) before fading as the fluid redistributes. The degree of pitting that occurs may be quantified and described by the following scale:

0 = none present
+1 = trace – disappears rapidly
+2 = moderate – disappears in 10–15 s
+3 = deep – disappears in 1–2 min
+4 = very deep – present after 5 min.

Cyanosis

Cyanosis describes the blue (cyan) discoloration imparted to the skin and mucous membranes due to low oxygen content of the blood. It appears that it only becomes visible when there is greater than 5% of reduced (i.e. oxygen-depleted) haemoglobin in the blood of the vessels being considered. Cyanosis may be peripheral or central. The former is observed in the nailbeds, lips and earlobes due to a higher degree of oxygen extraction at the peripheries. Central cyanosis, indicated by a bluish discoloration of the warm mucous membranes of the nose, mouth and under the tongue, is more significant in terms of evaluating the function of gaseous exchange in the lungs.

Body temperature

Body temperature is usually maintained between 36 and 37.5°C regardless of the environmental temperature. Various factors can cause fluctuations in temperature. These include:

- the body's circadian rhythms – the temperature is higher in the evening by 0.5–1.5°C
- ovulation results in fluctuations in temperature
- exercise and eating increases body temperature
- extremes of age affect a person's response to environmental change. In the elderly there is increased sensitivity to the cold and generally a lower body temperature.

Pyrexia is the term for a significant rise in body temperature. It is usually the result of infection although non-infectious causes include anticholinergic drugs, allergic reaction, hyperthyroidism,

malignancy and alcohol withdrawal. A low-grade pyrexia also occurs in most coronary patients as a non-specific response to myocardial necrosis. Pyrexia may also occur with the inflammatory response associated with pericarditis, usually some 24–72 h after the infarction.

The presence or absence of a pyrexia may help in diagnosis when the presenting history does not seem typical of ischaemia and it is necessary to eliminate the existence of an underlying infection.

Assessment of body temperature Although many nurses probably consider taking temperatures to be a mundane task requiring little skill or knowledge, several nurse researchers have, in the past, highlighted the need for more care and attention to be paid to the procedure (Takacs and Valenti 1982, Baker et al 1984).

A variety of thermometers are now in use including the clinical glass thermometer with oral or rectal bulbs, the electronic sensor thermometer, the chemical/disposable thermometer and the tympanic membrane thermometer.

The clinical glass thermometer containing mercury which expands with heat has been widely used in the past. However, they can be slow to respond to changes in temperature. The tympanic membrane thermometer which probes the ear canal has the advantage of providing rapid results, being easy to use and convenient for both the nurse and the patient (Burke 1996), although it can produce erroneous results if used incorrectly (White et al 1994). The electronic thermometer gives rapid and accurate measurements although they require regular calibration.

When recording trends in body temperature, the same site, instrument and technique needs to be used to limit the number of variables. The oral site is most commonly selected because it is convenient and thought to be sensitive to changes in temperature of the blood in the arteries. The maximum mouth temperature is obtained at the junction of the base of the tongue and the floor of the mouth either to the right or left of the frenulum. Other areas of the mouth are of a lower temperature and thus not an accurate reflection of the actual body temperature (Erickson 1980). People who wear lower dentures require relatively longer to return to a stable oral temperature after exercise. A hot drink will influence the oral temperature

Figure 4.2   Xanthelasma.

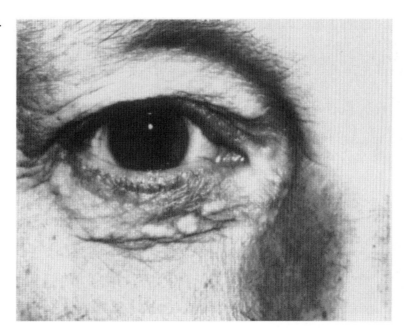

some 6 minutes after, and an iced drink will cool the mouth for 15 minutes after it has been drunk.

It appears that oxygen administration may have an adverse effect on accurate temperature assessment, as oxygen has a cooling effect (Dressler et al 1983). Unobserved mouth breathing may cause evaporative cooling of the oral cavity (Tandberg and Sklar 1983). Patients with a respiratory rate in excess of 20 breaths/min have lower recorded temperatures due to the ventilatory cooling of the mouth (Durham et al 1986). The mouth contains environmental air and the patient's lips need to be closed around the thermometer to allow the air to warm up to body temperature.

The length of thermometer insertion seems to affect temperature readings (Baker et al 1984), although there seems to be no clinical advantage in using a measurement time of longer than 3 min with mercury thermometers (Davies et al 1986).

The axillary site is often used for patients who are confused, restless or unconscious. The thermometer must be left in position for at least 9 min. Variations are apparent between the right and left arm of some individuals and the same side should be used for consecutive readings.

Alongside recording the actual temperature, assessment may involve asking the patient whether they feel hot, cold or uncomfortable, noting whether they seem flushed, warm or cold to the touch, and ascertaining when they last had a hot or cold drink.

Signs of hyperlipidaemia and coronary atherosclerosis

Many patients will be unaware that they have hyperlipidaemia even though they may have developed clinical manifestations of the condition. Observation of the patient can give cues but this needs to be confirmed with blood tests.

Corneal arcus is a white ring surrounding the cornea which is a particularly significant sign of hyperlipidaemia in those under the age of 50 years. In the elderly it is particularly common, often as a result of degenerative changes in the eye.

Xanthelasma are small, raised yellow plaques containing cholesterol which can be seen on the eyelids (Figure 4.2).

Tendon xanthomata are hard nodules found over the knuckles, in the Achilles tendon and the patella and with xanesthesia are an important clinical sign of familial hypercholesterolaemia (Figure 4.3).

Eruptive xanthomata are papules with yellow centres that appear over extensor surfaces and are a clinical indication of hypertriglyceridaemia (Jowett 2002).

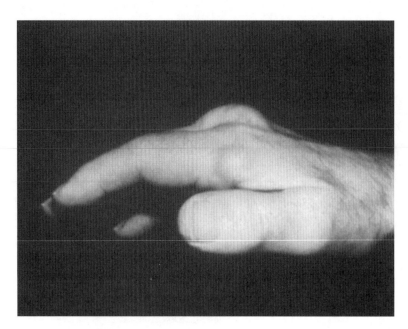

Figure 4.3   Tendon xanthoma.

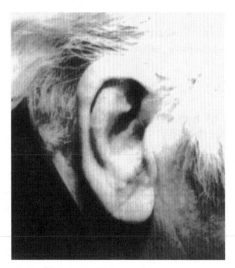

Figure 4.4   Diagonal earlobe crease.

Diagonal ear creases have been shown to have a high correlation with coronary atherosclerosis although the cause is unknown (Figure 4.4) (Patel et al 1992).

Emotional response

Patients with a suspected cardiac problem are likely to fear for their survival and worry about their families. Pain and other symptoms can also provoke emotional responses as can the response of the health care professionals they come into contact with.

Emotional disturbances are extremely common in the coronary care unit patient. A study of over 300 patients in hospital after a myocardial infarction (Mayou et al 2000) illustrated that 18.5% had anxiety that was probably clinically significant, with a further 19% identified as borderline cases. Almost 18% had clinically significant or borderline depression. If anxiety is unrelieved, then depression usually becomes apparent and may persist for long periods of time (Lane et al 2002). Certainly, emotional disturbances after myocardial infarction may adversely influence subsequent recovery and health outcome (Mayou et al 2000, Thompson and Lewin 2000).

Severe anxiety during the initial phase of the illness results in increases in heart rate, blood pressure and myocardial oxygen demand. These cardiovascular effects, mediated through the sympathetic nervous system, may result in life-threatening complications, including arrhythmias, heart failure and extension of the size of the infarct.

Assessment

The nurse is usually the first and perhaps the ideal person to identify and manage emotional responses that may affect the patient and his family. There is a need for skills that help recognize emotional distress and an understanding of the basic mechanisms of helping the patient to cope. Anxiety can be identified in a number of ways, such as subjectively by using a variety of self-report measures; objectively by measuring physiological and biochemical indices such as blood pressure, heart rate and plasma or urinary catecholamines; and by observing behaviour. Obviously, objective measures are often impractical, expensive, and time consuming to perform. Observation of behaviour can yield useful information. One study has concluded that six characteristics adequately discriminate anxious patients on cardiorespiratory wards (Shuldham et al 1995). These characteristics were: sweating, faintness, tendency to blame others, continual review of things on their mind, focus on self, and a lack of self-confidence. Simple self-report measures, such as VASs, can be practical and quick to use, and are valid and reliable instruments.

Several well-known and carefully formulated instruments are available to measure depression, including the Beck Depression Inventory (Beck et al 1961) and the Zung (1965) self-rating depression scale. As with anxiety, a VAS may prove more useful as an assessment tool. The Hospital Anxiety and Depression Scale (Zigmond and Snaith 1983) is a 14-item self-assessment scale that measures both anxiety and depression. It is based on the psychic symptoms of anxiety and depression and not on emotional or physical disorders. It is increasingly being used for cardiac patients, although careful consideration is needed before giving questionnaires to patients in the acute stage of their illness. All measures have their strength and weaknesses and it may be worth combining methods.

Inspection, palpation, auscultation and percussion

Observing and talking to the patient will give an indication as to his physical and emotional state. An assessment of blood pressure, pulse and temperature will add to the picture. However, a more formal physical examination of the cardiovascular system will supplement this information.

A comprehensive examination of the cardiovascular system needs to include inspection, palpation, auscultation and percussion. The first three are generally more helpful than the latter in determining the cardiac state of the patient.

In the UK, it is unusual for nurses to perform palpation, percussion or auscultation and there is comparatively little literature that looks at the development or impact of nurses undertaking these roles. In the USA advanced physical assessment skills are expected of nurses in many settings and physicians depend on the nurses' report of breath and heart sounds (Metral 2000). Despite the fact that the cardiac physical assessment skills were included in UK cardiac nursing text books over 20 years ago (Thompson 1982), they have still not become established as part of the cardiac nurses' day-to-day role. The skills are not taught in basic training or in most post-registration post-basic courses. There are courses offering post-registration physical assessment skills training, but these tend to offer limited opportunity for developing skills in the clinical situation. The reasons why UK nurses have not incorporated the physical assessment skills used everyday by medical colleagues are complex. However, this situation may change as nurses become more established in roles that necessitate sound clinical decision making without recourse to a medical opinion. Even before that time, it is important for them to understand what is involved in these methods of cardiac examination, particularly for explanations to the patient.

Inspection

This should include general observation of the patient's body build, skin, chest symmetry, neck vein pulsations, chest (precordial) movement and the extremities. The apical pulse, which is caused by left ventricular contraction, may be visible in the mid-left clavicular line at the fifth interspace, in about half of normal adults.

Palpation

Information gathered from inspection is augmented using the technique of palpation. This consists of a systematic examination of the chest.

The location, size and character of the apical pulse should be identified. This may be difficult if the patient is obese or has a hyperinflated chest. The apex beat may be displaced by abnormalities of the lungs or rib cage. It is described as a double or rocking beat if there is left ventricular aneurysm or heaving or thrusting with left ventricular hypertrophy. The apex beat tends to be weak and diffuse with left ventricular dilatation and has a tapping quality with mitral stenosis.

Thrills are palpable murmurs caused by abnormal blood flow and may be observed as a sort of purring sensation. Palpation with the palmar aspect of the base of the fingers best picks up vibrations, while palpation with the fingertips best discloses pulsations.

Auscultation

Auscultation means listening to the heart sounds. Sound is a wave motion that has four characteristics:

1 intensity: force of the amplitude of the vibration
2 pitch: frequency of the vibrations per unit of time
3 duration: length of time that the sound persists
4 timbre: quality that depends on overtones that accompany the fundamental tone.

Sound waves are initiated by vibrations. The heart sounds are produced by vascular walls, flowing blood, heart muscle and heart valves. The transmission of the heart sounds depends on the position of the heart, the nature of the surrounding structures, and the position of the stethoscope in relation to the origin of the sound. The auscultatory sites are the points on the chest to which the sounds are best transmitted, not the anatomical location of the valves.

Percussion

This is less helpful than other techniques of examination in determining cardiac state. Formerly, percussion was used to determine heart size. However, it is of no real value today. Dullness in the second intercostal space suggests the possibility of an aneurysm of the aorta or enlargement of the pulmonary artery.

Heart sounds

The *first heart sound* (S1) is created by vibrations from the closing of the mitral and tricuspid valves. The *second heart sound* (S2) represents the closing of the aortic and pulmonary valves. Using the diaphragm of the stethoscope and starting at the second right intercostal space, one can hear these heart sounds. S1 may be louder at the apex, while S2 may be louder at the base of the heart in the second intercostal space. During inspiration, there may be normal physiological splitting of S2 into two components, A_2 and P_2. This is caused by increased venous return to the right side of the heart during inspiration and by a prolonged delay in the closing of the pulmonary valve.

A loud first sound will be heard with abnormally high left atrial pressure (such as occurs with mitral stenosis) during tachycardias and if the atria contract very soon before ventricular systole. A soft first heart sound occurs with poor left ventricular contraction, calcification of the mitral valve or if the valve has poor movement.

The second heart sound is louder in pulmonary or systemic hypertension and may be a feature of pulmonary embolism.

A *third heart sound* ('ventricular gallop') occasionally occurs after S2, and is produced by vibrations of the ventricles due to rapid distension during rapid filling in the first phase of diastole. It is low-pitched and best heard at the apex. It may be normal in the young and during pregnancy. In those over the age of 40, a third heart sound suggests heart failure or the widely open mitral valve found in mitral regurgitation. A third heart sound is found in 5–10% of those with myocardial infarction and is a poor prognostic sign.

A *fourth heart sound* ('atrial gallop') occasionally occurs in late diastole and is thought to result from vibrations of the valves, supporting structures or ventricles during the atrial systolic ejection of blood into the non-distending ventricles found in ventricular hypertrophy or hypertrophic obstructive cardiomyopathy.

A *pericardial friction rub* may be heard when inflamed visceral and parietal pericardia rub against each other. It is heard best when the patient is sitting forward and produces a scratchy sandpaper like sound which may be localized, generalized, short term or long lasting.

Heart murmurs

Murmurs are caused by:

1 increased flow through normal structures
2 forward flow across a stenotic valve
3 backward flow through an incompetent valve
4 flow from a high-pressure chamber or vessel through an abnormal passage
5 flow into a dilated chamber.

Murmurs are evaluated according to their:

- timing
- location
- intensity
- pitch
- quality
- radiation.

The timing of a murmur may be systolic or diastolic, and it may be present through all or part of the cycle. Murmurs heard throughout systole are called *holosystolic* or *pansystolic*. They may be of equal intensity throughout or may exhibit a crescendo–decrescendo pattern. The intensity is graded on a scale of 1–6, with 1 being very faint and 6 being audible even when the stethoscope is slightly raised from the chest. Pitch may be high, medium or low. The quality may be harsh, blowing, rumbling or musical. Locations of murmurs are described according to the intercostal position and the distance from the mid-sternal, mid-clavicular or one of the axillary lines.

Jugular venous pressure and pulse

Examination of the jugular venous pressure (JVP) and pulse will provide information about the function of the right heart. Both the internal and external jugular veins may be examined, but the former is a more reliable indicator. When the patient is standing or sitting upright, the internal jugular vein is collapsed and when the patient is lying flat, it is completely filled. When the patient lies supine at approximately 45°, the point at which the jugular venous pulsation becomes visible is just above the clavicle and this is the position chosen for examination of the jugular venous pulse. In patients with very high JVP (e.g. pericardial tamponade) the jugular vein may be completely filled with the patient lying at 45° and it may be necessary to sit the patient bolt upright to see the top of the pulsation.

The JVP is measured by observing the number of centimetres above the sternal angle that venous pulsations can be seen. The sternal angle is a relatively constant distance of 5–7 cm above the right atrium. Confirmation of the level can be made by pressing on the liver, which temporarily increases venous return to the heart via the hepatojugular reflex. Normally, the JVP should not exceed 3 cm above the level of the sternal angle, with the head of the patient elevated to 30–45°. The most common cause of an elevated JVP is right ventricular failure secondary to left heart failure, pulmonary embolism or cor pulmonale. Increased blood volume and increased pressure within the pericardium are other possible causes.

Jugular venous pulsations consist of several components owing to various physiological events in the cardiac cycle. Clinical interpretation of these events is often difficult but in theory they are seen as diffuse undulating movements and are not palpable. They may increase or decrease with a change in body position.

The components of the jugular venous pulsations consist of three positive waves, a, c and v, and two negative waves, x and y. The 'a' wave is produced by a rise of pressure due to atrial systole. The negative 'x' wave is produced by a fall of pressure due to atrial diastole. The 'c' wave is a carotid artefact and is not usually possible to see in the jugular pulse. Blood continues to flow into the atrium during atrial relaxation, causing a rise in atrial pressure which produces the positive 'v' wave. When the tricuspid valve opens in early diastole, the atrial pressure falls producing the negative 'y' wave.

Large 'a' waves, known as cannon waves, can be seen when the right atrium closes against a closed tricuspid valve which can occur when the atria and ventricles are not synchronized (may occur in complete heart block). If the patient has atrial fibrillation there will be no 'a' waves, as the atria do not contract.

Cannon waves   If the atrium contracts when the tricuspid valve is closed (as in ventricular systole), a jet of blood is forced into the jugular veins and a visible 'cannon wave results. These waves occur intermittently in complete heart block and in ventricular tachycardia when atrial and ventricular systoles coincide. In junctional rhythms, atrial and ventricular contractions are synchronous and cannon waves are therefore regular with every heart beat.

Central venous pressure

The central venous pressure (CVP) is the pressure in the right atrium, and it serves as a guide for assessment of right heart function. As the CVP is a direct measurement of the venous pressure, it is one of the earliest parameters to alter if there are changes in the fluid status.

Measurement of CVP will:

- establish the pressure in the right atrium (filling pressure or preload)
- establish blood volume deficits
- evaluate circulatory failure
- act as a guide in fluid replacement
- reflect response to treatment.

Although a non-invasive technique for measuring CVP would be ideal, attempts have proved unsuccessful in practice. The invasive procedure involves inserting a flexible polyvinyl radiopaque catheter into the subclavian vein and advancing it along the vein until its tip is in or near to the right atrium. Electronic measurements of CVP will give continuous monitoring of changes in pressure at the catheter tip. Water manometry using solutions of saline or dextrose is another method.

The catheter is usually inserted at the patient's bedside using an aseptic technique under local anaesthesia. The subclavian route is most commonly used, although other veins such as the jugular, brachial, femoral and median basilic can also be used. Guidelines from National Institute for Clinical Evidence (2002) recommend two-dimensional (2D) imaging ultrasound guidance as the preferred method for insertion of central venous catheters into the internal jugular vein in elective situations and this is likely to have implications for the choice of vein.

The patient needs to be advised that the insertion site will be cleansed with a cool solution, that the procedure may be uncomfortable but not painful, and that the bed may be tipped slightly head downwards during catheter insertion. The procedure usually takes between 10 and 15 min.

After insertion, the catheter is usually connected to a three-way stopcock that connects to an intravenous solution and to a manometer which acts as a measuring device. The catheter is sutured in place at the skin surface and a sterile dressing is applied.

The ideal position for taking CVP reading remains controversial, particularly in assessment of circulatory volume depletion (Amoroso and Greenwood 1989). As a general rule it is often better to attempt measurements from the level of the right atrium itself so that posture does not affect the CVP. A position should be established where the patient feels comfortable to act as a baseline for subsequent CVP readings. A zero point is identified, usually the sternal notch, a point halfway from front to back of the chest at the level of the fifth intercostal space (mid-axillary line), or some other point near the right atrium and the phlebostatic axis (intersection of the transverse plane of the body and the fourth intercostal space, with the midline from front to back of the chest) (Figure 4.5). This reference point needs to remain constant with subsequent readings. The zero point is aligned to the manometer scale using a spirit level. The stopcock is turned first, so that the manometer fills with intravenous solution, and then turned so that this fluid flows into the patient. The level at which the solution stabilizes is the CVP. The fluid level may rise and fall significantly with venous pulsation and respiration and so readings should ideally be taken at the end of respiration.

If it does not prove practical for the patient to be in the same position for all readings, then the new zero point needs to be identified for each reading, and the fact that the patient is in a different position needs to be considered when interpreting the reading.

The normal CVP range is about 4–10 cmH$_2$O. The value in centimetres of water can be converted to millimetres of mercury by dividing the former by 1.36, since 1 mmHg is equal to 1.36 cmH$_2$O. The CVP rises in conditions such as right ventricular failure and fluid overload, and falls with a decrease

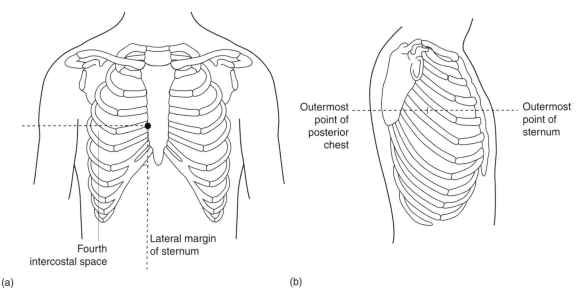

Figure 4.5   The phlebostatic axis. The crossing of two imaginary lines defines the assumed position of the monitoring catheter tip within the body, i.e. right atrial level. (a) A line that passes from the fourth intercostal space at the lateral margin of the sternum down the side of the body beneath the axilla. (b) A line that runs horizontally at a point midway between the outermost portion of the anterior and posterior surfaces of the chest.

in circulatory volume. CVP reflects changes in the venous system and right heart, but may not reflect changes in the left ventricular end-diastolic pressure (LVEDP) if the lungs and heart valves are normal. Thus, left heart failure following acute myocardial infarction may be undetectable. CVP monitoring is therefore not always an accurate guide to fluid replacement. It is important that CVP be regarded as a serial measurement, i.e. the pattern or trend of recordings considered rather than a single result.

Technical difficulties and complications   Complications include:

- pain
- anxiety
- air embolism
- infection
- trauma
- conduction disturbances
- arrhythmias
- bleeding.

The correct technique for catheter insertion is all important. As with any invasive procedure, adequate analgesia is required and diazepam may alleviate anxiety not helped by psychological support.

Tipping the patient's head during catheter insertion helps to minimize the likelihood of air embolism, particularly if the subclavian or jugular routes are chosen.

A full aseptic technique is essential, and the insertion site should be observed for inflammation or haematoma, covered with a clear adhesive dressing and changed as necessary. A chest X-ray taken after the procedure will confirm whether the catheter tip is correctly positioned and if there has been any damage, such as pneumothorax. The patient needs to be advised to report any pain or discomfort at the catheter insertion site or in the location of the catheter route, as this may indicate an infection or injury to peripheral nerves and veins.

The longer the catheter is left in place, the more likely it is that fibrin deposits will form along its surface with the danger of subsequent embolism. Thus, the catheter should only be left in place while management is being monitored and affected by the CVP readings.

PATIENT INTERVIEW

The patient interview is an important step in the data collection process. Its purpose is to gather pertinent information about the patient's present complaint or problem, health history and family and social history.

When the patient is stable it is possible to elaborate on an initial assessment in conjunction with a nursing history, to build a more detailed framework on which to base nursing care. Potential disorders in other body systems may exacerbate a cardiac problem. Pre-existing problems that the patient copes with adequately at home may become real problems in hospital. New problems may emerge as a result of the heart attack and its management. A knowledge of the patient and their behaviour before admission will enable the nurse to tailor care so that a near to normal lifestyle can be maintained in hospital.

The physical assessment needs to be accompanied by an appraisal of the patients' psychological, social and spiritual background and the extent of their knowledge, understanding and support services.

The patient's own interpretation of their illness and problems is important, so that goals can be formulated with their wishes and expectations taken into account. Establishing the implications the patient places on having suffered a heart attack, as well as level of knowledge and understanding, will help in planning recovery and avoiding misconceptions. Assessing the need, desire and ability to absorb further information will determine which method of giving information is likely to have greatest impact. Knowledge of any actions the patient may have taken in the past to modify their lifestyle in order to promote health gives an indication of their perceptions and motivation and the impact of this behaviour on plans for recovery. Thus, the likelihood of success with behaviour modification and compliance can be assessed.

Being aware of any religious, cultural or other personal practices that the patient would like to continue in hospital shows careful consideration and may reduce fear and anxiety. Formulating a picture of the patient's social background will help in identifying key areas such as work, leisure and family life on which to focus rehabilitation efforts and enable social supports such as family and friends to be mobilized effectively. A psychological assessment will hopefully identify the patient's response to admission to hospital, the

heart attack, its management and likely outcome, so that inappropriate methods of coping can be made amenable to modification.

History–taking

Traditionally a medical history involves a question and answer type session in order to provide data whereas the nursing assessment is less formal and aimed at getting to know the patient (Brown 1995). As nurses' roles have evolved to encompass initial patient assessments and involvement in medical management decisions, their style of assessment has shifted towards the medical approach. This more focused and abrupt style may have implications for how the nurse–patient relationship develops. It has been argued (Brown 1995) that a conversational interview, which combines elements of the data-collection interview with the more person-orientated style of conversation may be the best approach for nurses taking a patient history.

History-taking improves with experience and the style adopted will depend on specific patient circumstances. Certainly at some point there should be an opportunity for the patient to relate their problem(s) spontaneously in a calm, unhurried atmosphere. Information should be recorded as soon as it is gathered, to minimize omission and distortion of facts. Ideally, the patient should be comfortable, relaxed and in an environment that is private, free of distraction and conducive to interviewing. Unfortunately, such an ideal situation is far from reality. On admission, the patient may be extremely ill and the relatives too distressed to contribute much information, and so returning to talk at a later time may often be more appropriate. In any event, history-taking needs to be a continuing accumulation of information throughout the patient's stay in hospital. Too often it is seen as paper filling exercise and a formality to be completed as quickly as possible (Holt 1995). Often the written information from patient assessments is filed away and not referred to again. To make the process more relevant, the information collected needs to become an integral part of planning patient care.

During history-taking, the nurse should be sensitive and considerate, especially with regards to the amount of questioning and discussion the patient and family can tolerate, particularly if the patient is anxious or in pain. Ideally, the nurse should sit at the patient's bedside while eliciting the history, observing the patient's general appearance, manner of speaking, breathing, and evidence of agitation, pain or distress. Touch is useful here and permits a recording of the pulse as well as noting the condition of the skin. The patient is likely to benefit from perceiving that the nurse is listening to them and 'being with them' throughout the assessment rather than feeling that the nurse is undertaking a series of tasks on them in a manner that is impersonal and distant (Fredriksson 1999).

In order to establish the nurse–patient relationship, it is helpful to:

1   conduct the interview in privacy
2   introduce yourself to the patient
3   address the patient by their preferred name
4   inform the patient of the purpose of the interview
5   probe and listen for the patient's concerns and beliefs about their condition
6   show care and concern for the patient
7   be non-judgemental in response to the patient
8   use language that is appropriate for the patient's educational, cultural and psychological background
9   observe the patient's non-verbal behaviour.

A mixture of verbal and non-verbal communication skills are used, but it is important for the nurse to check with the patient that they are making the correct inferences from non-verbal cues.

Emotional responses to the symptoms related to cardiovascular disease may manifest themselves as fear, anxiety, depression or denial, which could be detrimental. Particular care should be shown towards the coronary patient who is elderly, confused or has a poor memory and may be unable to give a good history. The nurse should be alert to handicaps or other limitations of the patient.

The patient interview can be guided as follows:

1   use open-ended questions and statements
2   clarify words, phrases or statements
3   summarize information during and after the interview to ensure accuracy
4   reflect words, phrases, statements and feelings
5   use silence to organize your thoughts and allow the patient time to answer questions
6   use supportive statements and gestures
7   focus the interview on the current topic.

In making the patient assessment, information is supplemented by facts gathered from the family, significant others, past and existing data in nursing, medical or social reports, in addition to that from other health professionals who have cared for the patient. Therefore, it will include data from a detailed physical examination and laboratory investigations.

The goal of the assessment process is to obtain complete and accurate information. In order to do this it is sensible to use a systematic method of evaluation, such as the following.

Identification of the patient

This is a brief description of the patient, and the data base should include:

1   Name.
2   Sex.
3   Age and date of birth.
4   Race, nationality and religion.
5   Marital status and next of kin.
6   Address and telephone number.
7   Occupation (does it involve physical or emotional stress; if retired what was their work?).
8   Source of referral.
9   Chief complaint or concept of illness.
10 Other pertinent characteristics.

Essentially, the assessment consists of the following components:

1   Reason for admission.
2   History of present illness or problem.
3   Previous history.
4   Activities.
5   Family history.
6   Psychosocial history.

Spiritual assessment may form a part of some nursing assessments and there has been increasing literature around this in the past decade (McSherry and Ross 2001, Draper et al 2002).

1 Reason for admission Emphasis should be placed on the reason for the present admission to hospital (chief complaint). The nurse can provide valuable insight into the patient's health problem by collecting and recording several facts of why the patient is here. Adopting the patient model of Kleinman et al (1978) there are nine questions which may help elicit information about the patient's view of the problem:

1   What brings you here?
2   What do you think has caused your illness?
3   Why do you think it started when it did?
4   What do you think this illness does to you?
5   How severe is your illness?
6   What kind of treatment do you think you should receive?
7   What are the most important results you hope to receive from treatment?
8   What are the chief problems your illness has caused for you?
9   What do you fear most about your illness?

The patient should be encouraged to describe their own problems and expectations with little or no direction from the nurse. The coronary patient will often have more than one complaint, and these problems need to be identified.

Response to symptoms

Finding out how the patient responded to their symptoms is a useful way of putting their problem into perspective, exploring the patient's perception of the event and possibly identifying gaps in knowledge that will inform future patient education strategies.

The time it takes for patients with possible cardiac chest pain to seek professional help is particularly important in the era of time dependent reperfusion strategies. Several studies have examined patients' help seeking behaviour. Birkhead (1992) in an audit of 1934 patients with suspected myocardial infarction found that the time between symptom onset and the call for help was dependent on where the patient was at the time and whom they decided to call. The delay was longer when the patient was at home as opposed to a public place or at work and whether they decided to call the general practitioner (GP) rather than the emergency service. In this study most patients waited for more than 4 hours before seeking help. Several other studies have reported

even longer delays in seeking medical help (Yarebski et al 1994, Dracup et al 1995, Gurwitz et al 1997) with median time from onset of symptoms to presentation of between 2 and 6.5 hours. Interestingly, having a previous history of an acute cardiac event does not seem to be linked with a shorter response time. Patient characteristics also appear to be significant, with older patients (Maynard et al 1989, Yarebski et al 1994, Tresh 1998), women (Clark et al 1992, Meischke et al 1992), those from minority ethnic groups (Crawford et al 1994) and people experiencing social and economic deprivation (Ghali et al 1993) taking longer to come under medical care.

Symptom severity may influence patient delay: patients experiencing sudden onset, severe chest pain are likely to call for help sooner (Schmidt and Borsch 1990) as are those with left ventricular function (Rawles et al 1990, Trent et al 1995). Patients who call the emergency services in preference to their GP have been shown to have more severe symptoms and complications (Quinn et al 1999). Developing symptoms in the presence of a family member (particularly the partner) has been associated with additional delay, possibly a result of a range of emotional factors including denial (Alonso 1986).

One of the contributory factors to patient delay in seeking medical help is what they do once they start to experience symptoms. One study has shown that patients who did not seek the advice of family members and undertook limited diversionary tactics such as drinking tea or coffee or walking about to try and ease the symptoms took less time to decide to call for help than those who took measures to try and relieve the symptoms such as indigestion remedies and seeking reassurance from partners and other family members (Ruston et al 1998).

A knowledge of the above factors should help inform how patients are advised to respond to possible cardiac symptoms. Partners need to be included in the information giving as they may inadvertently delay the response to symptoms. Knowledge of symptoms may not be enough to promote action in the event of an acute coronary event. Cognitive and emotional processes, individual beliefs and values and the context of the event need to be considered (Pattenden et al 2002).

2 History of present illness This is a detailed description of the patient's problem. It should begin with an elaboration of the chief complaint and include a detailed history of the present problem from the time of onset to the present. Does the patient relate their present problem (heart attack) to associated factors in lifestyle (e.g. smoking, stress, diet), failure to comply with drug regimens, or failure or delay in seeking help?

The history provides subjective information relative to the severity of the disease process or health problem and its effect on the patient's activities of daily living. Thus, relevant information would include details of the onset of the problem, the presence or absence of cardiac risk factors, drugs (side effects may be responsible for some current complaint), diet and physical activity (functional capacities and limitations in terms of activities of living). When information is sought about symptoms that are induced by exercise, it is important to determine whether the patient performs the necessary activity sufficient to induce them.

Symptoms should be described according to specific factors:

1 body site/location: origination, location and radiation
2 quality: properties of the symptom
3 quantity: extent, severity, frequency, duration and intensity
4 chronology: onset and sequence
5 setting: situation, time, active/resting, emotionally upset/relaxed and alone/with someone
6 predisposing, aggravating and alleviating factors: change in position, extremes of temperature, deep breathing and GTN
7 associated symptoms.

3 Previous history Knowing that the patient has a previous history of CHD, particularly a previous admission with an acute cardiac event, will make it more likely that the current episode is also the result of a cardiac problem. Although it is known that patients forget what they have been told and may have misconceptions about their condition, a previous cardiac diagnosis may influence their understanding of their condition and this needs to be taken into account when giving information and advice.

A patient history also needs to determine any change in the patient's normal pattern of living that may or may not be caused by illness and to identify clues that may aid in eliciting the present problem. Information about symptoms relating to normal cardiac and respiratory problems in particular will help put the present situation into perspective. It is important to obtain data about previous hospital admissions, illnesses, accidents, allergies, immunizations and any treatment that may not necessarily seem to be related to the present problems already identified. If it is determined that the patient is receiving specific medications, their level of knowledge and compliance should be assessed.

4 Activities This should be a description of the patient's daily pattern of activity. It will usually be based on a model of activities of daily living which has been used in nurse education and practice for almost three decades. This assessment needs to include detailed information on:

1 dietary patterns, e.g. normal dietary intake, knowledge of blood cholesterol level, calorie intake and use of supplements
2 sleep habits, e.g. hours per day, sleep patterns, naps and use of sedatives
3 elimination habits, e.g. normal patterns and use of diuretics or aperients
4 hygiene practices, e.g. preference for bath or shower and frequency
5 rest and activities, e.g. work, leisure, sexual and social activities and rest periods.

Whether there have been any recent changes in the activities and the amount of help the individual needs with any activity should be incorporated into the assessment.

5 Family history This is obtained to provide a picture of the patient's family health, especially that of his parents, grandparents and siblings. This should include details of disease, age and cause of death and the presence of any familial diseases which are pertinent, e.g. hypercholesterolaemia, diabetes mellitus and hypertension. Knowing that an individual's father died from a heart attack at a young age may also be of help in understanding their coping responses.

6 Psychosocial history It is necessary to obtain accurate psychological and social data to help identify problems which may have a bearing on the patient's present condition or may affect the course of his illness. The psychosocial history should include information on five main areas (McGurn 1981):

1 coping mechanisms of the patient and family: the changes that the patient's heart attack imposes and the responses the patient and family are making to them
2 interpersonal relationships: the type and strength of interpersonal relationship and whether other people will help the patient cope with his illness and changes to his life
3 lifestyle: how the patient likes to spend his time and money, his general way of life, and the probable effect the illness will have
4 support system: the family, work companions, peers and neighbours, and the support that may be available
5 family/community assets: positive attributes the family and community agencies may have to offer.

7 Spiritual assessment The International Council of Nurses Code of Ethics for Nurses (ICN 2000) indicates that the nurse needs to promote an environment in which the human rights, values, customs and spiritual beliefs of the individual, family and community are respected. The UKCC (2000) guidelines on pre-registration education highlighted that nurses be taught how to undertake and document a comprehensive, sensitive and accurate nursing assessment of physical, social and spiritual needs of patients. The revised version of the patients' charter (DoH 2001) also highlights the importance of care that respects the spiritual needs of patients. However, undertaking an assessment of an individual's spiritual beliefs and how these impact on illness and recovery is likely to be a sensitive and skilled process for which nurses are likely to have received little if any preparation. Key issues surrounding spiritual assessment have been identified as (McSherry and Ross 2001):

- defining spirituality – concept of God/deity; its significance; sources of hope and strength;

religious practices; relationship between spirituality and health
- having clear motives for undertaking the assessment – what is the information used for
- the timing and detail of the assessment – one-off vs on-going
- how to assess – direct questioning vs observation
- determining who should assess – nursing does not have the monopoly
- ethical issues – is an assessment appropriate or needed? Impact on those assessing/confidentiality issues.

Some people take comfort from and re-examine their own spirituality in times of illness and some cultures may seek to find spiritual reasons for their illness and recovery (Webster et al 2001). Others may feel that their lives do not contain a spiritual dimension (Draper et al 2002).

It can be seen that assessment of the coronary patient is not simply a matter of noting a few facts, but is a comprehensive review of the patient and family and how the patient interacts with the environment and responds to a change in circumstances.

If nursing implies focusing on health rather than illness, the patient should be assessed in relation to health or wellness. Bauman (1961) states that health can he judged on:

- the subjective feeling of well-being
- the absence of any symptoms
- the ability to perform activities which those individuals in good health are able to perform.

Wellness can be considered a feeling of wholeness and uniqueness and depends on various factors, including cultural and experiential variables. The nurse and patient may be aiming to achieve wellness for the patient, but may have different ideas as to what wellness is.

References

Airaksinen KE (2001). Silent coronary artery disease in diabetes – a feature of autonomic neuropathy or accelerated atherosclerosis? *Diabetologia*, 44: 259–266.

Alonso AA (1986). The impact of the family and lay others on care seeking during life threatening episodes of suspected coronary artery disease. *Social Science and Medicine*, 22: 1297–1311.

Amoroso P, Greenwood RN (1989). Posture and central venous pressure measurement in circulatory volume depletion. *Lancet*, 1: 258–260.

Baker NC, Cerone SB, Gaze N, Knapp TR (1984). The effect of type of thermometer and length of time inserted on oral temperature measurements of afebrile subjects. *Nursing Research*, 33: 109–111.

Bauman B (1961). Diversities in conceptions of health and physical fitness. *Journal of Health and Human Behaviour*, 2: 39–46.

Beck AT, Ward CH, Mendelson M, Mock J, Erbaugh J (1961). An inventory for measuring depression. *Archives of General Psychiatry*, 4: 561–571.

Benner P, Tanner C (1987). How expert nurses use intuition. *American Journal of Nursing*, 87: 33–31.

Benner P, Tanner C, Chelsa L (1992). From beginner to expert: gaining a differential clinical world in critical care nursing. *Advances in Nursing Science*, 14: 13–28.

Birkhead JS (1992). Time delays in the provision of thrombolytic treatment in six district hospitals. *British Medical Journal*, 305: 445–448.

Bondestam E, Hourgren K, Gaston-Johansson F et al (1987). Pain assessment by patients and nurses in the early phase of acute myocardial infarction. *Journal of Advanced Nursing*, 12: 677–682.

Bourbonnais F (1981). Pain assessment: development of a tool for the nurse and the patient. *Journal of Advanced Nursing*, 6: 277–282.

Brown SJ (1995). An interview style for nursing assessment *Journal of Advanced Nursing*, 21: 340–343.

Burke K (1996). The tympanic membrane thermometer in paediatrics: a review of the literature. *Accident and Emergency Nursing*, 4: 190–193.

Cambell NR et al (1990). Accurate, reproducible measurement of blood pressure. *Canadian Medical Association Journal*, 143: 19–24.

Campbell S (1988). Silent myocardial ischaemia. *British Medical Journal*, 297: 751–752.

Carney SL, Gillies AH, Smith AJ et al (1995). Hospital sphygmomanometer use: an audit. *Journal of Quality in Clinical Practice*, 15: 17–22.

Caturvedi N, Rai H, Ben-Shlomo Y (1997). Lay diagnosis and health-care seeking behavior for chest pain in south Asians and Europeans. *Lancet*, 350: 1578–1583.

Cioffi J (2000). Nurse's experiences of making decisions to call emergency assistance to their patients. *Journal of Advanced Nursing*, 32: 108–114.

Clark LT, Bellam SV, Shah AH et al (1992). Analysis of pre-hospital delay among inner city patients with symptoms of myocardial infarction: implications for therapeutic intervention. *Journal of the National Medical Association*, 84: 931–937.

Closs SJ, Cheater F (1999). Evidence for nursing practice: a clarification of the issues. *Journal of Advanced Nursing*, 30: 10–17.

Crawford SL, McGraw SA, Smith KW et al (1994). Do blacks and whites differ in their use of health care for symptoms of coronary heart disease? *American Journal of Public Health*, 84: 957–964.

Crow R, Chase J, Lamond D (1995). The cognitive component of nursing assessment: an analysis. *Journal of Advanced Nursing*, 22: 206–212.

Davies SP, Kassab JY, Thrush AB, Smith PHS (1986). A comparison of mercury and digital clinical thermometers. *Journal of Advanced Nursing*, 11: 535–543.

Department of Health (1999). *Making a Difference: Strengthening the Nursing, Midwifery and Health Visiting Contribution to Health and Health Care*. Department of Health, London.

Department of Health (2000). *Towards a strategy for Nursing Research and Development. Proposals for Action.* Department of Health, London.

Department of Health (2001). *Your Guide to the NHS.* Department of Health, London.

Devon HA, Zerwic JJ (2002). Symptoms of acute coronary syndromes: are there gender differences? A review of the literature. *Heart and Lung*, 31: 235–245.

Dracup K, Moser DK, Eisenberg M et al (1995). Causes of delay in seeking treatment for heart attack symptoms. *Social Science and Medicine*, 40: 379–392.

Draper P, McSherry W (2002). A critical view of spirituality and spiritual assessment. *Journal of Advanced Nursing*, 39: 1–2.

Dressler DK, Smejkal C, Ruffalo ML (1983). A comparison of oral and rectal temperatures on patients receiving oxygen by mask. *Nursing Research*, 32: 373–375.

Durham ML, Swanson B, Paulford N (1986). Effect of tachypnoea on oral temperature estimation: a replication. *Nursing Research*, 35: 211–214.

Eraut M, Alderton J, Boylan A et al (1995). *Learning to Use Scientific Knowledge in Education and Practice Settings: An Evaluation of the Contribution of the Biological, Behavioral and Social Sciences to Pre-registration Nursing and Midwifery Programmes*. Research Report series no 3. English National Board for Nursing, Midwifery and Health Visiting. London.

Erickson R (1980). Oral temperature differences in relation to thermometer and technique. *Nursing Research*, 29: 157–164.

Field MJ, Lohr KN (1990). *Clinical Practice Guidelines: Directions for a New Program*. National Academy Press, Washington.

Fredriksson L (1999). Modes of relating in a caring conversation: research synthesis on presence, touching and listening. *Journal of Advanced Nursing*, 30: 1167–1176.

Gassner L-A, Dunn S, Piller N (2002). Patients' interpretation of the symptoms of myocardial infarction: implications for cardiac rehabilitation. *Intensive and Critical Care Nursing*, 18: 342–354.

Ghali JK, Cooper RS, Kowalty I et al (1993). Delay between onset of chest pain and arrival to the coronary care unit among minority and disadvantaged patients. *Journal of the National Medical Association*, 85: 180–184.

Gray JAM (1997). *Evidence-based Healthcare: How to Make Health Policy and Management Decisions*. Churchill Livingstone. Edinburgh.

Gurwitz JH, McLaughlin TJ, Willison DJ et al (1997). Delayed hospital presentation in patients who have had an acute myocardial infarction. *Annals of Internal Medicine*, 126: 593–599.

Hams S (1998). Intuition and the coronary care nurse. *Nursing in Critical Care*, 3: 130–133.

Helman CG (2000). *Culture, Health and Illness*, 4th edn.

Henderson V (1960). *Basic Principles of Nursing*. International Council of Nurses, Geneva.

Holt P (1995). The role of questioning in patient assessment skills. *British Journal of Nursing*, 4: 1145–1148.

International Council of Nurses (1973). *Code for Nurses: Ethical Concepts Applied to Nursing*. ICN, Geneva.

International Council of Nurses (2000). *Code of Ethics*. ICN, Geneva.

Junnola T, Eriksson E, Salantera S (2002). Nurses' decision making in collecting information for the assessment of patients nursing problems. *Journal of Clinical Nursing*, 11: 186–296.

Kleinman A, Eisenberg L, Good B (1978). Culture, illness and care. *Annals of Internal Medicine*, 88: 251–258.

Lane D, Carroll D, Ring C et al (2002). The prevalence and persistence of depression and anxiety following myocardial infarction. *British Journal of Health Psychology*, 7: 11–21.

Markandu ND, Whitcher F, Arnold A, et al (2000). The mercury sphygmomanometer should be abandoned before it is proscribed. *Journal of Hypertension*, 14: 31–36.

Maslow AH (1970). *Motivation and Personality*, Harper and Row, New York.

Mason D (1981). An investigation of the influences of selected factors on nurses inferences of patient suffering. *International Journal of Nursing Studies*, 251–259.

Maynard C, Althouse R, Olsufka M et al (1989). Early versus late hospital arrival for acute myocardial infarction in the Western Washington thrombolytic therapy trials. *American Journal of Cardiology*, 63: 1296–1300.

Mayou R, Gill D, Thompson DR et al (2000). Depression and anxiety as predictors of outcome after myocardial infarction. *Psychosomatic Medicine*, 62: 212–219.

McCaffery M (1990). Nursing approaches to non-pharmacological pain control. *International Journal of Nursing Studies*, 27: 1–5.

McCaughan D, Thompson C, Cullum N et al (2002). Acute care nurses' perception of barriers to using research information in clinical decision making. *Journal of Advanced Nursing*, 39: 46–60.

McSherry W, Ross L (2001). Dilemas of spiritual assessment: considerations for nursing practice. *Journal of Advanced Nursing*, 38: 479–488.

Meischke H, Eisenberg MS, Larsen MP et al (1993). Pre-hospital delay interval for patients who use emergency medical services: the effect of heart related medical conditions and demographic variables. *Annals of Emergency Medicine*, 22: 1579–1601.

Melzack R, Wall PD (1965). Pain mechanisms: a new theory. *Science*, 150: 971–979.

Melzack R, Torgerson WS (1971). On the language of chest pain. *Anaesthesiology*, 34: 50.

Melzack R (1975). The McGill Pain Questionnaire: major properties and scoring methods. *Pain*, 1: 277–299.

Metral CT (2000). Nursing – then and now. *Journal of Emergency Nursing*, 26: 575–576.

Meurier CE (1998). The quality of assessment of patients with chest pain: the development of a questionnaire to audit the nursing assessment records of patients with chest pain. *Journal of Advanced Nursing*, 27: 140–146.

Meurier CE, Vincent CA, Palmer DG et al (1998). Perception of the causes of omissions in the assessment of chest pain. *Journal of Advanced Nursing*, 38: 1012–1019.

Miller CL (2002). A review of coronary artery disease in women. *Journal of Advanced Nursing*, 39: 17–23.

Morrow DA, Antman EM, Giugliano RP et al (2001). A simple risk index for rapid initial triage of patients with ST-elevation myocardial infarction: an InTIME II substudy. *Lancet*, 358: 1571–1575.

National Institute for Clinical Excellence (2002). *Guidance on the Use of Ultrasound Locating Devices for Placing Central Venous Catheters*. Technology Appraisal Guidance No 49. NICE, London.

O'Connor L (1995). Pain assessment by patients and nurses, and nurses notes on it, in early acute myocardial infarction. Part 1. *Intensive and Critical Care Nursing*, 11: 183–191.

Panju AA, Hemmelgarn BR, Guyatt GH et al (1998). The rational clinical examination. Is this patient having a myocardial infarction? *Journal of the American Medical Association*, 280: 1256–1263.

Patel V, Champ C, Andrews PS et al (1992). Diagonal earlobe creases and atheromatous disease: a postmortem study. *Journal of the Royal College of Physicians of London*, 26: 274–277.

Pattenden J, Watt I, Lewin R et al (2002). Decision making processes in people with symptoms of acute myocardial infaction: qualitative study. *British Medical Journal*, 324: 1006–1012.

Quinn T, Allan TF, Thompson DR et al (1999). Identification of patients suitable for direct admission to a coronary care unit by ambulance paramedics. *Pre-hospital Immediate Care*, 3: 126–130.

Rawles J, Metcalfe MH, Shirreffs C et al (1990). Association of patient delay with symptoms, cardiac enzymes, and outcome in acute myocardial infarction. *European Heart Journal*, 11: 643–648.

Rebenson-Piano M, Hoim K, Foreman MD, Kirchoff KT (1989). An evaluation of the indirect methods of blood pressure measurement in ill patients. *Nursing Research*, 38: 42–45.

Reeves J, Boothroyd V, Feather CL (1998). *Audit to Establish the Knowledge Base of Health Professionals Working in Primary and Secondary Care in the Procedure of Blood Pressure Measurement*. Bradford Health Authority, Bradford.

Reischman R, Yarandi H (2002). Critical care cardiovascular nurse expert and novice diagnostic cue utilization. *Journal of Advanced Nursing*, 39: 24–34.

Roper N, Logan WW, Tierney AJ (1980). *The Elements of Nursing*. Churchill Livingstone, Edinburgh.

Ruston A, Clayton J, Calnan M (1998). Patients' action during their cardiac event. Qualitative study exploring differences and modifiable factors. *British Medical Journal*, 316: 1060–1065.

Sackett DL, Haynes RB, Guyatt GH et al (1996). *Clinical Epidemiology – A Basic Science for Clinical Medicine*. Little Brown, London.

Schmidt SB, Borsch MA (1990). The pre-hospital phase of acute myocardial infarction in the era of thrombolysis. *American Journal of Cardiology*, 65: 1411–1415.

Scott J, Huskisson EC (1976) Graphic representation of pain. *Pain*, 2: 175–184.

Shuldham CM, Cunningham G, Hiscock M (1995). Assessment of anxiety in hospital patients. *Journal of Advanced Nursing*, 22: 87–93.

Standing J (1997). Chest pain assessment tools. *Journal of Clinical Nursing*, 6: 85–92.

Sternbach RA (1968). *Pain: A Psychophysical Analysis*. Academic Press, New York.

Takacs KM, Valenti WM (1982). Temperature measurement in a clinical setting. *Nursing Research*, 31: 368–370.

Tandberg D, Sklar D (1983). Effect of tachypnoea on the estimation of body temperature by an oral thermometer. *New England Journal of Medicine*, 308: 945–946.

Then KL, Rankin JA, Fofonoff DA (2001). Atypical presentation of acute myocardial infarction in 3 age groups. *Heart and Lung*, 30: 285–293.

Thomas LH, McColl E, Cullum N et al (1999). Clinical guidelines in nursing, midwifery and the therapies: a systematic review. *Journal of Advanced Nursing*, 30: 40–50.

Thompson DR (1982). *Cardiac Nursing*. Nurses' Aides Series. Ballière Tindall, London.

Thompson DR, Lewin RJP (2000). Management of the post-myocardial infarction patient: rehabilitation and cardiac neurosis. *Heart*, 84: 101–105.

Thompson DR, Webster RA, Sutton TW (1994). Coronary care unit patients' and nurses' ratings of intensity of ischaemic chest pain. *Intensive and Critical Care Nursing*, 10: 83–88.

Thompson DR, Quinn T, Stewart S (2002). Effective nurse-led interventions in heart disease. *International Journal of Cardiology*, 83: 233–237.

Torrance C, Serginson E (1996). Student nurses' knowledge in relation to blood pressure measurement by sphygmomanometry and auscultation. *Nurse Education Today*, 16: 397–402.

Treasure T (1998). Pain is not the only feature of a heart attack (letter). *British Medical Journal*, 317: 602.

Trent RJ, Rose EL, Adams JN et al (1995). Delay between the onset of symptoms of acute myocardial infarction and seeking assistance is influenced by left ventricular function at presentation. *British Heart Journal*, 73: 125–128.

Tresh DD (1998). Management of the older patient with acute myocardial infarction: difference in clinical presentations between older and younger patients. *Journal of the American Geriatrics Society*, 46: 1157–1162.

UKCC (2000). *Requirements for pre-registration nursing programmes*. UKCC London.

Webster J, Newnham D, Petrie JC, Lovell HG (1984). Influence of arm position on measurement of blood pressure. *British Medical Journal*, 288: 1574–1575.

Webster RA, Thompson DR, Mayou R (2001). The experiences and needs of Gujarati Hindi patients and partners in the first month after a myocardial infarction. *European Journal of Cardiovascular Nursing*, 1: 69–76.

White JE, Nativio DG, Kobert SN et al (1992). Content and process in clinical decision making by nurse practitioners. *Journal of Nursing Scholarship*, 23: 153–158.

White N, Baird S, Anderson DL (1994). A comparison of tympanic thermometer readings to pulmonary artery catheter core temperature readings. *Applied Nursing Research*, 7: 165–169.

Williams B, Poulter NR, Brown MJ et al (2004). British Hypertension Society guidelines for hypertension management 2004 (BHS-IV): Summary. *British Medical Journal*, 328: 634–640.

Yarebski J, Goldberg RJ, Gore JM et al (1994). Temporal trends and factors associated with extent of delay to hospital arrival in patients with acute myocardial infarction: the Worcester Heart Attack Study. *American Heart Journal*, 128: 255–263.

Zigmond AS, Snaith RP (1983). The hospital anxiety and depression scale. *Acta Psychiatrica Scandinavica*, 67: 361–370.

Zung WW (1965). A self-rating depression scale. *Archives of General Psychiatry*, 12: 63–70.

Chapter **5**

Diagnostic procedures

Certain diagnostic tests may be useful in collecting objective data regarding the clinical state of the acute coronary patient. Indeed, electrocardiography and cardiac marker studies are routinely performed to confirm the diagnosis of myocardial infarction and to determine the evolution and extent of myocardial damage as part of a formal risk stratification strategy. Plain chest radiography and full blood count, glucose, urea and electrolytes are also routinely performed. Other common diagnostic investigations include echocardiography, cardiac catheterization, coronary angiography and nuclear imaging studies. Whatever the complexity of the test it is fundamental that it involves suitably qualified personnel both to perform the test and interpret and report on the results obtained (Halstead et al 2002).

The results of diagnostic tests are correlated with data obtained from the patient interview and the physical examination. From this complete data base, decisions can then be made regarding the nature of the patient's problem and the plan of management. It is important to remember that test results are not a guarantee of a diagnosis and that it is possible to get both false-positive and false-negative results. The accuracy of a test will depend on its *sensitivity* and *specificity* and test results can often only demonstrate the *probability* of disease. For a more detailed explanation of these terms, the reader is referred to Halstead et al (2002).

Identification of a potential cardiac problem needs to incorporate accepted parameters of normality and include consideration of the following (Halstead et al 2002):

- Can a positive assumption of a real problem be made?
- What are the differential diagnoses under consideration?
- What is likely to be the underlying pathology and probable causes and risk factors?
- What is the likely degree of severity of the condition?
- What courses of action need to be taken to treat the problem?

CARE OF THE PATIENT UNDERGOING DIAGNOSTIC TESTS

The acute coronary patient is likely to undergo a variety of medical investigations as an aid to diagnosis and to monitor the progress of therapy and recovery. These investigations may range from simple non-invasive procedures, such as serial blood pressure recording, to complex invasive procedures such as cardiac catheterization and angiography.

For the vast majority of coronary patients the hospital admission is sudden, unexpected and unplanned. For many it will be their first experience of being a patient. The hospital setting often depersonalizes patients and their families as well as staff, and technical and organizational decisions affect the delivery of nursing care. These factors do little to help the patient undergoing an investigation, who often feels helpless, anxious and at times very frightened (Thompson and Bowman 1985).

Diagnostic tests and medical investigations are increasingly more complex, rigorous and precise. Unfortunately, they are often very routinized, with little consideration being given to accommodate individual patient's needs. In order to remedy this neglected area the nurse needs to be familiar with certain fundamental issues, for instance, legal, moral and ethical implications.

The nurse's prime responsibility is to protect and enhance the well-being and dignity of each individual in their care, although they also have a responsibility to the profession, to colleagues and themselves.

Patients' rights

The code of ethics of the International Council of Nurses (1973) emphasized certain fundamental rights and freedoms of individuals: respect for dignity of the individual; and respect for the patient's right to privacy, competent care, and protection from unethical and incompetent practice. These principles still hold true today and may in fact have more relevance as treatment options become more complex and patients are potentially sicker.

The basic rights of the patient are:

- the right to know
- the right to privacy
- the right to treatment.

The Nursing and Midwifery Code of Professional Conduct (2002) reinforces these principles, highlighting that patients are entitled to receive safe and competent care; their individual preferences, interests and dignity needs to be respected and that they need to be helped to access information and support relevant to their needs.

Every patient therefore has a right to be adequately informed about the medical investigation or diagnostic test to be performed, as well as the rights to privacy and treatment. Each patient may choose to exercise their rights differently. Patients are now beginning to have a clearer concept of their rights and should not have to expect platitudes and lack of information. There is a danger that in an environment such as a coronary care unit, where there is an emphasis on practical skills and technology, that consideration of the patient's needs for psychological support and information may assume second place.

Planning investigations

Rapid scientific and technological advances have made the diagnosis of heart disease much more refined. As a consequence, the nurse's role in the preparation of patients for diagnostic tests has become more subtle than giving simple explanations. Nurses are expected to help the patient understand what the investigation means and how useful information will be obtained, as well as giving a full explanation of the risks and potential benefits of the procedure.

Ideally, investigations should be planned well in advance, with both the patient and nurse being fully aware of what is intended. Unfortunately, in coronary care, circumstances will often dictate that little warning is given, and this may provoke anxiety and stress. Hopefully, primary-style nursing as a method of organizing work will help minimize the perception of care being a series of tasks and will allow the opportunity for effective nurse–patient interaction. Although there is obviously little time for preparing the patient for the routine tests and procedures performed on admission, such as an ECG and venepuncture, the nurse needs to ensure close and continuous care. The patient may be in pain or distress or drowsy from the effect of narcotic analgesics and therefore not in the best condition to absorb information and understand what is happening. A careful, but brief, initial assessment of the patient's physical and psychological state will give an indication of the amount and type of information likely to be required immediately and that which can be postponed. Investigations carried out later in the patient's stay, such as cardiac catheterization or stress testing, allow ample time for a structured approach to preparation.

Interviews with patients who have previously undergone the procedure will provide subjective descriptions of physical sensations experienced. This information can be used in giving information to other patients preparing for the same procedure (Clark and Gregor 1988). The patient may benefit from talking with a patient who has undergone the procedure and from being shown the place where the test is to be performed. In some instances it may be beneficial for the patient to see and touch the materials and instruments to be used in the procedure.

Routine daily investigations need to be coordinated so that the patient has ample opportunity to rest. Attention needs to be focused on individual needs and any decisions made should follow considerate discussions with the patient.

The need for information

Providing information to assist the patient's understanding of the procedure is a fundamental nursing function. Unfortunately, the quality, quantity and manner in which information is given to the patient and relatives is often unsatisfactory. It is unfortunate that patients are still given information in a haphazard, unstructured and inflexible fashion. Yet, because the patient does not have accurate knowledge about their illness, and is having to adjust both socially and emotionally to a novel and difficult situation, they need accurate, relevant and comprehensible information.

Information is valuable because it reduces stress, thus giving the patient the ability and means to control their environment and enabling cooperation and participation in their care (Wilson-Barnett 1979). Nursing intervention should be designed to give the patient relevant information which can be comprehended and retained.

Wilson-Barnett and Fordham (1982) note that, in medical wards at least, the patient's need for information is most acute prior to investigations. They also cite evidence showing that undergoing diagnostic tests is the most stressful event during a patient's stay in hospital, yet few receive information about what will happen.

Giving information

Wilson-Barnett (1987) provides a useful set of headings under which the nurse can consider the preparation of patients undergoing a diagnostic test:

1 purpose
2 how and where it is done
3 preparation for the procedure
4 delay or variation in the procedure
5 sensations involved
6 length of the procedure
7 who will be there
8 after-effects.

The patient may worry that the investigation will indicate a poor prognosis, or that the procedure is dangerous and have unpleasant after effects. Janis (1965) states that the ability to cope with impending stressful situations requires:

1 preparatory communications regarding the sensations to be experienced and the probable change
2 reassuring statements indicating how the changes will be kept under control or mitigated

3 recommendations of what can be done to protect the individual or reduce the damaging impact of the potential change
4 the benefit or expectation that these recommendations will be effective in reducing the threat.

Nurses, by nature of their work, are ideally placed to communicate basic information to patients. However, most appear to have had little specific guidance on the amount, content, and methods of communication (Ashworth 1980). Attention needs to be focused on individual needs and there is something to be gained by asking the patient what they think is likely to happen and correcting any misconceptions. The patient may wish to ask questions and the nurse should be ready to answer them. Information needs to be simple and often a 'less is more' approach is effective (Stanley et al 1998).

The use of a detailed nursing history and establishing the patient's past experience, knowledge and anxiety levels will help in identifying individual needs.

Giving information may help some patients work out a coping mechanism in advance through 'rehearsing in their mind' the event that is about to take place. Many patients are dissatisfied with the information given as to why investigations are carried out, how to prepare for them and how the actual investigation will be performed (Engstrom 1984). Yet studies such as those of Johnson (1973) and Finesilver (1979) demonstrated that patients need to know what they will experience, for how long, and in whose company. Hartfield et al (1982) have also demonstrated that patients receiving information about the sensations to be experienced reported significantly less anxiety, and expectations more congruent with their actual experiences, than did subjects receiving information concerned only with the actual procedure.

In recent years there has been an increase in the production of health related written information although the evidence for its effectiveness is limited (Arthur 1995). The use of written material has increased partly as a result of increased patient turnover and shorter hospital stays, thus leaving less time for face-to-face patient education (Walsh and Shaw 2000). Written material can be a valuable tool for reinforcing the verbal messages, but it is only useful if the patient can understand it (Mumford 1997). Some individuals, including some from ethnic minorities (Hussein and Partridge 2002), may have difficulty understanding written material that is not targeted to their specific needs. Pictorial representation of the information may help some patients (Lloyd et al 1997).

Patients are also increasingly using the internet to source information, although the quality of what they find there may be variable and hunting this down is time consuming (Gilliam et al 2003).

Patient anxiety

Patients who are anxious retain less information (Ley 1988) and so increased attention needs to be focused on what information to give and how to present it. For example, it has been shown that people recall best the information they are given first and which they consider to be most important (Ley 1972). Initial information needs to be simple and direct, proceeding to a more detailed discussion according to the patient's needs and level of comprehension. The patient needs to know from the outset the reason why the test is being performed, what it entails, how long it will last, whether it will be painful, the personnel involved, what the benefits and the risks may be, and if there are any alternatives. It is vital that both nursing and medical staff are in agreement as to what is to happen to the patient and why, and that coherent and consistent information is given. It does not matter how often the information is reiterated to the patient as, under stress, there is a tendency to forget it.

The nurse has a role in identifying the patient's individual learning needs and formulating plans to give information that is applicable and relevant. The nature of the information, the way it is presented, the timing, frequency, method of repetition and reinforcement need to be appropriate for that patient.

People have different ways of coping with perceived stressful events, and this will be influenced by culture, past experience and personality. Byrne (1964) identified two coping styles: 'repressors' and 'sensitizers'. The former use defence mechanisms of avoidance and denial to deal with the hypothetical threat, whereas the latter approach threatening stimuli by the use of intellectualization and obsessive behaviour to neutralize threats.

Reassurance

Preparing the patient for an investigation necessitates a sensitive and structured approach. French (1979) noted that the phrase 'reassure the patient' frequently occurs in care plans, and he made the plea to avoid using the term 'reassure' because of its ambiguity. In the care plan the nurse should describe exactly the type of behaviour indicated, based on the assessment of the patient's needs, such as information (verbal and non-verbal), familiarization, touch, clarification of facts, and encouraging the patient to talk about their fears.

The main purpose of reassuring the patient is to give them confidence that those caring for them at a vulnerable time are dependable and supportive. Being dependent on other people renders the patient more vulnerable and less able to make rational judgements.

Consent

Over the past 20 years the culture of the NHS has shifted from one of medical paternalism and 'doctor knows best' towards a culture of 'partnership in care'. Obtaining appropriately informed and well-documented consent helps the process of developing trust between the patient and the professional carrying out the procedure. To succeed in law, claimants may not have to do more than demonstrate that on the balance of probability, they have not been adequately counselled, and that had they been so counselled, they would not have undergone the intervention in question (Beresford 2001). It is part of the Nursing and Midwifery Code of Professional Conduct (NMC 2002) that the nurse needs to obtain consent before giving any treatment or care. This code goes into further detail about the nature of the consent process stating that it is important to be sensitive to individual needs and respect the wishes of those who refuse care or who are unable to receive information about their condition. Patients have a right to decide whether or not to undergo any health care intervention, even where refusal may result in harm or death to themselves, unless a court rules to the contrary. It is important to assume that every patient is legally competent unless otherwise assessed by a suitably qualified practitioner. Those who are competent may give

consent in writing, orally or by cooperation. They may also refuse consent. All discussions associated with obtaining consent need to be documented in the patients' notes. Previous decisions that are applicable to the current situation need to be respected when patients are no longer legally competent. In emergencies, where treatment is necessary to preserve life the Code of Conduct states that it is acceptable to give care without the patient's consent, if they are unable to give it, providing it can be demonstrated that action is in the patient's best interests. It is best if the person obtaining consent is the person who will give the care or treatment to the patient. However, this is not always practical and it is acceptable for another individual capable of carrying out the care to obtain consent on behalf of a colleague and, of particular relevance to nurses, for an individual who has been specially trained to obtain consent for particular procedures they are unable to undertake themselves (DoH 2001b).

Care for cardiac patients can be complex and it may be particularly difficult for patients to assimilate information (Beresford 2001). Information needs to include how the intervention is carried out and what is expected of the patient, and the benefits, risks, side effects and details of any alternative treatment. Patients also need to be aware of the likely consequences if they do not have the intervention. The legal standard of informing the patient is defined with respect to the Bolam test, namely, information of the amount and quality that a reasonable body of medical opinion would consider appropriate.

Information needs to be given to the patient as soon as possible before the intervention so that they have opportunity to formulate questions. There is evidence that information, particularly about the risks of a procedure, is best given in written format in order for patients best to be able to retain it (Seymour et al 2000). The terminology also needs to be such that the patient will understand the implications. Individuals in interventional research trials are particularly vulnerable and often appear to lack sufficient knowledge to make an autonomous choice (Argard et al 2001). Research has reportedly shown that individuals find it hard to comprehend magnitude of risk and that the definition of high and low risk may vary between patients (Kurbaan and Mills 2001). Some have advocated using easily understood contexts to describe the scale of risk, such as the National Lottery (Barclay et al 1997).

ELECTROCARDIOGRAPHY

Introduction

Electrocardiography is the graphic recording from the body surface of the potential of electrical currents generated by the heart, as a method of studying the action of heart muscle. This recording may be displayed on special graph paper or on an oscilloscope (monitor).

An electrocardiograph is a machine, basically a recording galvanometer, which detects major electrical events, i.e. atrial and ventricular activation. With the modern electrocardiograph, the current that accompanies the action of the heart is amplified 3000 times or more. An electrocardiogram (ECG) is a graphic record of these changes plotted against time.

Waller (1887) recorded the first ECG in man and, although this technique was impracticable for clinical use, this observation led to the introduction by Einthoven of his string galvanometer as a clinical instrument (Cooper 1986, Krikler 1987).

Electrocardiography is an essential part of the examination of the cardiovascular system. It may be used for baseline or serial assessment. Like any other diagnostic test it should be considered in relation to all other relevant data, and not in isolation. The main value of the ECG is in the interpretation of cardiac arrhythmias, diagnosis of coronary heart disease and assessment of ventricular hypertrophy.

Cardiac electrophysiology and the conducting system of the heart have been described. Essentially, the heart is unique among the muscles of the body in that it possesses the property of automatic rhythmic contractions. The impulses that precede contraction arise in the conduction system of the heart. These impulses result in excitation of the muscle fibres throughout the myocardium. Impulse formation and conduction produce weak electrical currents that spread through the entire body. The electrodes of a galvanometer in an electrocardiograph are arranged so that when a wave of depolarization moves towards a recording electrode, an upright (positive) deflection is obtained; an electrode of the opposite side of the body shows a downward (negative) deflection.

The sequence of waves produced at each heart beat has arbitrarily been labelled P, Q, R, S, T and U. The P wave is associated with atrial activation, the Q, R and S waves with ventricular activation, and the T and U waves with ventricular recovery. Depolarization occurs before myocardial contraction, and repolarization follows myocardial contraction. Atrial activation begins normally at the sinus node and spreads through the thick muscle bundles of the atria, initiating atrial depolarization which is represented on the ECG as a P wave. The width of the P wave represents the time necessary for the atrial activation process. Following atrial depolarization, an absence of electrical activity is noted on the ECG for a brief period, representing passage of the impulse from the atria through the atrioventricular (AV) junction to the ventricular myocardium. This flat baseline, *isoelectric line*, further represents the early phase of repolarization. The passage of time is labelled as the P–R interval and is measured from the beginning of the P wave to the beginning of the QRS complex (Figure 5.1).

Ventricular depolarization is represented on the ECG by waveforms labelled QRS. The Q wave is always the first downward (negative) deflection,

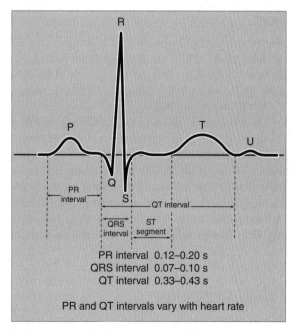

PR interval 0.12–0.20 s
QRS interval 0.07–0.10 s
QT interval 0.33–0.43 s

PR and QT intervals vary with heart rate

Figure 5.1   Deflections of a normal ECG showing nomenclature and time intervals.

and the R wave is always the first upward (positive) deflection. If a negative deflection follows an R wave, it is labelled an S wave. During this period of the QRS complex, atrial repolarization occurs.

Following ventricular activation, ventricular repolarization begins. The ST segment – a flat, isoelectric line between the S wave and the T wave – represents the early phase of ventricular muscle recovery. The T wave represents the actual recovery, or repolarization, of the ventricular muscle.

Occasionally, a U wave can be observed following the T wave. The origin of the U wave is not well understood, but it is considered significant in a state of hypokalaemia.

To be within normal limits the conduction impulse arising in the sinus node must pass from the atria through the AV junction to the ventricular myocardium within a given period of time. The P-R interval normally ranges from 0.12 to 0.20 s. Ventricular depolarization should normally occur within 0.12 s; thus the QRS interval (measured from the beginning of the Q wave to the point at which the S wave ends on reaching the baseline – ST segment), normally ranges from 0.08 to 0.11 s.

Lead systems

Leads

The standard ECG consists of tracings from 12 or more leads. They are three bipolar (standard) leads – I, II and III; three unipolar (limb) leads – aVR, aVL and aVF; six precordial (chest) leads – V_1, V_2, V_3, V_4, V_5 and V_6.

The term 'lead' refers to the ECG obtained as a result of recording the difference in electrical potential between a pair of electrodes. All the leads record the same electrical activity of the heart, but since they view it from different positions on the body surface the deflections are different in appearance in the various leads. The standard ECG therefore has 12 points of reference for recording electrical activity.

Bipolar (standard) leads

The galvanometer of the electrocardiograph carries two poles or terminals. Each of these poles is connected through a lead selector switch to electrodes placed on various parts of the body. The recorded deflections represent the difference in voltage applied across these poles. The bipolar (standard) leads represent differences between the limbs. Lead I equals the voltage of the left arm minus the voltage of the right arm, lead II equals the voltage of the left leg minus the voltage of the right arm, and lead III equals the voltage of the left leg minus the voltage of the left arm:

lead I: LA − RA;
lead II: LL − RA;
lead III: LL − LA.

The zero points are located midway between the extremities. The limbs behave simply as conductors away from the trunk. All electrodes placed at a distance greater than 15 cm from the heart are considered to be electrically equidistant.

The arms and left leg function as the three angles of an equilateral triangle in the frontal plane. If the sides of the triangle are displaced centrally but parallel to their normal positions, so that their zero points coincide, it will be seen (Figure 5.2) that:

- lead I occupies a horizontal position running between 0° on the left and 180° on the right intersection, with a circle inscribed around the original triangle
- lead II runs between +60° at its positive end and −120° on the negative
- lead III is positive at +120° and negative at −60°. The galvanometer is arranged to record an upstroke if the potential at the positive pole exceeds that of the negative pole.

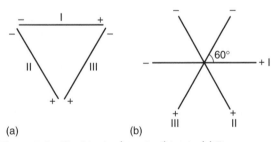

(a)   (b)

Figure 5.2 The bipolar (standard) leads. (a) The standard lead axes forming the Einthoven triangle. (b) The lead axis shifted to the centre of the triangle, forming a triaxial reference system.

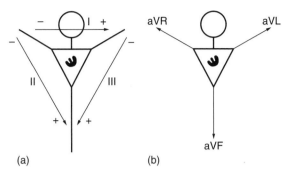

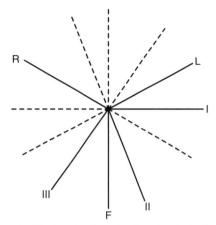

(a)   (b)

Figure 5.3   The (a) bipolar and (b) unipolar leads.

Figure 5.4   The bipolar (standard) and unipolar leads in relation to the hexaxial reference system.

Unipolar (limb) leads

In these leads the galvanometer is arranged to record the potential variations on each limb separately, instead of recording the algebraic sum of two as in the standard leads. One pole of the galvanometer is connected to a central terminal which is connected to all three limbs. The sum of the potential variations of these three leads is zero, so that the central terminal is zero. This corresponds to the centre of the chest and coincides with the conjunction of the zero points of the bipolar leads. The other pole of the galvanometer is connected in turn to each of the three limbs. The three unipolar limb leads are VR (right arm), VL (left arm) and VF (left leg or foot). An electrode is also placed on the right leg or foot, but this is not used for recording purposes and serves only to earth the patient. V stands for voltage. The voltages recorded are too low to be satisfactorily recorded and so are increased (augmented) to make them comparable with those from other leads: they are therefore designated aVR, aVL and aVF (Figure 5.3).

In effect, the three standard leads and the three limb leads arranged in the frontal plane with coinciding zero points constitute a hexaxial reference system (Figures 5.4 and 5.5), with each frontal plane lead being 30° apart.

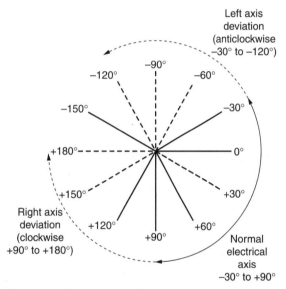

Figure 5.5   The hexaxial reference system.

Precordial (chest) leads

The six chest leads (V_1–V_6) are influenced by electrical activity throughout the whole heart, but especially by the area of the heart nearest to the recording electrode. Owing to the close proximity

of an electrode to the heart, the changes in electrical potential are greater than those recorded in the limb leads. The six chest leads are positioned as follows (Figure 5.6):

- V_1: fourth intercostal space immediately to the right of the sternum
- V_2: fourth intercostal space immediately to the left of the sternum
- V_3: midway between V_2 and V_4
- V_4: fifth intercostal space in the left mid-clavicular line

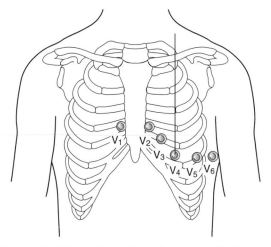

Figure 5.6 Electrode positions of the precordial leads (MCL, mid-clavicular line).

- V_5: directly lateral to V_4 in the left anterior axillary line
- V_6: directly lateral to V_4 and V_5 in the left mid-axillary line.

In women, the left-sided leads are placed under, not over, the left breast. The six chest leads provide detailed information about the heart. V_1 and V_2 face the free wall of the right ventricle. V_3 and V_4 are opposite the interventricular septum, and V_5 and V_6 face the free wall of the left ventricle. Many other additional recordings can be taken such as V_7 and V_8 (further lateral positions) or V_3R and V_4R (V_3 and V_4 positions on the right side of the chest).

Orientation of leads

The 12 leads of the standard ECG are orientated toward the various surfaces of the heart:

- leads I, aVL and V_5 and V_6 reflect electrical events occurring on the lateral surface of the left ventricle
- leads II, III and aVF reflect electrical events occurring on the inferior surface of the left ventricle
- leads V_1 to V_4 are orientated to the anteroseptal surface of the left ventricle
- leads V_1 and V_2 are orientated toward the right ventricle and reflect electrical changes

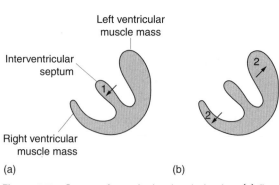

Figure 5.7 Stages of ventricular depolarization: (a) first stage; (b) second stage.

occurring in the anterior surface of the left ventricle
- leads V_5 and V_4 reflect electrical events occurring in the septal region of the left ventricle.

There are no leads that directly reflect the electrical activity on the posterior surface of the heart.

Activation of the ventricles

Depolarization of the ventricles begins in the left lower side on the interventricular septum and spreads through the septum from left to right (Figure 5.7). Depolarization then spreads outwards simultaneously through the free walls of the left and right ventricles, from endocardial to epicardial surfaces (Figure 5.7). As the free wall of the left ventricle has a much greater muscle mass than that of the right ventricle, the larger left ventricular forces counteract the smaller right ventricular forces, resulting in essentially a single force directed from right to left.

The left ventricle is the greatest mass of myocardium and dominates the ECG. If an electrode is placed over this area (e.g. V_6), the P wave will occur due to atrial activity. Because the first part of the ventricle to be activated is the interventricular septum from the left bundle, a Q wave will follow due to the electrical force moving away from the electrode. When the mass of the ventricle is activated, the wave of excitation moves towards the electrode resulting in a positive deflection (R wave).

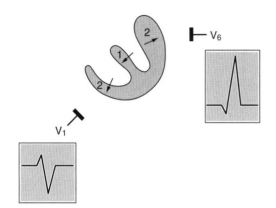

Figure 5.8 Representation of the basic form of ventricular depolarization and its effect on leads V_1 and V_6.

- Movement of an electric current predominately towards a lead produces a positive (upward) deflection.
- Movement of an electric current predominately away from a lead produces a negative (downward) deflection.

If an electrode is placed over the right side of the heart (e.g. V_1), then a small R wave ensues, due to the spread of excitation moving across the septum towards the electrode (the septum usually depolarizes first and from left to right). A negative deflection (S wave) occurs as the main muscle mass is then depolarized, the bigger left ventricle (where depolarization is spreading away from the electrode – hence the downward deflection) outweighing the effect of the right ventricle (where depolarization is spreading towards the electrode). As the left ventricle dominates the right ventricle it will affect the ECG; therefore in V_1 the main QRS deflection is negative, whereas that in V_6 is positive (Figure 5.8).

Cardiac vectors

A vector is a term used in physics to express the magnitude and direction of an electrical force in the three planes of space. The heart can be thought of as a source of electromotive force in the centre of an equilateral triangle. The portion of the electrical vector recorded in an individual lead depends on the angle between the vector and the direction of the lead: if the vector is parallel to the lead, it will be fully recorded in that lead; if the vector is perpendicular to the direction of the lead, no potential difference will be recorded in that lead; if the vector is intermediate to those just stated, a corresponding vector will be recorded in that lead.

The total electrical activity at any one time can be summated and represented as the *instantaneous vector*. All the instantaneous vectors occurring throughout the cardiac cycle form the *cardiac vector*.

The mean frontal plane QRS axis

The cardiac vector is described as the mean QRS vector or axis. It is customary to measure the mean QRS axis in the frontal plane. To describe the axis more precisely, the hexaxial reference system is used (see Figure 5.5).

If leads I, II, III, aVR, aVL and aVF are produced through their centres, there are then 12 leads each at 30° to the adjacent lead. A quick and accurate method of determining the mean QRS axis is to inspect the six frontal plane limb leads to find the one in which the algebraic sum of all deflections within the QRS complex is most nearly equal to zero (i.e. all negative deflections are subtracted and all positive deflections are added). It is convenient to use the small squares on the ECG paper for doing this. The smallest mean QRS deflection will always be in a lead at right angles to the axis. Thus, if the lead showing the smallest net QRS size is lead II, then the lead at right angles is lead aVL. The axis must then be directly along the lead (in this case aVL) or directly away from it, both of these positions being at right angles to the lead with the smallest net QRS size (in this case lead II). To determine which of these two possibilities is correct, the ECG is inspected (in lead aVL). The QRS must have a large dominant positive wave, or alternatively a large dominant negative wave. If the former, the axis of the heart is along the lead (aVL); if the latter, the axis is directed away from the lead.

The normal range for the mean frontal plane QRS axis in adults is from −30° to +90°. Leads I and II are normally both positive.

Right axis deviation is present when the axis ranges from +90° to +180° (lead I usually negative, lead II positive).

Left axis deviation ranges from −30° to −120° (lead I usually positive, lead II negative).

ECG paper and recording technique

In order to differentiate between normal and abnormal cardiac events, the nurse must be familiar with ECG recording paper and understand that horizontal movement across the paper denotes time. In order to standardize the recording of electrical events, a number of conventions are applied. The ECG recording paper moves under the recording pen at a uniform speed of 25 mm/s. The special standard ECG recording paper is divided by bold lines into 5 mm squares, subdivided by faint lines into 1 mm squares. As there will be 25 small squares moving under the pen each second, one large square (five small squares) is equal to 0.20 s (a fifth of a second) and one small square represents 0.04 s in time (Figure 5.9). The ECG is also standardized in terms of amplitude of electrical wave deflection. A vertical deflection of 1 cm (10 mm) is equal to 1 millivolt (mV). Thus, each 1 mm line represents 0.1 mV. The ECG is calibrated to 1 mV for standardization.

Voltage of upright deflections is measured from the upper border of the baseline (isoelectric line) to the peak of the wave. Downward deflections are measured from the lower border of the baseline to the lowest point (nadir) of the wave.

Correct recording technique is essential in order to obtain a good-quality ECG. Errors in lead placement or connection, paper speed selection, standardization and incorrect lead labelling are not uncommon.

Before recording proceeds, the patient needs to be informed of what is entailed in clear simple terms. It should be stressed that the electrocardiograph will not cause any harm and is merely a machine for recording small amounts of electrical activity in the heart. The patient should not be unduly anxious and should preferably be comfortable, warm and relaxed, because any fine muscle tremor due to discomfort, cold and anxiety may distort the ECG record. The nurse should also check for any electrical equipment nearby that may cause electrical interference.

The electrode leads (correctly labelled) are attached to the patient's limbs and chest after a special conducting gel has been applied to the skin surface (shaved if necessary, and clean and dry).

Calculating the heart rate

The heart rate may be calculated by using a specially designed ruler (usually available from pharmaceutical companies) or by using the ECG graph paper. Provided that the ventricular rate is regular and the ECG paper speed is 25 mm/s, one can divide the number of small (1 mm) squares on the paper between the R waves of the ECG into 1500. Alternatively, one can divide the number of large (5 mm) squares into 300. If the rhythm is irregular, however, one can count the number of R waves in 6 s and multiply by 10.

The ECG in acute myocardial infarction

The ECG is a major diagnostic tool in the evaluation of the coronary patient and indeed acute myocardial infarction is now categorized according to the presence or absence of ST segment elevation. Elevation of the ST segment helps identify a group of patients who clearly benefit from thrombolytic therapy.

It is reported that less than half the patients presenting to hospital with acute myocardial infarction will have the typical and diagnostic electrocardiographic changes present on their initial trace and as many as 20% of patients will have a normal or near normal electrocardiogram (Channer and Morris 2002). Therefore, serial recordings should be obtained, carefully studied and correlated with other clinical and diagnostic findings.

In acute myocardial infarction three pathophysiological events occur, either in sequence or simultaneously: ischaemia, injury and infarction. The electrocardiographic manifestations of these processes (Figure 5.10) involve changes in the

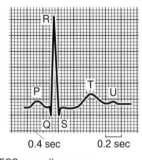

Figure 5.9 ECG recording paper.

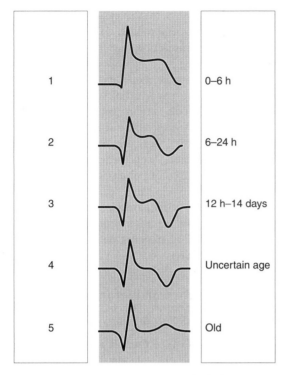

1   0–6 h

2   6–24 h

3   12 h–14 days

4   Uncertain age

5   Old

Figure 5.10   ECG changes of myocardial infarction.

T wave (ischaemia), ST segment (injury) and Q wave (infarction of the full thickness of the myocardium).

The infarction process progresses through three phases:

- the hyperacute phase
- the fully evolved phase
- the phase of resolution.

Hyperacute phase

This occurs within the first few hours of the onset of acute myocardial infarction. The transition from this to the fully evolved phase usually occurs within 24 h, and so it is frequently missed.

One of the first and most subtle changes in ischaemia is ST segment flattening, resulting in a more obvious angle between the ST segment and T wave. More obvious signs of ischaemia comprise ST segment depression that is usually down sloping or horizontal. Total occlusion of the artery supplying the myocardium under the recording lead, without any collateral circulation, usually results in ST segment elevation. There are also tall and widened T waves (at times exceeding the height of the R wave). The pathological Q wave does not occur until this large T wave has regressed. There is also increased ventricular activation time, i.e. the time from the beginning of the QRS complex to the apex of the R wave is increased.

Changes in the ST segment and T wave are not specific for ischaemia, they also occur in association with other disease processes including left ventricular hypertrophy, hypokalaemia and digoxin therapy.

Fully evolved phase

Myocardial necrosis is reflected by a broad, deep Q wave (pathological Q wave) in leads facing the necrotic area. Necrotic tissue is electrically inert – it cannot be depolarized or repolarized. If there is necrosis of the full thickness of a substantial amount of myocardium (transmural infarction), this can be described as a 'window' or 'hole' in the muscle wall. An electrode placed over this 'window' reflects activity of other muscle as 'seen' through this 'window'. If an electrode is placed over an area of dead muscle in the left ventricular wall, depolarization occurs as usual from the left side of the septum to the right. Thus, a small negative deflection will be inscribed on the ECG. Subsequently, depolarization spreads to affect the right ventricle, resulting in a further negative deflection on the ECG: the pathological Q wave of myocardial infarction. Pathological Q waves are wide (0.04 s or longer in duration), deep (usually greater than 4 mm in depth), usually associated with a substantial loss in the height of the ensuing R wave and usually present in several leads. It is, however, important to note that Q waves sometimes occur normally in leads III or aVF and are likely to diminish or disappear on deep inspiration. Q waves may also occur normally in aVR and with a vertical heart position or right axis deviation, as well as in leads I and aVL as a result of left axis deviation or a horizontal axis. Acute myocardial infarctions were commonly classed as Q wave or non-Q wave, but these terms have little utility in decision making as they describe the ECG after the infarct is complete (Smith et al 2002).

Myocardial injury is reflected by displacement of the ST segment. In most infarctions, myocardial injury is dominantly epicardial and this is present on the ECG with elevated ST segments in the leads facing this surface. The ST segment in the fully evolved phase of the infarction is coved (or convex upward).

Myocardial ischaemia is reflected by an inverted T wave. T-wave inversion occurs in those leads facing the ischaemic surface. The T waves are characteristically 'arrowhead' in appearance, being peaked and symmetrical. In patients with previous infarction producing a Q wave, the hallmark of new ischaemia is often ST segment elevation. This is thought to be associated with a wall motion abnormality or bulging of the infarcted segment. It rarely indicates reinfarction in the same territory (Channer and Morris 2002). If there is persistent T wave inversion with the changes of a previous myocardial infarction, ischaemia in the same area can produce 'normalization' of the T wave (return to an upright position).

The infarcted area consists of necrotic tissue surrounded by a zone of injured tissue which is in turn surrounded by a zone of ischaemic tissue. The typical infarct pattern consists of the pathological Q wave, the raised coved ST segment and the inverted pointed T wave (see Figure 5.10).

Phase of resolution

This phase follows on from the fully evolved phase. During the following weeks there is a gradual return of the elevated ST segment to the baseline. The inverted symmetrical T waves gradually return to a normal, or near normal, configuration, but they may persist for several months. The only evidence of a myocardial infarction may be a pathological Q wave.

Sustained ST segment elevation of 3 months or longer after acute myocardial infarction usually indicates a ventricular aneurysm.

When electrocardiographic abnormalities occur in association with chest pain but in the absence of definite infarction, they confer prognostic significance. About 20% of patients with ST segment depression and 15% with T wave inversion will experience severe angina or myocardial infarction within 12 months of their initial presentation, compared to 10% of patients with a normal trace (Channer and Morris 2002).

Location of myocardial infarction

Anterior myocardial infarction

The anterior surface of the left ventricle is orientated towards the chest leads. The anterolateral surface of the left ventricle is orientated towards lead aVL and the positive pole of lead I. Therefore, an anterior infarction will be reflected by the typical infarct pattern in leads I, aVL and V_1–V_6 (Figure 5.11). Anterior infarction can be subdivided into:

- *extensive anterior myocardial infarction:* infarct pattern in leads I, aVL and V_1–V_6
- *anteroseptal myocardial infarction:* infarct pattern in leads I, aVL and V_1–V_4
- *anterolateral myocardial infarction:* infarct pattern in leads I, aVL and V_4–V_6.

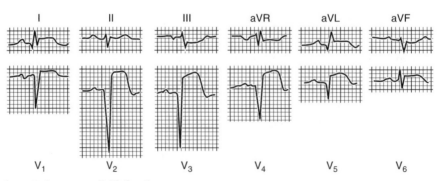

Figure 5.11   An anterior myocardial infarction.

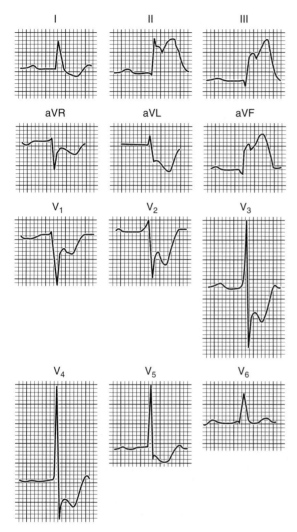

Inferior myocardial infarction

The inferior surface of the left ventricle is orientated towards leads II, III and aVF, and an inferior infarction will be reflected by the typical infarct pattern in these leads (Figure 5.12).

Posterior myocardial infarction

True posterior infarction is less common but may be missed or misdiagnosed. Although none of the 12 leads has a positive electrode close to the posterior myocardium, the process of infarction here can sometimes be seen in leads V_1 and V_2 (Figure 5.13). These leads show tall and slightly widened R waves, tall, wide and symmetrical T waves, and slightly depressed, concave-upward ST segments. The combination of these changes in the right chest leads is often described as a mirror image of the typical changes of infarction.

Subendocardial myocardial infarction

A subendocardial infarction may cause ST-segment depression and T-wave inversion. However, pathological Q waves are absent.

Further ECG leads may be required for infarctions in unusual sites. In high anterior and lateral infarctions, V_7 and V_8 and leads recorded in the second or third intercostal spaces may be useful.

The recognition of acute myocardial infarction on the ECG may prove difficult if there has been previous infarction which has resulted in persistent Q waves, ST-segment elevation or T-wave inversion. It is important to emphasize that ST-segment

Figure 5.12   An acute inferior myocardial infarction with anterior reciprocal changes.

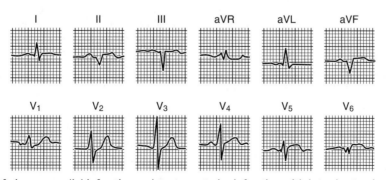

Figure 5.13   Old inferior myocardial infarction and acute posterior infarction with lateral extension.

and T-wave changes should never be interpreted as definitive signs of acute myocardial infarction, but should be placed in context with any other ECG changes and clinical findings including pattern of release of cardiac markers.

Most coronary patients demonstrate at least a modest change in the ECG, usually reflecting left ventricular events, although right ventricular infarction is strongly suggested by ST-segment elevation in leads V_4R or V_1-V_4.

EXERCISE TESTING

Exercise testing is often used to provide information about the likely prognosis of patients recovering from myocardial infarction. The test is based on the theory that patients with coronary heart disease will produce marked ST-segment depression on the ECG when exercising.

Indications

The main indications for exercise testing include:

1 Evaluation of chest pain.
2 Evaluation of arrhythmias.
3 Stratification of high-risk patients.
4 Assessment of cardiac reserve and functional capacity.

A low-level exercise test can be performed safely as early as 4 days after myocardial infarction. Such testing prior to the patient's discharge home is important for determining the immediate short-term prognosis. Low-level exercise testing takes a predicted level of 60–75% of the patient's maximal heart rate as being the end-point of the test. However, exercise tests are generally performed 4–6 weeks after the myocardial infarction when the patient can be safely exercised to the limit of his symptoms.

Patients who have persistent heart failure or angina that occurs at rest or minimal exertion should not be exercised. The presence of left bundle branch block, hypertension or valvular heart disease limits the interpretation of exercise-induced ST-segment changes on the ECG. The presence of atrial fibrillation or cardiomegaly are contraindications to exercise testing post-acute infarction. Relative contraindications include situations where

the risks of performing the procedure may exceed the benefits (White and Evans 2001).

Exercise testing is important in the diagnosis of chest pain and for indicating the extent of coronary heart disease in the patient with known myocardial ischaemia. However, false-negative tests may be obtained because ST-segment changes are not always present during exercise in patients with angiographically defined ischaemic heart disease. False-negative tests may also be found if the exercise test has been submaximal or the patient is taking beta-blockers which reduce cardiac workload. False-positive results may be obtained in up to a quarter of patients who have normal resting ECGs. Hyperventilation and increased sympathetic tone may be causative factors.

The three common methods of exercise testing include:

- climbing the stairs
- pedalling a stationary bicycle
- walking a treadmill.

The ideal components of an exercise protocol are shown in Table 5.1.

The ECG, heart rate and blood pressure are recorded while the patient engages in some form of exercise (stress). There are many different exercise protocols for different circumstances (American College of Cardiology/American Heart Association 1997). They are all similar in that the patient begins at a low level of exercise which gradually increases at 2–3-minute intervals. The aim of the testing is to

---

Table 5.1   Ideal components of an exercise protocol

1   An initial workload well within the patient's anticipated physical capacity
2   A gradually increasing workload maintained for a sufficient length of time to achieve a physiological steady state
3   An exercise level which does not cause excessive mental or physical stress
4   Continuous ECG monitoring with the facility to record rhythm and ECG changes during exercise, in conjunction with continuous evaluation of symptoms and signs
5   Medical supervision to ensure that the patient stops exercise when necessary, at the same time allowing for sufficient diagnostic information to be obtained

Table 5.2 Electrocardiographic changes during exercise

Normal exercise ECG
Shortened PR interval
Taller P wave
Downward displacement of the PR junction
Amplitude of QRS complex, R and T wave tend to decrease
Steady upsloping convex ST segment that returns to the baseline (PQ junction) within 0.04–0.06 s

Myocardial ischaemia and the ECG
ST-segment depression of 1.0 mm (0.1 mV) which is horizontal or downsloping for 0.08 s – normally develops during exercise and becomes more severe as the exercise progresses

increase the heart rate to just below maximal levels (i.e. about 160–200 beats/min in adults).

The principle is that coronary arteries that may be occluded will be unable to meet the heart's increased oxygen demand during exercise, resulting in chest pain, fatigue, dyspnoea, excessive tachycardia, a fall in blood pressure or arrhythmias. Symptomatic, haemodynamic and electocardiographic parameters can be assessed during the test. The rate of oxygen uptake (VO_2) from the body is also significant and is expressed in metabolic equivalents (METS). One MET is the oxygen uptake of the body at rest which is about 3.5 ml/kg/min. Cardiac patients will average about 21 ml/kg/min (6 METS). Those who can achieve 13 METs have an excellent prognosis regardless of other symptoms during the test.

On the ECG, ST-segment displacement may occur during or immediately after the test. The test is considered negative when there are no significant ECG abnormalities and the patient experiences no significant symptoms. The test is often considered positive when the depression of the ST segment exceeds 1 mm (0.1 mV) below the baseline for 0.08 s (Table 5.2), although this criterion can produce false-positive results in up to two-thirds of tests. A poorer prognosis than average is associated with:

- an ST-segment depression of 2 mm or more
- a limited duration of exercise tolerance for age and sex
- a failure of blood pressure to increase with exercise
- the presence of ventricular ectopic beats.

The benefits of exercise testing are:

1   It is non-invasive.
2   It is relatively quick and easy to perform.
3   It is relatively inexpensive.

Exercise testing performed early after infarction can reassure low-risk patients and their spouses about the capabilities of the patient to resume his customary activities. Taylor et al (1985) found that wives tended to judge their husbands' cardiac capabilities as being severely diminished and as being unable to withstand physical and emotional strain. They also found that when wives actually completed the exercise test alongside their husbands, their expectations of their husbands' ability was more realistic and their confidence increased.

The results of an exercise test are dependent on factors such as age, sex, and ethnic origin, current medication regimen, the fullness of the test applied and the criteria set for a positive result as well as the extent of the underlying cardiac condition.

Patient preparation

The exercise laboratory should be kept at a comfortable temperature and there should be ample space for staff, equipment and post-exercise treatment, i.e. drugs and resuscitation facilities.

The patient is asked to avoid a heavy meal and stimulants such as caffeine, alcohol and tobacco in the 4 hours prior to the test. Eating too close to the time of testing can cause the cardiac output to be distributed more towards the splanchnic bed, compromising the volume of blood available for the exercising muscles, and producing a less than optimal exercise response. Smoking prior to exercise testing also decreases the optimal exercise response because carbon monoxide has a higher affinity for haemoglobin than oxygen and thereby decreases the oxygen-carrying capacity of the blood.

The procedure should be explained in detail and, if the patient is unfamiliar with the exercise machine, a demonstration of its use will be of value. The term 'stress test' may be best avoided as it may sound ominous and increase patient anxiety.

The patient may fear that the test may induce pain or shortness of breath or exacerbate his condition and they should be reassured that the test will be stopped immediately at their request. The patient needs to be instructed to report dizziness, chest pain or breathlessness developing during the test, but that these symptoms are not necessarily an indication for immediate termination of the test.

The procedure takes about 30–45 min to perform. Men usually perform the test wearing only trousers and shoes, but women usually feel more comfortable wearing a loose-fitting gown. In women with large breasts, artefacts due to excessive movement of the chest ECG electrodes can be minimized by a suitable supporting garment.

Lead systems

The different recommended lead systems for detecting regional myocardial ischaemia use between 2 and 20 electrodes. The simplest and most useful lead for recording is MCL_5 (positive lead in the V_5 intercostal space, and the negative lead on the manubrium), which will demonstrate up to 90% of detectable abnormalities. However, the commonest lead system uses the normal 12-lead recording positions. The torso rather than the limbs are used for the limb leads to prevent entanglement and to reduce movement artefact. Precordial mapping techniques using more than 12 leads are really only research tools.

A standard resting ECG and blood pressure recording should be obtained before the test to provide baseline data. Any current medication the patient is receiving should be noted. During the test the patient should be encouraged to exercise for as long as possible, depending on the protocol used, but signs of fatigue, pain, syncope and breathlessness should be noted, especially in the stoical patient. The patient should be instructed to breathe normally and, if walking a treadmill, warned not to look down as this may produce dizziness. Automatic blood pressure and ECG recorders will usually obtain readings at predetermined time intervals, and the test is continued until completion or another end-point has been reached (Table 5.3).

Ideally, the test should be stopped gradually to prevent any sudden change in blood pressure resulting in dizziness. At the end of testing the

Table 5.3   End-points of an exercise test

Absolute	Relative
Patient's request	Chest pain without ECG changes
Fall in blood pressure or heart rate	Fatigue, anxiety, dizziness, cramp
Progressive angina	Attainment of predicted maximal heart rate
Ventricular tachycardia or fibrillation	Marked ST-segment depression (5 mm)
Severe dyspnoea or faintness	Increasing ectopic activity or heart block
Equipment failure	Marked elevation of blood pressure (unless patient is an athlete)

level of the test achieved (with timing) should be recorded with the reason for stopping. All symptoms and blood pressure readings should be recorded on the ECG. Patients are advised to lie down for 3–5 min. They are likely to be interested in the test results and these, together with any implications for the future, should be discussed with them. Close monitoring of patients with abnormal test results is necessary. Sudden death is a possible but rare complication up to 2 h after the test.

Although ECG changes are important, they need to be interpreted in the context of symptoms during the test and the recovery period. In general, early onset of angina symptoms, widespread marked ST depression, poor blood pressure response and slow recovery are indicative of severe coronary heart disease.

BLOOD TESTS

Biochemical cardiac markers

When myocytes are damaged, large intracellular proteins are able to leak out through the membrane walls and can be detected in the blood. There are a variety of serum cardiac markers that are used in the diagnosis of acute coronary syndromes. Using different combinations of tests at different times may help in diagnosis. Almost all cases of myocardial infarction can be detected within 90 min of presentation by measuring troponin I, CK-MB and myoglobin (Ng et al 2001).

Cardiac troponins

The cardiac troponins are proteins that are bound to the thin filaments of the contractile apparatus of the myocytes in muscle. There are three cardiac troponins (troponin T, I and C) and it is now becoming routine to measure levels of cardiac troponin T (cTnT) or cardiac troponin I (cTnI) in clinical practice. Both these cardiac troponins are released into the blood within 3 hours of myocardial injury, peaking at 12 hours and remaining elevated for up to 14 days. Troponins have a 100% sensitivity for diagnosing myocardial damage 12 hours after presentation to hospital.

The consensus document published by the European Society of Cardiology and the American College of Cardiology (Alpert and Thygesen 2000) considered the best biochemical marker for detecting myocardial necrosis to be a concentration of cardiac troponin exceeding the decision limit on at least one occasion during the first 24 hours after the onset of the clinical event. As with any new diagnostic test, issues around which troponin to use, the concentration level at which a test becomes positive, agreement on test protocols and cost take a while to resolve. Laboratory and/or manufacturers' literature should be consulted for guidance as reference ranges, and cut-off values differ between the assays currently being used in practice. Troponin levels greater than the 99th percentile for a given reference control are defined as being high.

The use of cardiac troponin is also facilitating risk stratification enabling high-risk patients to be identified and appropriately targeted for therapy. Troponins are particularly useful for late diagnosis (Fromm et al 2001) and are of prognostic value in acute coronary syndromes. Individuals with chest pain, abnormal ECG and a positive troponin test have a 30-day mortality of 11.9% compared with 3% in those with comparable presentation but with a negative troponin and troponin levels (Collinson 1998).

Myoglobin

Myoglobin is a small haem protein found in skeletal and cardiac muscle. Its small molecular weight allows it to escape easily from damaged tissue. It is the marker that most fits the role as an early marker (Pateghini et al 1999) and levels can be quickly measured at the bedside. It is detectable as early as 3–4 hours and peaks early at 6–12 hours, falling to normal level after 24 hours. It has particular value in the triage of patients presenting with chest pain as the negative predictive value of this marker for excluding early infarction 4 hours after admission is high. Two negative samples taken approximately 2 hours apart rule out the incidence of myocardial infarction in approximately 90% of cases. However, the fact that it is found in skeletal muscle means that it is not specific for cardiac damage. Normal myoglobin levels are reported as $<100\,\mu g/l$.

Creatinine kinase

Creatinine kinase (CK) is found in high concentrations in skeletal and cardiac muscle and also in the brain. It has been the gold standard for detecting myocardial infarction for many years, although levels are affected by events such as cardiac surgery and strenuous exercise and levels may remain normal in 10% of infarctions. CK levels rise and fall within 72 hours, reaching their peak at 24 hours. Normal values are 33–145 iu/l for adult females and 33–186 iu/l for adult males. The more specific CK-MB iso-enzyme may be measured. CK-MB has two isoforms: MB1 found in serum and MB2 from myocardial tissue. A ratio of MB2:MB1 of >1.5 is taken as diagnostic of myocardial damage. With conventional testing, this raised ratio becomes elevated before total CK-MB levels rise (Swanton 1998). The normal value for CK-MB is 1–12 iu/l. CK-MB is particulary useful for detecting reinfarction. (The prolonged elevation of the troponins limits their use in this context.) Measurement of CK-MB is also a better indicator of infarct size than measurement of troponin levels.

Lactase dehydrogenase (LDH)

Lactase dehydrogenase levels were used for detecting myocardial damage in patients who presented late. Levels begin to rise within 24–48 hours after infarction, peaking at about 4–5 days. It can also rise in renal disease, liver disease and in haemolysed blood samples. Normal values are 266–500 iu/l.

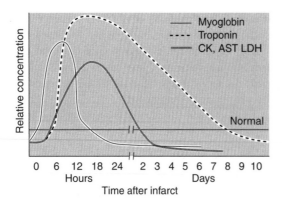

Figure 5.14 Time-activity curves for diagnostic enzymes following acute myocardial infarction.

Aspartate aminotransferase (AST)

Aspartate aminotransferase is also known as serum oxaloacetic transaminase (SGOT). Levels rise after 8–12 hours, peaking at 24 hours. It is less specific than CK-MB and is less widely used. The normal value is 10–45 iu/l.

Full blood count

The white cell count is usually elevated in acute myocardial infarction, peaking at about 15 000 cells/mm^3 after 2–4 days. Higher levels are indicative of infection or pericarditis. The erythrocyte sedimentation rate (ESR) usually rises after the first few days following acute infarction and may remain elevated for many weeks.

Urea and electrolytes

A knowledge of serum sodium and potassium is particularly important in patients who are receiving diuretics and digoxin. Since electrolytes can have a major effect on cell excitability, and since acute coronary patients are already at high risk of arrhythmias secondary to altered cell excitability, it is vital that serial measurements are obtained.

Potassium

The effects of *hyperkalaemia* on the myocardium may result in cardiac arrest. The common ECG changes that suggest hyperkalaemia include prolonged PR interval, wide QRS complex, tall tented T wave, or ST depression. Supraventricular tachycardia, ventricular ectopic beats, atrial fibrillation or, in severe cases, ventricular fibrillation or asystole may result.

Drugs, including thiazide diuretics and insulin may cause *hypokalaemia*, which also impairs myocardial contractility. Flattened T wave, ST depression, prominent U wave, or ventricular ectopic beats on the ECG, suggest hypokalaemia. The more profound the hypokalaemia, the greater the propensity for the occurrence of ventricular ectopic beats. The ECG changes are reversed by administration of potassium. Maintaining a serum potassium of over 4 mmol/l is recommended.

Calcium

Hypercalcaemia, suggested by a shortened QT interval on the ECG, increases myocardial contractility. *Hypocalcaemia*, suggested by a prolonged QT interval on the ECG, depresses myocardial contractility.

Sodium

Most diuretics decrease sodium levels by promoting sodium excretion, whereas corticosteroids elevate sodium levels by promoting retention. Antihypertensive agents such as methyldopa and hydralazine may cause sodium and water retention.

Magnesium

A deficiency of magnesium is known to predispose to the evolution of cardiac arrhythmias, mainly ventricular ectopic beats, and an increased sensitivity to digitalis-induced arrhythmias. A knowledge of magnesium levels is particularly relevant if the patient has been on high doses of diuretics.

Blood glucose level

Stress-related hyperglycaemia is common in the acute phase following infarction. Although glucose tolerance frequently returns to normal, about two-thirds of patients with an initial blood sugar exceeding 10 mmol/litre will be diabetics who have been previously undiagnosed (Husband et al 1983). Patients with diabetes who present with acute coronary syndromes have an in-hospital and long-term mortality of almost twice that of non-diabetics (McGuire et al 2000). Much of the excess mortality in patients with diabetes occurs as a result of a higher incidence of heart failure in this group, attributed to a specific diabetic cardiomyopathy (Francis 2001) or early metabolic changes producing increased myocardial oxygen requirements and depressed myocardial performance, as it does not seem to be related to heart size or the size of the infarction.

Blood glucose levels will be measured initially by a blood sample sent to the laboratory. Subsequent capillary samples may then be taken by the nurse to monitor response to therapy. It is important that this is done accurately (Rumley 1997). The Department of Health (DoH 1996) highlights the need for standardization in the training, reliability and quality control of near patient blood glucose monitoring. Correct technique includes:

- checking the meter is calibrated correctly
- check test strips are in date
- ensure patient washes their hands to encourage blood flow and remove any sugar from the skin surface – do not use alcohol wipes
- avoid site near to iv glucose, avoid frequent use of the same finger
- use disposable lancet to prevent cross infection
- obtain ladybird-sized drop of blood from the side of the finger and apply to test strip in one application
- clean meter at end of session and dispose of waste appropriately.

Serum lipid levels

Cholesterol concentrations are reduced and triglyceride concentrations elevated for about 3 months following a myocardial infarction, so unless done in the first 24 hours, after the onset of symptoms, random serum lipid level measurements will be inaccurate. For other patients, early assessment of serum lipid concentration will highlight pre-existing hyperlipidaemia.

CHEST X-RAY

The plain chest X-ray is an important part of the full cardiological assessment. X-rays, because of their short wavelength, can penetrate materials which do not transmit visible light. Materials of differing density will absorb varying degrees of radiation. Air has less density and causes dark images on the X-ray film, whereas bone has a high density causing light images. A great deal can be learned from a careful study of the cardiac contours and of the lung fields, as shown on a simple posteroanterior (PA) film of the chest. X-rays detect heart shape and size, lung vessel changes and interstitial oedema. Serial study of the chest X-ray is usually warranted.

The X-ray is likely to be unremarkable during an uncomplicated infarction, although common abnormalities observed during acute myocardial infarction are cardiac enlargement and signs of left ventricular failure (LVF). In roughly 40% of acute coronary patients who develop pulmonary oedema, there will be radiographic evidence of pulmonary congestion before other clinical signs are present. Radiographic findings usually correlate well with the patient's haemodynamic state, although there may be discrepancies as a result of a time lag caused by the fact that it takes some time for pulmonary interstitial fluid to accumulate to a level that is visible on the chest X-ray.

The patient who is unstable usually has a portable X-ray performed at the bedside to limit unnecessary workload on the heart. These films provide an anteroposterior (AP) view which tends to produce greater magnification of the thoracic structures and is not as accurate as the PA film, but nevertheless provides useful diagnostic information. Patients who are stable should have a PA chest X-ray which is preferred because it allows better observation of the bases of the lung and gives a more accurate representation of heart size.

The main problem with X-rays for the patient is fear of the radiography equipment and the possibility of a serious condition being shown on the film. Patients in pain and discomfort may find it difficult to cooperate with the radiographer.

Acute cardiac nurses are increasingly being required to be able to interpret the chest X-ray. A systematic approach to basic chest X-ray interpretation can be found in Hatchett (2002).

ECHOCARDIOGRAPHY

Echocardiography is a non-invasive technique which uses pulses of high-frequency sound waves (ultrasound) emitted from a transducer to evaluate cardiac anatomy, pathology and function. The ultrasonic waves in echocardiography have a frequency range of millions of cycles per second. Ultrasound will travel in straight lines unless it is reflected or refracted by an interface between two different structures or tissues. More sound waves will be reflected if the ultrasound beam is directly perpendicular to the plane of the structure. Various areas within the heart may be identified by their characteristic patterns of motion.

Echocardiography is a very convenient, safe and relatively inexpensive investigation and the information obtained from it is frequently used to influence management. A study of 300 referrals for echocardiography found that additional information pertinent to patient management was obtained in 81% of cases (McDonald et al 1988). This study also revealed that echocardiography has a role in reassuring patients regarding the structure and functioning of their heart, especially when there is some doubt with diagnosis.

Patients may be anxious about the actual procedure and this should be allayed by careful preparation, including an explanation of the procedure and its purpose. For instance, the patient should be informed that the procedure involves the operator applying a lubricant to the skin surface of the chest wall and moving a transducer or probe back and forth by hand across the surface. The only preparation required is that the patient is asked to undress to the waist, if able, and then assisted onto the examining table asked to lie initially in the supine position and later on their side. Echo cardiography can also be performed at the patient's bedside.

The two main techniques used are M-mode and cross-sectional echocardiography. The Doppler shift of ultrasound can be combined with these to provide information on the velocity and direction of blood flow. Echocardiography is used in coronary care for a variety of purposes, particularly:

- supporting the diagnosis of ischaemic chest pain
- assessing complications of myocardial infarction

- assessment of cardiac failure
- assessing prognosis.

M–mode echocardiography

This is essentially a graph of depth of tissues against time. A single beam of ultrasound is directed towards the heart, usually from the fourth left intercostal space, producing a columnar view of cardiac structures. By rotating the transducer, a sweeping view may be obtained. It is a useful technique for obtaining measurement of chamber size, wall thickness and assessing left ventricular function in patients who do not have areas of myocardial dysfunction. It may also be used to demonstrate mitral and aortic valve disease and pericardial effusions.

Cross–sectional echocardiography

An arched ultrasonic beam sent to the heart produces a fan-shaped cross-sectional image of cardiac structures, showing how the structures relate spatially. Up to 60 pictures are produced each minute to produce a moving real-time image which is anatomically recognizable. Multiple views from different sites are used to build up a complete picture of the heart. The images are stored on a computer floppy disc, and the computer can aid evaluation by accurately measuring ejection fractions and valve diameters.

M-mode and cross-sectional echocardiography enable the physician to estimate global and regional left ventricular function in the coronary patient. They are valuable for detecting a mural thrombus in the left ventricle.

Doppler echocardiography

The Doppler effect refers to the change in apparent frequency of a sound wave as a result of relative motion between the observer and the source. This effect can be used with red cells to calculate blood velocity, either by continuous wave or pulsed ultrasound. Continuous-wave Doppler emits a constant stream of ultrasound along a single line and superimposes all velocities along that line. Pulsed wave Doppler assesses the velocity of blood at one site and can measure flow at precise depths in conjunction with the two-dimensional image.

Colour flow echocardiography

Colour flow echocardiography assigns a colour to the image depending on the direction and velocity of the blood flow. This information is calculated using the Doppler effect and is displayed over two-dimensional or M-mode image. The flow towards the transducer is displayed as red and the flow away in blue. This technique is very sensitive and can detect the small degree of regurgitation that occurs through normal valves and is particularly useful in detecting abnormal blood flow within the heart and the great arteries.

Stress echocardiography

Stress echocardiography involves imaging during periods of increased myocardial workload induced by exercise or pharmacological stress. Drugs used include dobutamine, arbutamine and coronary dilators such as adenosine and dipyridamole. Stress echocardiography allows imaging areas of altered myocardial contractility and can be used to diagnose coronary heart disease. It is particularly useful for differentiating between infarcted and hybernating myocardium in order to make decisions about revascularization. Stress echocardiography has also been used in the triage of patients with atypical chest pain from the emergency department (Colon et al 1998).

Contrast echocardiography

Contrast echocardiography involves injecting a contrast medium containing microbubbles into the blood stream. These bubbles produce echoes as they pass through the heart that are picked up by the transducer and can be used to detect defects in wall motion, septal defects and to define the endocardial border of the left ventricle.

Transoesophageal echocardiography (TOE)

In transoesophageal echocardiography the ultrasound transducer is mounted on a flexible endoscope and passed orally down the oesophagus to lie adjacent to the posterior aspect of the heart. This enables the use of a higher frequency transducer which produces better quality pictures. Patients may find this procedure uncomfortable and it can be performed with or without sedation. Additional care must involve pulse oximetry, oral suction and oxygen therapy.

MYOCARDIAL PERFUSION IMAGING

Non-invasive imaging techniques can provide useful additional information about coronary artery blood flow and ventricular size and wall motion, using special cameras, computers and radioisotopes. Myocardial perfusion imaging is the only non-invasive method of assessing myocardial perfusion and is based on the principle that the radioisotope is distributed throughout the myocardium in proportion to blood flow. The isotopes give off gamma-rays, a computerized scintillation camera takes pictures which, when fed into a computer, produce an image that shows the agent's concentration in a particular area. The most common radionuclide imaging methods include thallium scanning and technetium-99 (^{99m}Tc) pyrophosphate scanning.

Thallium scanning

This is also known as 'cold spot' imaging and involves the intravenous injection of thallium-201, a radioactive isotope that emits gamma-rays and resembles potassium. It is used to determine areas of ischaemic myocardium and infarcted tissue and can evaluate coronary artery and ventricular function. Abnormal tissue does not take up the tracer and therefore appears as a light area or 'cold spot' on the scan. Thallium scanning does not distinguish between infarction and ischaemia, nor old and new infarctions. However, exercise testing with thallium is more successful in detecting residual ischaemia post-infarction than the conventional ECG exercise test.

^{99}Tc pyrophosphate scanning

In contrast to thallium scanning, this is known as 'hot spot' scanning and uses technetium-labelled pyrophosphate which is taken up by damaged myocardial cells. In general, this imaging method can identify and locate acute myocardial infarction. It is particularly useful in right ventricular infarctions.

The radioisotope is administered intravenously, the dose being low, resulting in only a small amount of radiation to the patient. The scan is performed by a technician or physician and a consent form is usually required to be signed prior to the procedure. The patient should be advised that there may be a waiting period between the administration of the radioisotope and the scanning, and that he should remove any clothing and jewellery from the site to be scanned.

RADIONUCLIDE VENTRICULOGRAPHY

Radionuclide ventriculography is sometimes performed following acute myocardial infarction to assess global myocardial performance. There are two main techniques: first-pass scanning and multiple gated acquisition (MUGA) scanning.

First-pass scanning

A radioisotope (usually ^{99m}Tc) is injected into a peripheral vein and its radioactivity counted on its first passage through the heart.

MUGA scanning

Technetium is used to label the patient's red cells which are then reinjected. A period of equilibrium is then allowed and radioactivity is measured within the heart as it beats and recorded frame by frame on a videotape activated by the ECG (one frame per cycle).

Both of these methods can be used to obtain radioactive counts during the cardiac cycle, from which an ejection fraction (the percentage of residual volume that is expelled from the heart during ventricular systole) is calculated with the aid of a computer. The normal ejection fraction is $65 \pm 12\%$. Because of the substantial daily variation in the ejection fraction during the first few days following acute myocardial infarction, and because the left ventricle may later recover function, it is

advisable to wait until the patient has recovered before evaluating myocardial function with this technique.

POSITRON EMISSION TOMOGRAPHY

Positron emission tomography is the most effective non-invasive imaging technique to detect myocardial viability. The commonest method uses N-13 ammonia as a short-lived tracer of blood flow combined with the fluorine-18-labelled glucose analogue fluorodeoxyglucose (FDC) as a metabolic imager. The scan is able to distinguish between normal myocardium which takes up the FDC with normal contractility; infarcted myocardium which does not take up the FDC and has impaired contractility; and hybernating myocardium that has impaired contractility but still takes up the FDC.

MAGNETIC RESONANCE IMAGING (MRI)

Magnetic resonance imaging is a safe and non-invasive imaging technique that uses a strong magnetic field to produce a three-dimensional image of the body, including the heart. Cardiac MRI is increasingly being used to provide information on cardiac morphology, perfusion and left ventricular function. Specific contrast agents can be used to differentiate between infarcted and ischaemic myocardium and also to determine the size of infarction.

Rapid-sequence cine MRI is being used to assess graft patency post-bypass surgery, and flow contrast techniques enable the estimation of coronary blood flow through vein grafts.

Three-dimensional magnetic resonance coronary angiography (MR-CA) has been shown to be an accurate non-invasive way of identifying narrowing in the proximal and middle coronary artery segments, particularly in left main stem and three vessel disease. Its advantages over conventional angiography include the fact that it is non-invasive, takes less time to perform and has no risk of stroke, myocardial infarction or sudden death.

Other developing non-invasive techniques for assessing the coronary artery lumen include electron beam computed tomography and multislice computed tomography. As yet image quality of these new techniques prevents them being a viable alternative to conventional angiography (deFeyter and Nieman 2002).

CARDIAC CATHETERIZATION AND CORONARY ANGIOGRAPHY

Cardiac catheterization

Cardiac catheterization can be defined as the insertion into one or more of the heart chambers (usually under screening) of a fine flexible radiopaque catheter. The catheter is inserted via a peripheral vein or artery under sterile conditions in a cardiac laboratory equipped with facilities for screening, cine-filming and videotape recording, multi-channel pressure recording, blood gas estimation, anaesthesia and resuscitation. The right and left side of the heart may be investigated separately or together. Cardiac catheterization is mainly performed to:

- visualize the heart chambers and vessels by means of radiopaque substances under X-ray control (angiography)
- measure pressure and record the waveforms from the cavity of the heart chambers and great vessels
- obtain blood samples from the heart for the measurement of cardiac output and the identification of intracardiac shunts through blood gas analysis.

Cardiac catheterization tends to be performed when a definite diagnosis of coronary atherosclerosis, and the extent of it, is required. Following myocardial infarction, an assessment of the functional severity of myocardial damage through cardiac catheterization can have an important predictive value in identification of the patient with high short-term mortality risk and the selection of patients who might benefit most from various management and therapeutic options. Cardiac catheterization will be performed on the patient who is a prospective candidate for coronary bypass surgery. It is also used to evaluate the effect of reperfusion therapy.

Right heart catheterization

A catheter is introduced into the right atrium via a basilic or saphenous vein. Once in the right atrium the catheter is manoeuvred through the tricuspid valve to the ventricle, then to the pulmonary artery and it is eventually wedged into a distal pulmonary artery where the pulmonary arterial wedge pressure is obtained. Blood sampling and pressures are obtained on the gradual withdrawal of the catheter. A balloon-tipped flow-directed catheter may also be inserted to facilitate measurement of the pulmonary artery wedge pressure: a record of indirect left atrial pressure.

Left heart catheterization

A catheter is introduced into the brachial or femoral artery and is advanced into the aorta and then into the left ventricle (retrograde aortic technique). Alternatively, a catheter is introduced into the right atrium using a stilette as a guide. The trans-septal needle perforates the inner atrial septum and the catheter is passed over the needle into the left atrium (trans-septal technique). Left heart catheterization is useful for recording pressures and estimating oxygen saturation of extracted blood samples. It is also used for diagnosing aortic valve stenosis.

Cardiac output determination

If the oxygen content of the blood in the pulmonary artery and brachial artery and the oxygen consumption are known, the cardiac output can be calculated from the Fick formula:

$$\text{Cardiac output (litres/min)} = \frac{\text{Oxygen consumption (ml/min)}}{\text{Arteriovenous oxygen difference (ml/litre)}}$$

Angiography

Selective coronary angiography was introduced in 1959, and is an invaluable specialist investigation for defining coronary circulation. Angiography involves injecting contrast medium into the heart during cardiac catheterization. Venography refers to the examination of the veins, and arteriography to examination of the arteries. The procedure shows the shape and size of the heart chambers and will pinpoint any stenosis or occlusion in the coronary arteries. Coronary obstruction is demonstrable in about 90% of cases thought to have coronary heart disease.

Angiography is usually recommended for:

- acute coronary syndrome patients, e.g. troponin positive
- patients with stable angina whose symptoms are significantly affecting their lifestyle
- patients with unstable angina following inpatient stabilization
- selected patients post-myocardial infarction.

Cine-angiography involves taking films of the dye injection at 80–200 frames/s to record the movement of the heart structures as the dye is ejected from the heart. This serves to show defects of myocardial contraction and also any valvular regurgitation. Cine-angiography has been used to measure the effects of exercise on myocardial function. The cine-film can be played back immediately through the use of video-recording facilities.

Coronary blood flow is graded by an internationally recognized system known as the TIMI flow grade (the name comes from its use in thrombolytic agent trials – **Thrombolysis In Myocardial Infarction**). The grades of flow are shown in Table 5.4.

Procedure

Cardiac catheterization is usually carried out under local anaesthesia, often with mild sedation as a premedication. A general anaesthetic is not normally given because it prevents the patient from indicating if he experiences any breathlessness or chest pain during the catheterization procedure. It also alters blood oxygenation and cardiac output measurements. However, the patient is normally asked to fast for 4–6h prior to the procedure to prevent aspiration should cardiac arrest occur. The catheterization is performed by the cardiologist and takes about 90 min.

Table 5.4 Grades of coronary blood flow

TIMI 0	No perfusion
	No antegrade flow beyond the point of occlusion
TIMI 1	Penetration with minimal perfusion
	Contrast fails to opacify the entire bed distal to the stenosis for the duration of the picture run
TIMI 2	Partial perfusion
	Contrast opacifies the entire coronary bed distal to the stenosis. However, the rate of entry and/or clearance is slower in the coronary bed distal to the obstruction than in comparable areas not perfused by the dilated vessel
TIMI 3	Complete perfusion
	Filling and clearance of contrast equally rapid in the coronary bed distal to stenosis as in other coronary beds

A consent form will need to be signed by the patient. They are asked to wear a gown and warned that they will have to lie flat on their back on a hard table in the catheter laboratory throughout the procedure. The skin over the selected site of incision is shaved and cleansed to minimize the risk of infection. The patient undergoing angiography needs to be warned to expect a sudden burning or bursting sensation when the dye is injected into the heart. If the dye or catheter evokes vasospasm, the patient will experience a searing pain in the affected vessel and the procedure will have to be stopped. Angina may be provoked as a result of the catheter blocking the artery or because of general haemodynamic changes.

Patients may have concerns about lying flat during and after the procedure, the insertion of the catheter, possible complications and the results of the test (Peterson 1991). The proximity and noise of the X-ray equipment, the semi-darkness, the masked and gowned staff, and the movement of the table during positioning, can add to the anxiety of the patient. Patients have described cardiac catheterization as an experience during which they were nervous and unable to relax. The procedure has been shown to increase heart rate, blood pressure, myocardial oxygen consumption, and plasma catecholamine concentration (Turton et al 1979).

Patient preparation

The patient will be fully informed about the purpose of the investigation and what to expect in order to allay anxiety (Finesilver 1979). Patients require different types of information tailored to their own needs and coping styles. Nurse-led pre-admission clinics are a way of promoting individualized information and advice, and ward-based nurses need to offer similar support to patients who have less time to prepare for the procedure. Cohen and Hasler (1987) recommended that sensory preparation in the form of cassette tapes and slides be used prior to the procedure. Other patients may benefit from booklets or leaflets (Dowling and O'Keefe 1990). Watkins et al (1986) found that some patients were less anxious if told what sensations to expect, whereas others responded better if they were not told in so much detail what the procedure would be like. Positive reappraisal techniques seem to help patients feel less emotional and physical distress during the procedure (Kendall et al 1979). Teaching the patient relaxation techniques prior to the procedure has been shown to reduce stress levels (Rice et al 1986).

After the procedure

Following the procedure the patient may require analgesia and should be given the opportunity to rest. Any heparin infusion should be stopped prior to removal of the femoral artery sheath and the ACT/APTT monitored for 1–4 hours depending on the last recorded ACT. After sheath removal, digital pressure should be applied over the femoral artery to help the puncture site to close. Protocols for the length of time this pressure is applied varies between centres but is generally between 5 and 10 min. Manual compression devices are available and tend to be fitted as a belt around the hips and then inflated to 20 mmHg above the systolic blood pressure to apply even pressure over the femoral area. A dressing needs to be applied to the wound site which should be observed for excessive bleeding. Pedal pulses, colour and movement of the feet should be checked for signs of adequate circulation. The limb needs to be kept straight for 1–2 hours to prevent turbulence of blood flow at the incision site. If the catheter is inserted in the femoral artery, the patient is advised to rest in bed, to prevent flexing the hip and possible artery occlusion. They should be advised to report any swelling or bleeding from the groin. The length of time the patient is in bed varies between centres, but can be as short as 2 hours (Vlasic and Almond 1999). Prolonged bed rest can result in back pain and difficulty with using a bedpan or urinal. The limb needs to be inspected regularly for presence of a pulse, warmth and sensation. The patient should be encouraged to drink to remove the radiopaque dye from the system. Lying at an angle of 30° may make this easier for the patient.

Some centres insert a sealing device such as the Angio-Seal via an introducer to promote wound closure once the sheath has been removed. The use of this device limits the discomfort of groin pressure and means the patient can move their limb freely and be mobilized sooner.

Complications

Angiography carries a small morbidity and mortality rate due to myocardial infarction, coronary artery dissection and arrhythmias, but this is less than 0.1% and increasingly, low risk patients are being treated as day cases. Transient cardiac arrhythmias, including ventricular ectopic beats, atrial ectopic beats, asystole, and ventricular fibrillation and varying degrees of heart block, although uncommon, may occur. Perforation of the heart or great vessels, syncope, and emboli to the brain, lungs or major vessels are also possible. The artery used for the procedure may become occluded by spasm or thrombosis, and embolectomy and atrial repair may be necessary if it does not respond to heparinization. A reaction to the dye may produce a variety of symptoms ranging from a rash to laryngeal spasm and anaphylaxis. Hydrocortisone and antihistamine may need to be given. The procedure becomes more complex if patients have had glycoprotein IIb/IIIa inhibitors and thrombolytic agents as is the case with patients being assessed for rescue angioplasty when the bleeding rate may be as high as 6% (GUSTO Angiographic Investigators 1993).

References

ACC/AHA (1997). American College of Cardiology/ American Heart Association guidelines for exercise stress testing. *Circulation*, 96: 345–354.

Alpert UJ, Thygesen K (2000) for the Joint European Society of Cardiology/American College of Cardiology Committee. Myocardial infarction redefined. A consensus document for the Joint European Society of Cardiology/American College of Cardiology committee for the redefinition of myocardial infarction. *Journal of the American College of Cardiology*, 36: 959–969.

Argard A, Hermeren G, Herlitz J (2001). Patient's experiences of intervention trials on the treatment of myocardial infarction: is it time to adjust the informed consent procedure to the patient's capacity? *Heart*, 86: 632–637.

Arthur VAM (1995). Written information: a review of the literature. *Journal of Advanced Nursing*, 21: 1081–1086.

Ashworth P (1980). *Care to Communicate: An Investigation into Problems of Communication between Patients and Nurses in Intensive Therapy Units*. Royal College of Nursing, London.

Barclay P, Costigan S, Divies M (1997). Lottery can be used to show risk. *British Medical Journal*, 316: 1242.

Bauman B (1961). Diversities in conceptions of health and physical fitness. *Journal of Health and Human Behaviour*, 2: 39–46.

Beresford NW (2001). Consent issues in cardiology. *Heart*, 86: 595–596.

Byrne D (1964). Repression-sensitization as a dimension of personality. *Progress in Experimental Personality Research*, 1: 169–220.

Channer K, Morris F (2002). ABC of clinical electrocardio- graphy. Myocardial ischaemia. *British Medical Journal*, 324: 1023–1026.

Clark CR, Gregor FM (1988). Developing a sensation information message for femoral arteriography. *Journal of Advanced Nursing*, 13: 237–244.

Cohen JA, Hasler ME (1987). Sensory preparation for patients undergoing cardiac catheterisation. *Critical Care Nurse*, 7(3): 68–73.

Collinson P (1998). Troponin T or Troponin I of CKMB (or none)? *European Heart Journal*, 19: N16–N24.

Cooper JK (1986). Electrocardiography 100 years ago. Origins, pioneers, and contributors. *New England Journal of Medicine*, 315: 461–464.

Colon PJ, Guarisco JS, Murgo J, Cheirif J (1998). Utility of stress echocardiography in the triage of patients with atypical chest pain from the emergency department. *American Journal of Cardiology*. 82: 1282–1284.

deFeyter PJ, Nieman K (2002). New coronary imaging techniques: what to expect? *Heart*, 87: 195–197.

Department of Health (1996). *Extra-laboratory Use of Blood Glucose Meters and Test Strips: Contraindications, Training and Advice to Users*. Medical Devices Agency Adverse Incident Centre Safety Notice 9616, June.

Department of Health (2001b). *12 Key Points on Consent: the Law in England*. Department of Health, London.

Dowling N, O'Keefe M (1990). Preparation for cardiac catheterisation. *Nursing Review*, 10: 15–19.

Engstrom B (1984). The patient's need for information during hospital stay. *International Journal of Nursing Studies*, 21: 113–130.

Finesilver C (1979). Preparation of adult patients for cardiocatheterization and coronary cineangiography. *International Journal of Nursing Studies*, 16: 211–221.

Francis GS (2001). Diabetic cardiomyopathy: fact or fiction? *Heart*, 85: 247–248.

French HP (1979). Reassurance: a nursing skill? *Journal of Advanced Nursing*, 4: 627–634.

Fromm R, Meyer D, Zimmerman J et al (2001). A double blind, multicentred study comparing the accuracy of diagnostic markers to predict short and long term clinical events and their utility in patients presenting with chest pain. *Clinical Cardiology*, 24: 516–520.

Gilliam AD, Speake WJ, Scholefield JH et al (2003). Finding the best from the rest: evaluation of the quality of patient information on the internet. *Annals of the Royal College of Surgeons of England*, 85: 44–46.

GUSTO Angiographic Investigators (1993). The effect of tissue plasminogen activator, streptokinase, or both on coronary artery patency, ventricular function and survival after acute myocardial infarction. *New England Journal of Medicine*, 329: 1615–1622.

Halstead F, Turner B, Wilson S (2002). Diagnostic procedures. In *Cardiac Nursing: A Comprehensive Guide* (R Hatchett, DR Thompson, eds). Churchill Livingstone, Edinburgh, pp. 127–146.

Hartfield MT, Cason CL, Cason GJ (1982). Effects of information about a threatening procedure on patients' expectations and emotional distress. *Nursing Research*, 31: 202–206.

Hatchett R (2002). Observation and monitoring devices. In *Cardiac Nursing: A Comprehensive Guide* (R Hatchett, DR Thompson, eds). Churchill Livingstone, Edinburgh, pp. 69–96.

Husband DJ, Alberti KG, Julian DG (1983). Stress hyperglycaemia during acute myocardial infarction: an indicator of pre-existing diabetes? *Lancet*, 2: 179–181.

Hussein S, Partridge M (2002). Perceptions of asthma in South Asians and their views on educational materials and self management plans. *Patient Education and Counseling*, 48: 189–194.

International Council of Nurses (1973). *Code for Nurses: Ethical Concepts Applied to Nursing*. International Council of Nurses, Geneva.

Janis IL (1965). Psychodynamic aspects of stress tolerance. In *The Quest for Self-Control* (S. Klausner, ed.). Free Press, New York.

Johnson JE (1973). Effects of accurate expectations about sensations on the sensory and distress components of pain. *Journal of Personality and Social Psychology*, 27: 261–275.

Kendall PC, Williams L, Pechacek TF, Gramm LE, Shissiak C, Herzoff N (1979). Cognitive-behavioural and patient education interventions in cardiac catheterization procedures. *Journal of Consulting and Clinical Psychology*, 47: 49–58.

Krikler D (1987). Electrocardiography then and now: where next? *British Heart Journal*, 57: 113–117.

Kurbaan AS, Mills PG (2001). Consent on cardiac practice. *Heart*, 86: 593–594.

Ley P (1972). Primacy, rated importance and recall of information. *Journal of Health and Social Behaviour*, 13: 311–317.

Ley P (1988). *Communicating with Patients*. Croom Helm, London.

Lloyd G, Cooper A, Jackson G (1997). Information delivery: the provision of written information for patients following coronary angiography and post-discharge management. *International Journal of Clinical Practice*, 51: 387–388.

McDonald IG, Guyatt GH, Gutman JM, Jelinek VM, Fox P, Daly J (1988). The contribution of a non-invasive test to clinical care. The impact of echocardiography on diagnosis, management and patient anxiety. *Journal of Clinical Epidemiology*, 41: 151–161.

McGuire DK, Emmanuelson H, Granger CB et al (2000). Influence of diabetes mellitus on clinical outcomes across the spectrum of acute coronary syndromes: findings from the GUSTO11b study. *European Heart Journal*, 21: 1750–1758.

Mumford M (1997). A descriptive study of the readability of patient information leaflets designed by nurses. *Journal of Advanced Nursing*, 26: 985–991.

Ng SM, Krishnaswamy P, Morrisey R et al (2001). Ninety-minute accelerated critical pathway for chest pain evaluation. *American Journal of Cardiology*, 88: 611–617.

Nursing and Midwifery Council (2002). *Code of Professional Conduct*. Nursing and Midwifery Council, London.

Pateghini M, Pagani F, Bonetti G (1999). The sensitivity of cardiac markers: an evidence based approach. *Clinical Chemical and Laboratory Medicine*, 37: 1097–1106.

Pateghini M (2002). Acute coronary syndrome. Biochemical strategies in the troponin era. *Chest*, 122: 1428–1435.

Peterson M (1991). Patient anxiety before cardiac catheterisation. An intervention study. *Heart and Lung*, 20: 643–647.

Rice VH, Caldwell M, Butler S, Robinson J (1986). Relaxation training and response to cardiac catheterization: a pilot study. *Nursing Research*, 35: 39–43.

Rumley A (1997). Improving the quality of near patient blood glucose measurement. *Annals of Clinical Biochemistry*, 34: 281–286.

Seymour L, Woloshynowych M, Adams S (2000). Patient perception of risk associated with elective heart surgery. *Health Care Risk Resource*, 33: 8–11.

Smith SW, Zvosec DL, Sharkey SW et al (2002). Terminology and ECG types in acute coronary syndromes. In *The ECG in Acute MI. An Evidence-Based Manual of Reperfusion Therapy* (SW Smith, DL Zvosec, SW Sharkey et al, eds). Lippincott Williams and Wilkins, Philadelphia.

Stanley BM, Walters DJ, Maddern GJ (1998). Informed consent: how much information is enough? *Australian and New Zealand Journal of Surgery*, 68: 788–791.

Swanton RH (1998). *Cardiology*, 4th edn. Blackwell Science, Oxford.

Takacs KM, Valenti WM (1982). Temperature measurement in a clinical setting. *Nursing Research*, 31: 368–370.

Taylor CB, Bandura A, Ewart CK, Miller NH, DeBusk RF (1985). Exercise testing to enhance wives' confidence in their husbands' cardiac capability soon after clinically uncomplicated acute myocardial infarction. *American Journal of Cardiology*, 55: 635–638.

Thompson DR, Bowman GS (1985). *Medical Investigations*. Baillière Tindall, London.

Turton MB, Deegan T, Coulshed N (1979). Plasma catecholamine levels and cardiac rhythm before and after cardiac catheterization. *British Heart Journal*, 39: 1307–1311.

Verweij J, Kester A, Stroes W, Thijs LG (1986). Comparison of three methods for measuring central venous pressure. *Critical Care Medicine*, 14: 288–290.

Vlasic W, Almond D (1999). Research-based practice: reducing bedrest following cardiac catheterisation. *Canadian Journal of Cardiovascular Nursing*, 10: 19–22.

Waller AD (1887). A demonstration on man of electromotive changes accompanying the heart's beat. *Journal of Physiology*, 8: 229–234.

Walsh D, Shaw D (2000). The design of written information for cardiac patients: a review of the literature. *Journal of Clinical Nursing*, 9: 658–667.

Watkins LO, Weaver L, Odegaard V (1986). Preparation for cardiac catheterization: tailoring the content of instruction to coping style. *Heart and Lung*, 15: 387–389.

White RD, Evans CH (2001). Performing the exercise test. *Primary Care*, 28: 29–43.

Wilson-Barnett J (1979). *Stress in Hospital: Patients' Psychological Reactions to Illness and Health Care*. Churchill Livingstone, Edinburgh.

Wilson-Barnett J (1987). Diagnosis and therapy. In *Nursing the Physically Ill Adult* (JRP Boore, R Champion and MC Ferguson, eds). Churchill Livingstone, Edinburgh, pp. 231–250.

Wilson-Barnett J, Fordham M (1982). *Recovery from Illness*. Wiley, Chichester.

Chapter 6

Acute care: intervention

CHAPTER CONTENTS

INTRODUCTION

Changes in diagnostic criteria and the emphasis on reperfusion strategies have dramatically changed the nature of the management of the acute coronary patient over the past decade. However, the principles of limiting the extent of the acute event, reducing the effect and the likelihood of complications, promoting comfort and well-being and working towards a return to previous lifestyle remain the same. There is also a need to look beyond immediate care and seek to establish the extent of the underlying coronary heart disease and determine what needs to be done to optimize prognosis.

Diagnosis

The main purpose of the assessment process is to establish a rapid diagnosis followed by early risk stratification to identify those patients who will benefit from early interventions. Nurses will also gain information about patient problems, including their response to symptoms and formulate strategies for planning nursing care. While it is important that these issues do not get lost in the medical management of the patient, it is perhaps inevitable that, at least in the acute phase, nursing care will need to be given in the context of the patient's medical diagnosis, as it is this that largely determines what happens to the patient.

Flow charts for the medical management of stable angina and myocardial infarction with ST elevation are given in Figures 6.1 and 6.2.

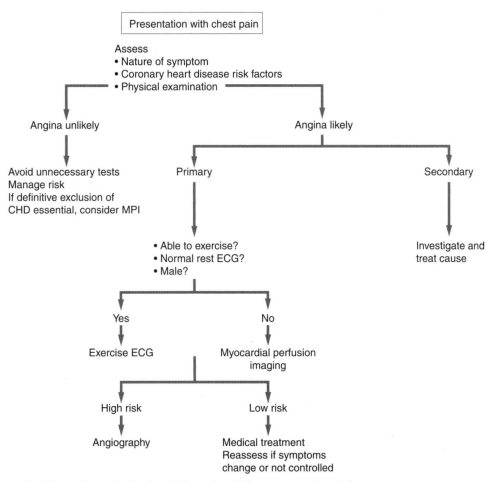

Figure 6.1   Algorithm of investigation in stable angina. CHD = coronary heart disease.

Diagnosis of myocardial infarction and acute coronary syndrome

It is generally accepted that the term myocardial infarction reflects death of cardiac myocytes caused by prolonged ischaemia (Van de Werf 2003). Acute myocardial infarction used to be defined by criteria based on typical symptoms of ischaemic chest discomfort, evolutionary changes in the ECG involving the development of Q waves, and an increase in the creatinine kinase level greater than twice the upper reference limit. At least two of these criteria had to be met to diagnose a myocardial infarction (WHO 1959). However, developments in the detection of small quantities of myocardial necrosis using markers that are more sensitive than creatinine kinase have prompted a new definition

of myocardial infarction which is likely to lead to an increase in the number of patients diagnosed, and confuse clinicians, epidemiologists and patients (McKenna and Forfar 2002). Some patients with acute coronary syndromes who would previously have been diagnosed as having unstable angina are now classified as having myocardial infarction (Pell et al 2003).

In 2000, the Joint European Society of Cardiology and American College of Cardiology Committee recommended changing the diagnostic criteria for acute myocardial infarction to include:

- a typical rise and fall of biochemical markers of myocardial necrosis such as troponin or CKMB with at least one of the following:
  - ischaemic symptoms

- development of pathological Q waves
- electrocardiographic changes indicative of ischaemia – ST segment elevation or depression
- coronary intervention.

From a practical point of view, patients with acute myocardial infarction may be classified as:

- ST elevation myocardial infarction (STEMI) – this group presents with the symptoms of myocardial ischaemia and ST elevation on the ECG which subsequently evolves to Q waves and includes those with new bundle branch block or posterior ECG changes. Cardiac enzymes are usually high.

- Non-ST segment elevation myocardial infarction (NSTEMI) – this group presents with symptoms of myocardial ischaemia but without ST elevation on the presenting ECG. The ECG usually has

some changes but it may be normal. Cardiac markers will be positive. NSTEMI may be considered together with unstable angina as their pathogenesis and presentation are similar, although they differ in the severity of the extent of ischaemia. The term 'unstable coronary syndrome' may be more useful to describe both unstable angina and NSTEMI.

The term 'acute coronary syndrome' defines a continuum of clinical manifestations of coronary artery disease classified by presenting ECG changes and concentrations of cardiac markers (Fox 2000). The definition includes STEMI, NSTEMI and unstable angina.

Unstable angina covers a range of clinical states falling between stable angina and acute (non-ST elevation) myocardial infarction, including angina at rest lasting more than 20 minutes, increasing

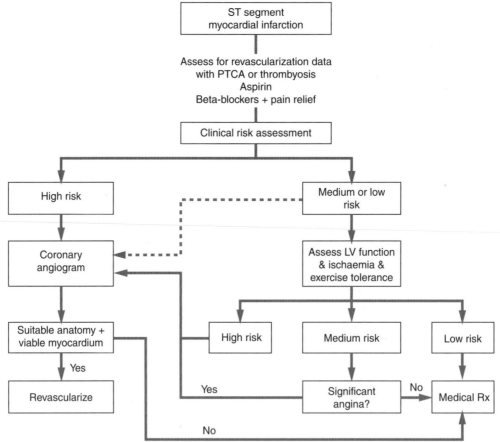

Fiugre 6.2   Algorithm for ST segment myocardial infarction.

angina and angina occurring more than 24 hours after an acute myocardial infarction.

Diagnosis of stable angina

Stable angina involves a fixed coronary artery lesion limiting oxygen supply at times of increased demand. Symptoms are therefore typically provoked by any activity that increases myocardial oxygen demand. Cardiac markers will be negative and the ECG may show signs of transient ischaemia.

Management according to risk

It is important to allocate treatment resources based on current best evidence and manage the patient according to their risk of mortality and morbidity. Hazards of acute coronary syndromes not diagnosed as myocardial infarction with ST elevation have been underestimated in the past and it has been shown that myocardial infarction or death will affect 12.2% of these patients within a 6-month period (Collinson et al 2000). Risk stratification provides important prognostic information and determines treatment strategy. Risk assessment can be complex and score cards are available (Antman et al 1999).

Features that define risk in acute coronary syndromes are shown in Table 6.1.

Several guidelines have been produced for the management of unstable angina and NSTEMI in the UK, Europe and America (ACC/AHA 2000, Bertrand et al 2000, British Cardiac Society 2001). Guidelines for the management of ST segment elevation have also been published by the Task Force on the Management of Acute Myocardial Infarction of the European Society of Cardiology (Van de Werf et al 2003). These guidelines present an 'ideal' framework based on the results of clinical trials from selected populations and tend not to represent subgroups such as the elderly, women and those from ethnic minorities. However, it is useful to have a consensus of opinion on which to base clinical judgement.

In summary:

- Patients with STEMI require prompt revascularization with pharmacological thrombolysis or mechanical intervention (PCI) accompanied by aspirin and pain relief.

- Patients with NSTEMI at high risk require intensive therapy with beta-blockers, clopidogrel, low molecular weight heparin and glycoprotein IIb/IIIa inhibitors. Coronary angiography should be performed prior to discharge from hospital.

- Patients at intermediate risk as indicated by a stress test and an absence of the features of high risk, or those with a mildly elevated troponin level, but with a stress test indicating a low risk, should have a low threshold for angiography.

- Patients at low risk are those with a negative troponin and stress test results that indicate a low risk. These patients can be discharged from hospital. Other investigations may be appropriate and outpatient follow up is required.

Risk assessment following treatment

After initial treatment, increased risk is indicated by:

- raised troponin levels
- recurrent ischaemic symptoms

Table 6.1 Some features that define risk in acute coronary syndromes

High risk	Medium risk	Low risk
Age over 70 years	History of myocardial infarction and/or	No high-risk features
ST depression on first ECG	left ventricular failure	Normal ECG
Refractory angina	Diabetes	Clinically stable
Haemodynamic instability	Recurrent ischaemia	No past history of coronary artery disease
Markedly raised troponin	Already on aspirin	Troponin not raised
	Mildly raised troponin	

- recurrent ischaemic ST segment changes – with or without symptoms
- a positive exercise test
- poor left ventricular function.

Evaluation of care

The climate of today's health system is one which encourages the measurement of processes outcomes. This can provide useful information on trends and verification as to whether set standards have been met. The Myocardial Infarction National Audit Project (MINAP) was established in response to the audit requirements of the National Service Framework for CHD (Birkhead 2000). It aims to collect comparable data on acute myocardial infarction from across the country. However, audit can only ever give part of the picture as not everything can be measured, complex cases do not fit neatly into the tick boxes of audit pro-forma and data will inevitably be misinterpreted, recorded incorrectly or lost. Relying on retrospective audit data makes it impossible to recognize deficiencies in care for the individual patient and care can not be rectified at the time. The value of nurses evaluating the care of individual patients should not be lost in the trend to streamline the process for audit purposes. Evaluation of care is ongoing and has three important functions:

- to determine whether the objectives have been met
- to provide information for reassessment of patient needs
- to discover what actions are most consistently effective in solving particular problems.

Pre-hospital care

Most deaths from acute myocardial infarction occur in the community (Norris 1998) and the ambulance service have a well-defined role in providing a rapid response (a current target of 8 minutes from the call for help) to anyone with suspected heart attack. Emergency calls are now triaged to ensure that life-threatening emergencies are given priority (NHS Executive 1996). Patients may still call their GP when they experience chest pain although this tends to prolong the time until they receive professional help (Birkhead 1992).

Whoever first attends the patient the priorities are: rapid assessment of vital signs, any immediate life-saving measures, symptom relief, oxygen and 300 mg of soluble aspirin (ISIS-2 1988) to suspected myocardial infarction patients and prompt transfer to hospital. Training ambulance crews to defibrillate has had a major impact on the reduction of out of hospital mortality. Direct communication between the ambulance crew and coronary care unit (CCU) staff has been shown to reduce the admission delays and facilitate patient triage (Millar-Craig et al 1997, Prasad et al 1997). Increasing numbers of paramedics are now trained to deliver thrombolysis (Quinn et al 2002).

Delays

The major delays to hospital assessment and appropriate treatment are:

- delay from the onset of symptoms to the patient calling for professional help
- delay in professional help getting to the patient
- delay in getting the patient to hospital
- delay in recording the initial ECG and patient assessment
- delay in the decision to administer treatment (most significantly thrombolysis)
- delay in commencing the therapy.

The time elapsing from the patient arriving at the hospital to them receiving appropriate thrombolysis is termed 'door to needle time'. The term 'call to needle time' refers to the time between the call for professional help and receiving thrombolysis and this should be no more than 60 minutes (DoH 2000). However, the most significant time interval is the time from when the symptoms first start to when the patient receives thrombolysis. A reduction in this 'pain to needle time' will require public education strategies but it is unclear what the 'key message' should be.

Pre-hospital thrombolysis

There is a growing interest in pre-hospital thrombolysis for appropriate patients (Quinn et al 2002). This can be given by paramedics, GPs or, rarely, hospital response teams. An overview of clinical trials of pre-hospital thrombolysis showed significantly lower all-cause hospital mortality compared with in-hospital thrombolysis (Morrison et al 2000). On average 1 hour was saved by pre-hospital treatment. If it is going to take longer than 30 minutes from the time the patient calls for help to get them to hospital, then it is probably wise to invest in training ambulance crew to administer thrombolysis. Pre-hospital thrombolysis may be of particular value in rural populations (GREAT Study Group 1992, EMIP Study 1993) and has been shown to be as safe in the hands of appropriately trained paramedics as with medical staff (Weaver et al 1993). Paramedics are authorized to administer streptokinase (NICE 2002a) and other thrombolytics under Patient Group Directions as highlighted in guidelines developed by the Joint Royal Colleges Ambulance Liaison Committee.

Nursing versus medical intervention

In the CCU, most registered nurses are able to initiate treatment in a crisis situation (for example defibrillation and the administration of certain drugs during an episode of ventricular fibrillation) and routinely to perform tasks normally designated as being of a medical nature in other situations and areas. Nevertheless, there is a real danger that the nurse may become engrossed in such tasks to the detriment of nursing activity. There is probably a need for more conscious decision making about the amount of medically-derived work undertaken and its repercussions on the unique role of the nurse. Medical tasks are often repetitive ones, requiring relatively little skill. If too much emphasis is placed on these technical and medical skills, the caring role of the nurse may be delegated to the less skilled and ultimately standards of care will deteriorate (McFarlane 1980).

Technical tasks tend to cluster around the admission period. This is also the time when the patient and family are likely to be in need of skilled and appropriate psychological support. Nurses need to determine where their time is best spent in terms of benefitting the patient. A diagrammatic representation of nursing activity when a patient is admitted to a CCU is shown in Figure 6.3.

For the benefit of the patient who may be in pain or at risk from sudden deteriorating health as a result of an arrhythmia, the nurse (often the only suitably experienced person available) needs to be able to perform certain procedures, such as recording an ECG and inserting an intravenous cannula. Such activities, however, can and should be performed as part of, and in concordance with, an underlying philosophy of nursing – providing information and support and establishing an effective nurse–patient relationship while such procedures are being performed. Meeting basic needs may be of the greatest significance to the patient who is not fully appreciative of the relevance of other more technical interventions.

Nursing care

Whatever the patients' diagnosis when they are first admitted to hospital with a suspected cardiac problem it is usually a nurse who is the first health professional with whom the patient and family come into contact, and it is their initial assessment and subsequent intervention, which has an important bearing on outcome.

The acute stage is a time when there is greatest potential for overlap between nursing and medical practice. There may also be difficulty delineating between what the patient feels is important and the nursing and medical goals. At times the coronary care nurse may assume a complementary role in an essentially medical arena. For example, their role during thrombolytic therapy is often one of explaining, coordinating, monitoring, and observing response.

Patient problems

The identification of problems for the coronary patient will depend on the depth and extent of the assessment. A knowledge of the patient's background, usual lifestyle and his perception of the present situation, together with a good interpersonal relationship, will help highlight problems which are specific and pertinent to the individual concerned. Possible patient problems include:

- pain and discomfort
- fear

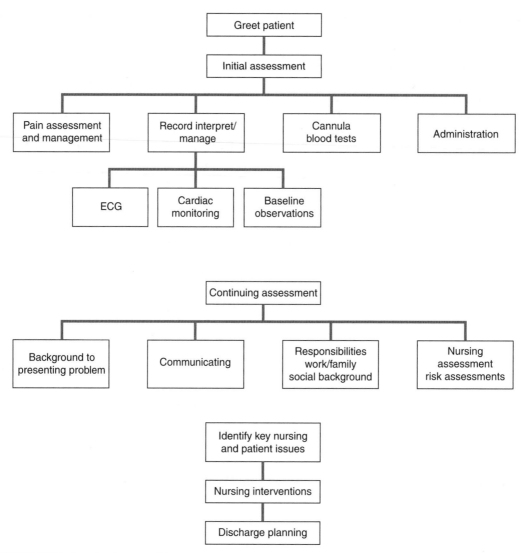

Figure 6.3 Admission algorithm for CCU nurses.

- anxiety
- decreased activity levels
- increased dependency
- lack of knowledge about the problem
- misconceptions
- unrealistic expectations
- altered activities of living
- loss of control
- ineffective or inappropriate coping responses.

The resolution of many of these problems lies solely within the remit of nursing, and nurses need to realize their potential for influencing outcome and promoting effective recovery alongside supporting other therapeutic management goals for the patient.

Nursing intervention

Nursing intervention is designed to help the patient overcome various physical and psychological insults. In the strange and, sometimes, frightening environment of the CCU, the nurse needs to establish a close rapport with the patient and family in order to be effective in reducing anxiety and fear, promoting the resolution of losses, encouraging adjustment to change, and planning together for a successful recovery.

Nursing intervention includes giving careful and detailed explanations about the significance of the diagnosis, including the nature of the disease, purpose of treatment, use of technology, need for rest, and allowances and limitations of activities. Encouraging independence, fostering a realistic but optimistic outlook and confronting inappropriate behaviour, are important facets. Although such intervention will involve the provision of flexible and individually tailored care, a number of key areas need to be considered:

1 *Minimization of stress*: aiming to reduce noxious physical (e.g. temperature and pain) and sensory (e.g. noise, lighting and invasion of territory and privacy) stimuli and specific stressors identified in the assessment.

2 *Preservation of patient routines*: planning care so that the patients' routines with which they are familiar are preserved. In the CCU, eating, toileting and resting habits are often dramatically changed and may have detrimental consequences. Changes in established routine may lead to disorientation with a perceived sense of loss of time; loss of control over planning daily events; and associated feelings of dependency and helplessness. Patients should be included in planning their daily activities: appropriate use of information gained in an accurate and thorough nursing history is needed.

3 *Prevention of non-concordance*: avoiding complex and difficult drug and dietary treatment regimens which are related to non-compliance. The nurse needs to ensure that patients assimilate information and check beliefs which may be incongruent with those of health professionals. They have the right to choose not to comply with advice, and the nurse has the responsibility to ensure that this choice is a decision based on a knowledge of the likely consequences of the action.

4 *Control of pain and discomfort*: ensuring that the patient is free from pain. In the CCU this often means the use of narcotic analgesics and nitrates, but other non-pharmacological interventions should be considered.

5 *Provision of adequate rest*: preventing needless disturbance of the patient and planning appropriate rest periods, as many patients are often seriously deprived of adequate sleep.

6 *Education and support of the patient and family*: ensuring that the patient and family understand what is happening and why, and encouraging patients to take responsibility for their own health.

Caring

Coronary care nursing contains both technological 'cure' elements and supportive, empathetic 'care' elements (Hudson 1993) and is a complex activity not fully understood (Beeby 2000). Caring activities have been described as those that consist of assisting and helping others and are accompanied by values which involve a particular way of perceiving the situation and emotional involvement in the provision of care (Woodward 1997).

Patients' and relatives' perception of good care has been shown to focus on interpersonal aspects of caring, characterized as individualized and patient focused, provided humanistically through the presence of a caring relationship (Atree 2001). Patients in acute environments have been shown to want someone to help them through a period when they are vulnerable (Hunt 1999). The increased throughput of patients, reduced junior doctors' hours and the increasingly technical environment can make it difficult for nurses to maintain parts of their role, such as patient comfort and dignity, that are fundamental aspects of caring (Quinn and Thompson 1995).

Organization of care

Organization of care delivery will depend on the number of staff, skill mix and the number and characteristics of the patients. It also depends on the underlying philosophy of care. Care delivery needs to be organized to maximize the quality of patient care and staff support. This is not always straightforward. Movement of experienced staff to roles away from bedside nursing and the variety of shift patterns contribute to this challenge.

Primary nursing

In the CCU the nurse–patient ratio has been traditionally higher than in ward areas. The majority of staff are also qualified and experienced; many will have undertaken post-basic specialist courses. These factors have facilitated the development of primary-style nursing as a method of organizing care to give maximum responsibility to the nurse and to foster the nurse–patient relationship. Primary nursing, originating in the USA in the early 1970s and coming to prominence in the UK in the early 1980s, simply means that one nurse is responsible for one patient, although in reality it usually means a small group of patients. Primary nursing has been viewed as both a model of care delivery and a nursing philosophy (Pontin 1999). The primary nurse is responsible for continually assessing the patient and planning care accordingly. When the primary nurse is not available, responsibility for care is delegated to an 'associate' nurse who aims to maintain continuity of care. The benefits of primary nursing have been identified as continuity and consistency of care; an improved nurse–patient relationship; increased nurse job satisfaction; a clearer role for the nurse in the multidisciplinary team; and an increased patient focused care. However, problems of perceived isolation and overwhelming work load can arise if the primary nurse is not appropriately supported. Organization of care around a primary nursing framework becomes increasingly difficult with flexible shift systems, increased patient throughput and reduced ratios of experienced to inexperienced staff.

Planning care

The traditional 'nursing process' approach to nursing involves the systematic cyclic approach to care incorporating patient assessment, care planning, implementation of the plan and subsequent evaluation of the care given to see if the identified problems had been resolved. Nurses are required to set achievable goals and set realistic time frames within which these goals will be achieved. However, in reality, and for a variety of reasons, nurses often focus on the care that has been given rather than on the care the patient needs and with an increasing emphasis on standardized protocols and the need to achieve targets, it is easy for individual patient goals to become lost. In the 1980s nursing models attempted to give a theoretical structure to the process of nursing and some were used effectively to support the delivery of nursing care to coronary patients. However, nursing models have tended to be superseded by care pathways which give a framework to care delivery often at the expense of an underpinning nursing theory. Development of care pathways around a nursing model may be one way forward (Chilcott and Hunt 2001).

Documentation of care

The Essence of Care document sets benchmarks for best practice for record keeping (DoH 2001). This emphasizes the need for patient records to demonstrate effective communications which support and inform high quality care and there are professional guidelines which offer nurses a framework on which to develop quality documentation (UKCC 1998).

The nursing record system is the record of care planned and/or given to the individual patient. In theory, the method chosen to record nursing care may have an influence on the quality of nursing practice, although any link is difficult to demonstrate (Currell et al 2002). The care plan, which is the traditional written record of the patient's care often fails to provide evidence of the quality of care that has actually been provided. Standardization and computerization of documentation has been an opportunity to describe patient care by naming and linking patients' needs with nursing interventions (Bowles 2000), although there is a danger that the standardization detracts from individualized care planning.

Care pathways

Care pathways, also known as critical pathways, are management plans that display goals for patients and aim to provide the sequence and timing of actions necessary to achieve these goals with optimal efficiency (Pearson et al 1995). They have been widely adopted, particularly in cardio-vascular medicine, as a method to reduce variation in care, decrease resource utilization and potentially improve health care quality (Every et al 2000). They can be useful tools for multidisciplinary records, providing guidance on care delivery and generating information for audit. They have been shown to encourage staff to focus on clinical care (de Luc 2000). In reality many patients will deviate from the 'normal' course and have coexisting problems which may not fit into a pathway. Individual patient factors should not be controlled by the system and not all variation from the pathway be seen as negative (Every et al 2000). It is also important that streamlining care does not have a negative impact on patient outcomes through limiting opportunities for clinical decision making.

INITIAL INTERVENTION

Conventional practice usually involves establishing a route for intravenous therapy and ECG monitoring, and administering drugs for the relief of pain and anxiety. These usually take place well before the patient reaches CCU. The priorities on admission to the CCU include:

- assessment of vital status and resuscitation as necessary
- effective handover from emergency staff
- assessment of appropriateness for reperfusion therapy (if not already given)
- immediate cardiac monitoring
- establishment of intravenous access
- relief of pain and anxiety
- decrease in myocardial work.

The order in which these are accomplished will depend on the patient and the decision-making processes of those undertaking the initial assessment.

CARDIAC MONITORING

The continuous monitoring of cardiac rate and rhythm provides the means to anticipate the occurrence of potentially fatal disorders of cardiac rhythm and conduction and to assess the response to any interventions. The success of cardiac

monitoring depends on the identification of such problems and tends to be reliant on vigilant staff who can interpret the significance of any arrhythmia. Monitoring systems are now sophisticated and incorporating computers that detect and interpret arrhythmias in great detail.

The nurse must be familiar with electrode placement and monitor operation, as well as being able to recognize and distinguish normal and abnormal cardiac rhythms.

Monitoring systems involve sensors, transmission links and processing devices. The sensors are small metal electrodes which are fixed to the skin to allow cardiac electrical activity to be detected and conveyed to the monitor (oscilloscope) for visual display. The electrodes are usually self-adhesive and disposable, and usually require minimal or no skin preparation. Nevertheless, a few steps can be taken if the signal is poor:

1 shaving of the skin to improve electrode contact and to facilitate easy and painless removal when required
2 wiping the skin with alcohol preparations to remove excess body oil and sweat
3 rubbing the skin with dry gauze to remove loose, dry skin and aid contact.

The electrodes are best placed on the patient's chest rather than the limbs to provide a clear signal with good definition of smaller ECG deflections such as the P wave. The electrode site should be observed daily for allergic reactions, but otherwise there is no need to change the electrodes routinely. Transmission of the signal takes place along wires from the patient to the monitor, although radiotelemetry, which allows the patient more freedom of movement, is useful for patients who are beginning to mobilize. The monitor cable should be long and flexible enough to allow the patient to walk around the bed area and for using a commode.

Processing of the signal requires amplification, after which it may be displayed on an oscilloscope, paper chart recorder, or on magnetic tape. The monitor should be placed in good view and not, for example, on a bedside table behind fruit and flowers. Time should be taken to inform the patient and family carefully about the purpose of cardiac monitoring and that although the heart is being monitored it does not necessarily imply that the patient is critically ill.

Electrocardiographic monitoring commonly requires three chest electrodes, usually two of which are placed in the right and left infraclavicular spaces and the third at the right sternal edge. In this position, a tracing with a configuration similar to lead I is obtained. Additionally, a clear site is left for application of chest electrodes for a 12-lead ECG recording, defibrillation and external cardiac massage should they be required.

The ECG tracing should be observed for the following features:

- rate
- rhythm
- P–R interval
- ectopic beats.

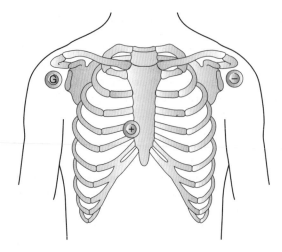

Figure 6.4 Modified chest lead 1: placement of the positive (+), and negative (−) and ground (G) electrodes.

Ideally, the lead that best displays an upright P wave and QRS complex is best for monitoring, but the exact configuration of the complexes is not particularly important unless they are changing from beat to beat.

A three-lead equivalent of lead V_1 and termed MCL-1 (modified chest lead 1) is the best position for recognizing arrhythmias and bundle branch block, and of particular value in differentiating between left ventricular ectopy and supraventricular impulses conducted with right bundle branch aberration. This is recorded by placing the positive electrode in the normal V_1 intercostal (fourth right), while the negative and the earth (ground) electrodes are located near the left shoulder and right shoulder, respectively (Figure 6.4).

Ambulatory cardiac monitoring

When the arrhythmia is frequent, documentation is easily accomplished with brief periods of static monitoring. However, if the arrhythmia is infrequent or transient, then extended monitoring is required. Ambulatory ECG monitoring is designed to document transient rhythm and conduction disturbances. It is commonly applied to the investigation of transient symptoms such as syncope, dizziness, chest pain and palpitations and is increasingly being used to assess antiarrhythmic therapy, detecting ischaemia and determining

prognosis (Mickley 1994). Recorders can be either continuous (loop recorders) or intermittent (sampling). They may also be activated by the patient in response to symptoms (event recorder). The standard ambulatory monitor was first developed by Holter (1961), and hence these recording machines are often known as 'Holter monitors' whatever their origin. The complete unit consists of a miniaturized tape recorder carried in harness. The recording electrodes are applied to the chest in the MCL-1 position. A cassette tape is inserted into the machine and the patient is asked to carry out his normal daily activities. A detailed diary for the period being studied should be kept by the patient, with records of episodes of sleep, exertion, watching television, etc., and clear descriptions of any symptoms. A typical 24-hour recording will provide about 100 000 complexes for analysis, which is, fortunately, performed by using a computerized high-speed ECG scanner.

Other recording devices include, transtelephonic recorder which makes use of the telephone line, and telemetry units.

Most patients do not seem to mind being attached to a cardiac monitor, nor mind being disconnected from it in preparation for transfer to a ward (Thompson et al 1986). Indeed, a significant proportion seemed to find the presence of the monitor reassuring. Nevertheless, there does seem to be a need to ensure that the patient and family understand the purpose of monitoring, including the fact that the monitor will not affect the patient's heart.

Telemetry units

Telemetry units are often used for patients who are well enough to mobilize or be transferred to another area, but still need to have their heart rhythm observed. They are often used in the early post-infarction period. Standard chest electrodes are fitted, attached to a small transmitter which is carried in the pyjama pocket or chest harness. The cardiac rhythm is transmitted continuously to a receiver where it is displayed and analysed in the same way as for static monitors.

It is important that those charged with observing the screen know where the patient is and how to contact the area concerned should any significant arrhythmias be observed.

Longer range telemetry units are increasingly being used by paramedics in the triage of patients with suspected cardiac chest pain. The ECG can be transmitted to the A&E department or CCU for advice and information.

INTRAVENOUS CANNULATION

Peripheral venous cannulation is a common procedure and the correct technique will improve the chances of success and patient comfort and safety. The indications for peripheral intravenous cannulation are:

- to administer parenteral drugs
- to introduce or replace fluids
- to obtain blood samples.

Devices available for peripheral venous cannulation include a range of metal needles with short lengths of narrow-bore plastic tubing ending in various plastic materials such as Teflon. A dual function device is usually available to permit continuous infusion and/or intermittent injections for drug therapy. Devices with ports are best avoided as the caps are often not replaced correctly increasing the risk of infection and air entry. Also they cannot be sterilized with a swab as there is no flat surface. The smallest, shortest gauge cannula should be used in any given situation.

Technique

The most convenient site for percutaneous peripheral venous cannulation is the back of the hand or in the forearm of the non-dominant side, so that the patient's hand is available for normal use. Veins at the elbow should not be used as they may result in joint embolization and kinking of the cannula. Veins chosen should feel bouncy and refill when pressed. They should also be straight and free from valves (felt as small lumps) to allow easy advancement of the cannula.

The procedure should be fully explained to the patient. After clothing has been removed from the limb, the vein should be engorged by applying a tourniquet. Warming or gentle slapping often promotes dilatation of constricted vessels. The skin is prepared by effective cleansing with 70% alcohol. A cursory wipe does more harm than good as it disturbs the skin flora. The skin needs to be allowed to dry for up to 30 seconds and not be retouched. Shaving the area may cause microabrasions and result in microbial growth. The skin is then carefully stretched so that it can be perforated a short distance away from the vein. The needle is then passed through the wall of the vein into the lumen. Once inside the vein the angle is reduced to prevent perforation of the posterior vein wall. A flashback of blood is often seen at the hub of the cannula. After a short distance the needle point is withdrawn into the cannula before it is fully advanced to reduce further risk of perforation. By placing a finger on the skin, over the end of the cannula, the needle can be completely withdrawn allowing blood to flow back only as far as the hub. If an infusion is required, the line may then be attached. After removing the tourniquet, the cannula should be flushed with normal saline.

Thrombophlebitis and cannula-related infections are common complications of the use of peripheral venous catheters, often causing pain and discomfort to the patient and necessitating removal and resiting of the cannula. In addition, septicaemia is a significant risk. Limiting the duration of catheter placement to 48–72 hours may minimize the problem (Royal College of Nursing 1999).

Cleanliness of the puncture site may be maintained by the application of a sterile, dry, non-occlusive dressing. The cannula must be secured, thus limiting movement and preventing damage which may lead to leakage or inflammation. Splints must be avoided, as movement of the limb discourages stasis of blood and possible thrombosis. The cannula should be flushed twice daily with saline to maintain patency.

PAIN RELIEF

Pain has a number of adverse effects including anxiety, sleeplessness, increased sympathetic tone, which may increase myocardial work, and decrease myocardial oxygenation, and increased vagal tone. Rapid and effective pain relief is essential to minimize the occurrence of such effects. Inadequate pain management will result in increased discomfort and suffering for the patient, and possibly contribute to extension of infarct size and inhibit recovery. Effective pain management builds on effective pain assessment which is discussed elsewhere. Nurses have the most contact with patients and yet various studies have illustrated that pain assessment and subsequent pain management are inconsistent (Thompson et al 1994, O'Connor 1995, Meurier 1998, Meurier et al 1998).

Patients are likely to have tried various measures to reduce their pain prior to hospital admission. Many believe their pain to be due to indigestion, and some coronary patients do in fact experience pain relief with the use of antacids. Some may have taken paracetamol or aspirin, while others may have been given drugs administered by intramuscular or intravenous routes by their family doctor.

Control of pain requires attention to psychological as well as physical variables. A calm relaxed atmosphere, a friendly concerned approach from the nurse, and keeping the patient fully informed are all ways that may help to minimize the pain.

The amount of analgesia required depends on the degree of pain, the size of the patient and the effect of previous doses. Typically, episodes of acute coronary pain last a relatively short time and there is little danger of addiction or dependency.

The nurse needs to make sure that the patient is aware that it is not necessary for the patient to be in pain and that it is important to report any discomfort. Nurses who physically distance themselves from the patient by sitting behind a central monitoring console for long periods are likely to inhibit communication of pain.

Patients may expect the nurse to know when they are in pain and when intervention is necessary. They may feel too ill to articulate their pain, or they may bear their pain due to stoicism or the fact that they consider suffering pain to be an intrinsic part of a heart attack. Some may wish to feel in control of their response to the heart attack and not want any outside intervention, or dislike the sense of loss of control that analgesia may produce.

Although it is usually the doctor who prescribes analgesia, it is invariably the nurse who has to decide when to give it and to teach the patient about it. Giving patients some control over their pain experience, such as deciding when they require analgesia and helping to evaluate its effectiveness, is an important nursing consideration.

Narcotic analgesics

Pain relief in the coronary patient initially necessitates pharmacological intervention. The most effective pharmacological agents are the opiates: morphine and diamorphine. Apart from reducing pain, fear and anxiety, and promoting sleep, a narcotic analgesic will reduce catecholamine release which may decrease the tendency to ventricular arrhythmias. The vasodilator effect will reduce afterload and may reduce infarct size and improve heart failure. Narcotic analgesics decrease ischaemic discomfort in three ways:

1 decrease anxiety through action on the central nervous system
2 dilate capacitance vessels (venules) in the peripheral circulation, so that blood pools in the periphery, decreasing left ventricular volume and systolic blood pressure and resulting in a decrease in myocardial oxygen consumption
3 produce central nervous system sedation and primary analgesia through stimulation of opiate receptors.

Diamorphine is the preferred drug for hospital use. Its actions are similar to those of morphine, but it is more potent as an analgesic. It should be given intravenously, both to achieve rapid action and avoid localized muscle damage with consequent enzyme release, which may interfere with subsequent laboratory diagnosis of the myocardial infarction. Intravenous administration should be accompanied with antiemetics, and the depressant effects on the respiratory centre in the medulla need to be borne in mind, particularly in patients with chronic chest disease. Diamorphine is usually administered in doses of 2.5–5 mg i.v., repeated every 5 minutes or so as necessary. Registered nurses may, under a patient group direction, administer it for the treatment of cardiac pain to a patient in CCU or A&E departments (Great Britain 2003).

Nurses tend to underestimate the amount of opiates required. For instance, Bondestam et al (1987) found that in over one-third of instances where opiates were given, patients reported no relief from pain. The reduction of anxiety diminishes the patient's restlessness and autonomic activity, with a consequent reduction in the metabolic demands of the myocardium. Intravenous diamorphine reaches its peak analgesic effect within 20 min of administration and maximum respiratory depression is reached within 5–10 min.

Patients can occasionally become hypotensive following the administration of narcotic analgesics, presumably as a result of capacitance vessel vasodilatation in the presence of hypovolaemia. They may also experience a dry mouth and a bradycardia as a result of decreased sympathetic activity. Hypotension and bradycardia usually respond to atropine. Nausea and vomiting due to stimulation of cerebral chemoreceptors and reduced gut motility are other side effects. The antidote, naloxone 0.4 mg i.v., should always be available for respiratory depression which is a further possible side effect due to the respiratory centre becoming less sensitive to $PaCO_2$.

Other anti-ischaemic agents, including beta-blockers and nitrates, will also reduce cardiac ischaemic pain as will thrombolytics. These are discussed later in the chapter.

Non–pharmacological methods of pain control

In addition to pharmacological intervention, there is a wide range of pain-relieving strategies that can be instituted by the nurse, such as ensuring peace and comfort, careful positioning of the patient, reassurance, protection from stressful situations, limitation of unnecessary activity, and promotion of sleep. Providing the patient with information about the cause of their pain may also reduce the amount of pain experienced (Johnson 1973).

Coping strategies such as therapeutic touch (Fredrikson 1999), relaxation and distraction (Day 2000) are useful if they are performed by a skilled nurse. Other useful methods for the relief of pain, which may be used alone or in conjunction with drugs, include guided imagery, hypnosis and transcutaneous electric nerve stimulation (Peric-Knowlton 1984, Wells 1984). However, the nurse needs to be aware of the limitations as well as the benefits of the interventions available.

Patients need to be prepared to cope with chest discomfort after their acute event, avoiding situations that might trigger angina, such as exercising after a heavy meal, going out in the cold, and emotional stress. Non-pharmacological approaches to symptom control in patients with frequent angina have included the use of transcutaneous electrical nerve stimulation (TENS) and spinal cord stimulation (Anderson et al 1999, Hautvast et al 1999).

Oxygen therapy

Oxygen is often administered to the coronary patient and should be given especially to those who are breathless or who have any features of heart failure or shock. The rationale behind oxygen therapy is that most patients will have a reduced PO_2, and inhaled oxygen will raise the level thereby increasing the diffusion of oxygen into the ischaemic myocardium and reducing pain.

The usual method of administration in the acute phase is by high concentration non-re-breathe mask, and later by nasal cannulae which, unlike masks, do not interfere with communication, eating or drinking. A flow rate of 2–4 l/min is recommended (Van de Werf 2003). Long-term oxygen therapy requires humidification and the patient may need relief from the irritation and discomfort from the prongs of the cannulae.

Oxygen is usually only given for a short period during episodes of acute pain. It needs to be given with caution to patients with chronic obstructive pulmonary disease associated with carbon dioxide retention, as correction of hypoxia may lead to respiratory centre depression (Murphy et al 2001).

Non-cardiac chest pain

A significant proportion of chest pain patients admitted to hospital are likely not to have non-cardiac causes (Erhardt et al 2002). These patients will still be concerned about the cause of their pain and need effective symptom relief with appropriate analgesia. Some patients with suspected cardiac chest pain will be referred for angiograms and found to have normal coronary arteries. These patients have been found to be uncertain about how to cope with their symptoms and often receive conflicting advice. They have been found to suffer from substantial psychological problems and reduced quality of life (Goodacre et al 2001). Patients with non-cardiac chest pain are likely to benefit from individualized support and advice in follow-up care (Potts et al 1999).

Syndrome X describes a particular syndrome in which patients experience angina with angiographically normal coronary arteries. It is also known as microvascular angina syndrome and is particularly common in women. Invasive studies often show abnormal myocardial contractility and the condition possibly reflects an early form of myopathy. Various metabolic and endocrine factors have also been implicated.

ANTI-ISCHAEMIC AGENTS

Beta-blockers

These agents diminish myocardial ischaemia by improving the balance between oxygen supply and demand. They act predominately on the beta-1 receptors. A decrease in sympathetic stimulation results in a decrease in heart rate, myocardial contractility, blood pressure and cardiac output. Beta-blockers may facilitate an increase in myocardial blood supply by redistributing coronary artery blood flow. Sympathetic blockade also influences the electrical component of the conducting system, producing decreased automaticity of the sinus node, decreased conduction time through the AV node and decreased atrial and ventricular excitability.

Beta-blockers are important in the management of unstable angina and reduce the risk of myocardial

infarction by 13% (Yusuf et al 1988). They should be given as early as possible, preferably intravenously unless there is severe left ventricular failure or significantly impaired left ventricular function.

Intravenous beta-blockers should also be given as soon as possible after the onset of acute myocardial infarction. They reduce pain, infarct size, incidence of fatal arrhythmia mortality and the risk of cardiac rupture (Freemantle et al 1999). They should be given in small frequent doses to reduce the pulse rate to around 60 beats/min. Agents with a short duration of action are the best choice, as it is not possible to predict which patients may have adverse reactions. A cardioselective agent is preferred such as atenolol or metoprolol. If tolerated, oral beta-blockers need to be continued for at least 3 years for maximum benefit.

Nitrates

Nitrates are used in angina and can also be used in left ventricular failure. Currently licensed in the UK are glyceryl trinitrate (GTN), isosorbide mononitrate, isosorbide dinitrate and pentaerithrityl tetranitrate. There is no evidence for their routine use in the acute phase of myocardial infarction (Van de Werf et al 2003). Nitrates release nitric oxide into vascular smooth muscle and improve myocardial oxygen supply while reducing oxygen consumption. They tend to dilate veins to a greater extent than arteries and therefore reduce preload more than afterload. This leads to decreased end-diastolic volume and ventricular wall tension which, in turn, results in decreased workload and oxygen consumption. Nitrates also dilate the large capacitance vessels and collateral channels, thereby increasing myocardial subendocardial blood flow and myocardial oxygen supply. For intravenous administration in unstable angina, the starting dose should be low (2–5 µg/min) and increased gradually until the relief of symptoms or the blood pressure is adversely affected. (This would reduce perfusion pressure and may worsen ischaemia.) Nitrates are often given in conjunction with a beta-blocker to offset the increase in heart rate that nitrate therapy can produce. Intravenous nitrates need to be weaned off rather than stopped abruptly to avoid rebound tachycardia. Dose-dependent tolerance can occur if patients receive nitrates for more than 24 hours and periodic reductions in infusion rates may be necessary. Side effects include headache, flushing, dizziness and hypotension.

Nicorandil is a potassium channel activator which works in a similar way to a nitrate although it does not produce tolerance.

Calcium channel blockers

Calcium channel blockers reduce the calcium flow through the slow channels of the active cell membranes and affect the myocardial cells, the specialized conduction tissue and the cells of the vascular smooth muscle. They produce vasodilatation and some affect the heart rate and atrioventricular function. They tend to be used for symptom relief in patients already on beta-blockers and nitrates. They may also be of benefit in patients who cannot tolerate beta-blockers. Verapamil should be avoided in patients taking beta-blockers as there is a risk of inducing asystole. Calcium channel blockers do not have a specific role in acute myocardial infarction but diltiazem may have a role in NSTEMI (Boden et al 2000) and the use of diltiazem and verapamil may be appropriate post-infarction in obstructive airways disease when beta-blockers may be contraindicated. The main groups of calcium channel blockers are the dihydropyridines (e.g. nifedipine), the phenyl alkylamines (e.g. verapamil) and the benzothiazepines (e.g. diltiazem). The short-acting dihydropyridines (e.g. nifedipine, nicardipine) need to be avoided unless the patient is on a beta-blocker as they can produce a tachycardia.

INTERVENTIONS TO LIMIT INFARCT SIZE

As acute myocardial infarction is a dynamic process occurring over a period of several hours, early interventions designed to interrupt the infarction process can salvage viable but jeopardized areas of myocardium. If reperfusion of the ischaemic myocardium is initiated within 6 h of coronary occlusion, necrosis may be limited or prevented (Tiefenbrunn and Sobel 1991).

Infarct size determination

Considerable research has been directed towards determining the extent of infarction and towards developing methods of limiting or decreasing the size of the infarcted area. This is generally based on three broad principles:

1   the mass of damaged myocardium determines the prognosis
2   the mass of damaged myocardium can be measured quantitatively
3   the damaged myocardium may be modified by appropriate treatment.

A number of techniques have been used to determine the evolution and extent of myocardial ischaemia, including:

- cardiac enzyme and other biochemical marker profiles
- electrocardiography: ST-segment elevation, loss of R-wave amplitude, pathological Q waves
- echocardiography
- thallium scanning
- radionuclide ventriculography
- positron emission tomography.

Interventions, whether pharmacological or mechanical, are designed to limit infarct size by either:

1   increasing myocardial oxygen supply to the hypoperfused area, e.g. by
    - thrombolytic therapy
    - percutaneous coronary interventions (PCIs)
    - reversal of coronary artery spasm
    - supplemental oxygen therapy; or
2   decreasing myocardial oxygen demand, e.g. by
    - mechanical myocardial support
    - cardiac depressant drugs to reduce cardiac workload
    - retarding inflammation at the infarct site.

Timing of interventions

Myocardial salvage may be impossible after several hours in those patients with abrupt, total occlusion, no collateral function or a high myocardial oxygen demand, but may be potentially possible after more than 6 h in patients with good collateral function, intermittent occlusion, a slow heart rate or a low blood pressure at the time of coronary occlusion (Pepine 1989).

Pharmacological interventions

Pharmacological interventions commonly include:

- thrombolytic agents
- beta-blockers
- nitrates.

Restoring coronary flow and myocardial tissue reperfusion

The primary aim in limiting infarct size is rapid recanalization of the occluded coronary arteries. In the vast majority of cases the occlusion is caused by coronary thrombosis, which usually occurs at the site of a ruptured atheromatous plaque.

For patients with the clinical presentation of myocardial infarction with persistent ST-segment elevation or new or presumed left bundle-branch block, early pharmacological or mechanical reperfusion should be performed unless there are clear contraindications.

Thrombolytic therapy

Thrombolytic therapy, also referred to as fibrinolytic therapy, is probably the single most important advance in coronary care since defibrillation. The aim of thrombolysis is to induce dissolution of the thrombus, establish recanalization and provide subsequent reperfusion to the ischaemic zone. Most thrombolytic agents activate plasminogen to form plasmin which degrades fibrin and breaks down fresh thrombus.

Acute myocardial infarction is a dynamic process, with necrosis occurring first in the subendocardial layer and spreading to the subepicardial layer as it evolves to a transmural infarction. Necrosis of the ischaemic myocardium is virtually complete within 6 h of coronary occlusion. Therefore, this time span seems to be the critical period in which to intervene to prevent necrosis and attempt reperfusion with the aim of salvaging the maximum amount of jeopardized myocardium. Optimal benefit results when thrombolysis restores patency promptly and persistently. Improved left ventricular function and survival are most marked when thrombolysis is instituted early after the start of symptoms. The fibrinolytic overview (Fibrinolytic Therapy Trialists' (FTT) Collaborative Group 1994) reported a progressive decrease of about 1.6 deaths per hour of delay per 1000 patients treated. It has been estimated that for every 1000 patients receiving thrombolysis within the first hour, 65 lives could be saved (Boersma et al 1996). It has been suggested that the most appropriate place for thrombolysis is the patients' home (Rawles 1997) and it may be given prior to hospital by the GP or an ambulance paramedic. The National Service Framework for CHD (DoH 2000) set a standard that 75% of A&E departments should be able to provide early thrombolysis.

Thrombolytic agents have no effect on the cause of thrombus formation or on underlying atherosclerosis and patients with underlying coronary stenosis may require PCI with either percutaneous transluminal coronary angioplasty (PTCA), stenting or surgical revascularization (coronary artery bypass surgery).

The thrombolytic agents currently available in the UK are streptokinase, alteplase (rt-PA), reteplase and tenecteplase.

Streptokinase is the most extensively tested and least expensive thrombolytic agent. It is a bacterial protein that combines with circulating plasminogen, and this complex converts additional circulating plasminogen to the proteolytic enzyme plasmin which brings about dissolution of the fibrin clot. Plasmin is also able to degrade fibrinogen and clotting factors V and VIII. Thus, the action of streptokinase results in a systemic lytic state that is characterized by low levels of circulating fibrinogen and plasminogen and high levels of fibrinogen degradation products. This predisposes to systemic bleeding as a complication of streptokinase therapy. Other problems include hypotension.

Streptokinase is usually only given on one occasion. This is due to antibody production to the first dose which builds up over a 5-day period following initial administration. A subsequent dose would therefore be ineffective.

Alteplase (rtPA) is a naturally occurring protein which has a greater clot specificity than streptokinase, thus fibrinogen and alpha-2 antiplasmin concentrations are less likely to become depleted and systemic bleeding is less likely. Cloning of the rtPA gene has provided large amounts of the drug for clinical use. The drug is usually given by a bolus. Accelerated rtPA is given as a 15 mg bolus followed by 50 mg over 30 minutes and the remainder over an hour. Protocols for thrombolysis vary, but alteplase is often used for treating anterior myocardial infarctions based on the results of the GUSTO-1 (1993) trial. Presentation with a low blood pressure is a further indication to use alteplase as it is less likely to decrease blood pressure further.

Thrombolytic therapy should not be given to those in whom the infarction has been established for more than 12 hours unless there is evidence of ongoing ischaemia with ECG criteria for thrombolysis.

Choice of agent will depend on an individual assessment of risk and benefit and on factors such as availability and cost. Practically, the best form of thrombolytic drug to give is one that can be given in the form of a bolus. This is likely to facilitate more rapid treatment both in and out of hospital and reduce the risk of medication errors. Tenecteplase and reteplase are both given as a bolus.

Contraindications

Table 6.2 gives contraindications for thrombolysis.

Patient selection

Nurses are in a key position to identify potential candidates for thrombolytic therapy within the

---

Table 6.2   Contraindications to thrombolytic therapy

Absolute contraindications
   Haemorrhagic stroke or stroke of unknown origin
      at any time
   Ischaemic stroke in preceding 6 months
   Central nervous system damage or neoplasms
   Recent major trauma/surgery/head injury (within
      preceding 3 weeks)
   Gastrointestinal bleeding within the last month
   Known bleeding disorder
   Aortic dissection

Relative contraindications
   Transient ischaemic attack in preceding 6 months
   Oral anticoagulant therapy
   Pregnancy or within 1 week post partum
   Non-compressible punctures
   Traumatic resuscitation
   Refractory hypertension (systolic blood
      pressure >180 mmHg)
   Advanced liver disease
   Infective endocarditis
   Active peptic ulcer

---

critical time period necessary for successful outcome. They have a role in educating prospective patients and relatives to recognize the early warning signs of myocardial infarction and stressing the importance of seeking immediate medical attention. Nurses also have a responsibility to help colleagues to keep up to date with the developments in thrombolytic therapy, including guidelines for its use and contraindications.

Possible candidates for thrombolytic therapy include patients with recent onset of chest pain of at least 20 min duration, but usually not longer than 6 h, that is not relieved by sublingual GTN. Patients need to have electrocardiographic changes reflecting definite acute myocardial injury, i.e. persistent ST-segment elevation of at least 0.1 mV in at least two contiguous leads or new or presumed new left bundle branch block. It is worth noting that posterior infarction may present with ST depression with prominent R wave in leads V_1 to V_2.

Although there is some controversy over the benefits of thrombolysis in the elderly (Thieman et al 2000), age should not be an exclusion criteria as the risk benefit ratio is probably in favour of treatment (Savage and Channer 2002).

Nurse-led and nurse-initiated thrombolysis

Nurses are often the first hospital staff to come into contact with the patient and there is evidence that experienced nurses can identify patients suitable for thrombolysis (Quinn 1995, Quinn et al 1998). Several authors have highlighted that nurse involvement in thrombolysis reduces the door to needle time (Caunt 1995, Hughes et al 1997). Currently in practice, nursing input tends to involve the nurse assessing patient suitability and then the actual prescribing of the thrombolytic is undertaken by the physician. However, nurse *initiated* thrombolysis is being developed in many areas, particularly A&E departments. Nurses are able to make a rapid assessment of the patient, interpret the ECG, and if appropriate administer thrombolysis against an agreed patient group direction before medical examination takes place (Wilmhurst 1999). There are guidelines for developing patient group directions (Royal College of Nursing 2000) which need to be developed by the multidisciplinary team and reviewed regularly. There are no educational pre-requirements for those planning to work with a patient group direction, but many trusts undertake some assessment of competency. If nurses can enhance patient assessment and expedite appropriate treatment then this has obvious benefits for all patients presenting with possible cardiac chest pain. However, the role should not be taken on lightly. Thrombolysis has potentially serious side effects and may do more harm than good if given inappropriately. While the employing trust is likely to assume vicarious liability, nurses taking on the role need to be prepared for the inevitable side effects associated with thrombolysis (Rhodes 1998). It has been argued that having a small nucleus of 'thrombolysis nurses' may lead to medical staff and other nurses becoming de-skilled and, if the service is not available 24 hours a day, that there will be inequalities in the service provided (Quinn and Morse 2000).

Complications

Possible complications that occur with thrombolysis are given below:

1 *Bleeding episodes*. The most frequent bleeding sites are at venous and arterial puncture sites. Haematuria is a frequent occurrence, whereas bleeding from recent cuts and abrasions and gingival bleeding are less common. The patient is usually monitored for signs of hypotension associated with internal bleeding, and needs to be advised about reporting any bleeding episodes and to avoid activities likely to result in cutting or bruising himself. Treatment will be stopped if bleeding is considered to be life-threatening. Interventions that need to gain venous access such as temporary pacing or haemodynamic monitoring need to make use of the antecubital fossa or the femoral vein to limit bleeding. Major intracranial haemorrhage complicates between 0.2 and 1% of cases and half of these will be fatal. Major systemic haemorrhage affects about 7 patients in every 1000 treated.

2 *Reperfusion arrhythmias*. Arrhythmias occur frequently with reperfusion, particularly with streptokinase and are not regarded as complications as such unless causing haemodynamic disturbances. Accelerated idioventricular rhythm is common, particularly with reperfusion of the left anterior descending coronary artery (anterior myocardial infarction). Sinus bradycardia, asystole and AV block are more frequent with reperfusion of the right coronary artery (inferior myocardial infarction).

3 *Allergic reactions*. The allergic reaction associated with streptokinase may incorporate fever, dry rash and anaphylaxis. Therefore, the patient needs to be closely observed following treatment.

4 *Hypotension*. This is particularly common with streptokinase and should be managed by temporarily stopping the thrombolysis infusion and lying the patient flat. Occasionally atropine may be required.

Reperfusion

Reperfusion after coronary thrombosis is a phenomenon that occurs naturally in many patients with myocardial infarction, but it tends to occur too late to confer immediate benefit. Thrombolytic agents are capable of achieving reperfusion within about 90 min of the start of treatment in vessels that would not otherwise have opened. Signs and symptoms of reperfusion usually develop within 30–60 min and may include:

- abrupt cessation of chest pain
- improved left ventricular function
- reperfusion arrhythmias or conduction disturbances
- resolution of ST-segment elevation
- characteristic release pattern of cardiac markers.

ST segment resolution has been found to correlate well with 30-day outcome (INJECT 1995). However, there is debate over which ECG leads to use and the timing after thrombolysis. In using the lead with the most significant ST elevation on admission, failed reperfusion has been defined as a less than 50% resolution of the ST segment elevation one hour after the initiation of treatment (Sutton et al 2000). Full restoration of coronary blood flow fails in up to 75% of cases and this is associated with a mortality of between 16 and 20% (de Belder 2001).

Coronary angiography is the most accurate method of assessment of reperfusion, as it can accurately assess epicardial coronary blood flow. However, many hospitals do not have direct and early access to catheterization facilities.

Management following failed thrombolysis

If reperfusion does not occur then the options are:

- further thrombolysis – there is limited evidence that this is effective
- rescue angioplasty – this incurs an increased risk of bleeding associated with glycoprotein IIb/IIIa inhibitors
- emergency coronary artery bypass surgery – this is more risky than angioplasty.

ANTI-THROMBIN THERAPY

Intracoronary thrombus is made up of fibrin and platelets. Thrombus breakdown can be facilitated by inhibition of thrombin, fibrinolytic drugs and anti-platelet agents.

Aspirin

Aspirin is an anti-platelet drug that acts inside the platelets and irreversibly blocks the production of thromboxane A2 from arachidonic acid. This results in a reduction (but not absolute prevention) of the platelets' tendency for aggregation for the lifespan of the platelet, which is 7 days. Aspirin reduces death and progression to myocardial infarction in patients with unstable angina by 36%. A low daily dose of 75 mg should be given as soon as the diagnosis of unstable angina has been made. It can be chewed, or dissolved in water to aid absorption.

Aspirin adds benefits when given alongside thrombolysis in acute myocardial infarction (ISIS-2 1988) and also been shown to produce about a 25% reduction in reinfarction and death when given to post-myocardial infarction patients (Antithrombotic Trialists Collaboration 2002). An initial dose of 300 mg is given, followed by a daily dose of 75 mg. Aspirin may occasionally trigger bronchospasm in asthmatics and it should not be given to those with known hypersensitivity, bleeding peptic ulcer, blood dyscrasia or severe hepatic disease.

Clopidogrel

Clopidogrel helps prevent platelet aggregation by inhibiting the expression of the GP IIb/IIIa inhibitor. It can be used as an alternative to aspirin (CAPRIE Steering Committee 1996). It has been shown that if clopidogrel is given with aspirin in unstable angina, then the risk of subsequent myocardial infarction and recurrent ischaemia is significantly reduced (CURE investigators 2001). Both drugs need to be started as soon as a diagnosis is made and continued for at least 9 months.

Heparin

Heparin is a naturally occurring polysaccharide which exerts its anticoagulant action by combining with antithrombin III. This complex, in the presence of thrombin, forms a reversible combination in which thrombin is inactivated and activated coagulation factors are blocked. Heparin prevents the initiation as well as the propagation of thrombi. Both intravenous unfractionated heparin and subcutaneous low molecular weight heparin (LMWH) are effective in reducing the risk of thrombus formation. Heparin also forms part of some post-thrombolysis regimens (de Bono et al 1992).

The LMWHs licensed in the UK are certoparin, dalteparin (Fragmin), enoxiparin and tizaparin. They have the advantage of having a more predictable anticoagulant effect than unfractionated heparin intravenous infusions. They are also easier to administer and do not require anticoagulation monitoring. They have also been shown to be superior in reducing mortality and serious ischaemic cardiac events (Cohen et al 1997, Antman et al 1999). LMWH is of greatest benefit in those with positive troponins and should be given for at least 2 days if there is recurrent ischaemia. In patients at particularly high risk, LMWH needs to be continued until the time of angiography or, if revascularization is not an option, for a period of not less than 2 weeks (Wallentin et al 2000).

Patients with myocardial infarction have an approximate 10–40% risk of developing deep vein thrombosis and a 1% risk of developing fatal pulmonary embolism. Low-molecular weight heparin should be given to all patients with myocardial infarction from admission until they are fully mobile

- to prevent or treat deep vein thrombosis and pulmonary embolism (less common due to early mobilization)
- to prevent or treat thromboembolism from the left side of the heart, mostly seen in large anterior infarcts, atrial fibrillation or ventricular aneurysm
- possibly to limit infarct size.

Full anticoagulation with heparin followed by warfarin, or prolonged subcutaneous high dose heparin is recommended in patients at increased risk of thromboembolic complications, including extensive anterior myocardial infarction, prolonged cardiac failure, atrial fibrillation, cardiogenic shock, left ventricular aneurysm and inability to mobilize.

Warfarin

As described above, warfarin should be used for anticogulation of selected high-risk patients post-myocardial infarction. Warfarin produces a deficiency in clotting factors II, VII, IX and X. It is not effective for 36–48 h and is therefore commenced during heparinization. Oral anticoagulation is monitored by prothrombin time (PT) estimation, expressed in terms of International Normalized Ratio (INR), essentially equivalent to the British Corrected Ratio (BCR). This ratio should be kept between 2 and 4.5, the higher end of the scale for those patients who are at greatest risk. Warfarin can interact with other drugs such as barbiturates, phenylbutazone, amiodarone and cimetidine. Bleeding is quite common, and vitamin K is used in severe cases. The patient receiving warfarin therapy at home should be advised to observe for bleeding gums, bruises and the presence of blood in the urine, stool and mucosa. They should also be advised to inform their doctor and dentist that they are taking warfarin, in case any interacting medications are prescribed; to avoid excessive alcohol intake; and of the need for frequent blood tests to monitor response to therapy.

Glycoprotein IIb/IIIa inhibitors

Glycoprotein IIb/IIIa receptors are found on the surface of the platelet. Platelets become activated by the release of various chemical messengers following endothelial damage and the receptors bind with fibrinogen molecules to form crosslinks with other activated platelets. A mesh of platelets rapidly forms. Inactivating the glycoprotein IIb/IIIa receptor blocks the final common pathway in platelet aggregation and therefore prevents the propagation of clots.

The guidelines on the use of glycoprotein IIb/IIIa inhibitors produced by the National Institute for Clinical Excellence (2002b) recommend that they should be considered part of the management pathway for unstable angina or NSTEMI, particularly those at risk of subsequent myocardial infarction and sudden death. Their use is also advocated as an adjuct to PCI, particularly for those patients with diabetes and in complicated procedures. The three glycoprotein IIb/IIIa inhibitors in widespread use are abciximab, eptifibatide and tirofiban. Abciximab is currently licensed for use in the context of PCI. It has a short plasma half life (30 minutes) but longer duration of action once bound to platelets and takes about 48 hours for platelet function to recover. Eptifibatide and tirofiban are licensed for the medical stabilization of unstable angina or NSTEMI. They are small molecules with very short half lives, necessitating prolonged or repeated infusions.

MECHANICAL INTERVENTIONS

Mechanical interventions in myocardial infarction

A major drawback with thrombolytic therapy is that, although clots are lysed, thrombolytic agents have no effect on the underlying cause of thrombus formation. At least 80–90% of patients are estimated to have an underlying high-grade stenosis that may require mechanical recanalization. Other mechanical devices offer support to the work of the heart.

Mechanical interventions include:

- percutaneous transluminal coronary angioplasty (PTCA) and/or stenting
- coronary artery bypass graft (CABG) surgery
- intra-aortic balloon counterpulsation
- ventricular assist devices.

Percutaneous coronary interventions (PCI)

The role of PCIs during the early hours of myocardial infarction can be subdivided into:

- primary PCI
- facilitated PCI
- rescue PCI.

Primary PCI is defined as angioplasty and/or stenting without prior or concomitant pharmocological thrombolysis. It is effective in achieving and maintaining coronary artery patency and avoids the risk of bleeding associated with pharmacological thrombolysis. The Task Force on the management of acute myocardial infarction of the European Society of Cardiology (Van de Werf et al 2003) reports that clinical trials have shown that primary angioplasty produces more effective reperfusion, less reocclusion, improved residual left ventricular function and better clinical outcome. Despite conflicting evidence of long-term benefits, primary PCI is the preferred option if it can be performed within 90 minutes after the first medical contact (Van de Werf 2003). It is not carried out routinely as it requires an experienced team and the necessary facilities. If a patient is admitted to a hospital without such facilities then it is recommended that a careful assessment is made of the patient's suitability for transfer to a tertiary centre for mechanical intervention. Primary PCI has been shown to be superior to hospital thrombolysis (within 3 hours of symptom onset) and is still regarded as an 'excellent' reperfusion strategy (Cucherat et al 2004).

Facilitated PCI describes a combined pharmacological and mechanical approach whereby the patient with acute myocardial infarction receives thrombolytic therapy with or without additional glycoprotein IIb/IIIa inhibitors, and is transferred for prompt angioplasty/stenting PCI (Dalby and Montalescot 2002).

Rescue PCI is PCI performed on a coronary artery which remains occluded after pharmacological

thrombolytic therapy. There is evidence that this can bring clinical benefit if the infarct-related artery can be recanalized at angiography (Ellis et al 1994) and that patients can be transferred to a tertiary centre for this intervention safely (Vermeer et al 1999).

Other candidates for mechanical reperfusion include those with evidence of continuing extensive ischaemia or symptoms that persist despite optimal medical therapy (DoH 2000). Some patients may be referred for prognostic reasons. The number of coronary revascularization procedures carried out in the UK has increased substantially in recent years. The amount of CABGs has almost doubled over the past 10 years with nearly 30 000 operations now being carried out each year. The number of PTCAs performed annually has increased at an even faster rate with around 40 000 being carried out each year (BHF 2003).

Percutaneous transluminal coronary angioplasty

PTCA is a well-established method of myocardial revascularization for alleviating symptoms and improving prognosis. The technique involves the introduction of a thin double-lumen balloon catheter into the coronary artery to the site of a coronary stenosis which is inflated there. This process produces clefts in the atheromatous lesion, compression and redistribution of its contents, endothelial desquamation and stretching of the media. In most cases, this results in a substantial increase in the arterial lumen.

PTCA, for the appropriate patient, compares favourably as an alternative treatment to CABG surgery in terms of risk, success rate and cost. The mortality rate for first-time angioplasty is less than 1%. Further advantages of PTCA are decreased length of hospital stay and the fact that neither a general anaesthetic nor thoracotomy are required. PTCA is particularly applicable for patients in whom CABG is not feasible or carries relatively increased risk. For instance, elderly patients with unstable or refractory angina can be treated with acceptable results.

Patients with occluded coronary arteries may be treated with PTCA, although the success rates are not as impressive as those in patients with patent but stenosed vessels. Patients with multiple coronary vessel disease are now contributing to a greater proportion of candidates suitable for PTCA. However, it is unclear whether PTCA should be used in an attempt to treat all coronary obstructions in patients with multivessel disease. For example, CABG may be more appropriate for patients with triple-vessel disease, as it has been shown to exert prognostic benefit in addition to symptom relief. The main problem with PTCA was restenosis that followed up to 50% of procedures. But this has been improved considerably by the widespread use of stents.

Stents

Coronary artery stents are small mesh cylinders placed in the arteries at the time of angioplasty. They help by increasing the vessel lumen, sealing dissections and tagging the intimal flap between the stent and the arterial wall. Threatened or abrupt vessel closure following angioplasty is the best indication for stenting. Although stents have addressed the problem of arterial recoil, they have not prevented in-stent stenosis, which affects about a quarter of cases. Repeat PTCA is the most usual way of clearing in-stent stenosis.

A logical approach to reducing restenosis and maintaining arterial patency is to use drugs that interfere with the process of restenosis. Coating stents with these drugs allows local drug delivery and these eluting stents have demonstrated a dramatic reduction in coronary restenosis (Morris et al 2002).

The success of PTCA largely depends on the nurse who is aware of the patient's specific needs in undergoing the procedure, aware of the potential complications and sufficiently skilled to minimize all risk to the patient. The importance of notifying the nurse of any chest pain or discomfort during or following the procedure should be stressed, so that immediate relief can be given. Mild chest discomfort is common immediately after PTCA, but should subside over the first couple of hours.

Sheaths should not be removed until the activated clotting time (ACT) is within the prescribed protocol range, to prevent haemorrhage and haematoma formation. The patient will generally stay in hospital for 24 hours with a PTCA procedure but this depends on presenting symptoms. The patient is usually routinely attached to a cardiac monitor for 24 hours and any arrhythmias noted and treated where necessary. Peripheral pulses are frequently checked for occlusive thrombus at the insertion site.

Laser-assisted angioplasty and atherectomy

Atherectomy involves cutting way the deposits inside the coronary artery. It is particularly useful for hard calcified lesions but cannot be used if there is an active thrombus. Directional atherectomy removes atherosclerotic plaques with a cylindrical rotating cup-shaped blade, the ablated tissue being collected in a chamber in the catheter nose. PTCA is carried out after the atherectomy. Rotational atherectomy drills into the plaque using a diamond-shaped burr. Laser assisted angioplasty uses ultraviolet, pulsed laser beams to ablate the plaque by vaporizing the tissue and disrupting the plaque with mechanical shockwaves. This method is particularly useful in completely blocked arteries. PTCA is performed once there is an adequate lumen diameter.

Coronary artery bypass grafting

Historically, coronary artery bypass surgery was performed 2–3 months after infarction in an attempt to prevent reinfarction. Now the possible benefit of surgical revascularization within a few hours of the onset of chest pain has been studied and it may be indicated when angioplasty has failed, there has been sudden coronary artery occlusion, or on selected patients with cardiogenic shock (Van de Werf et al 2003).

Mortality rates from CABG surgery in acute infarction are affected by the extent of necrosis at the time of operation. The earlier the bypass surgery is performed, the lower the mortality rate and the larger the area of functional myocardium. DeWood and Berg (1987) showed that when CABG surgery is performed within 6 h of the onset of chest pain, both postoperative and long-term mortality rates are lower for the acute coronary patient.

CABG is a surgical technique in which an occluded or stenosed section of a coronary artery is bypassed using part of a vein or an artery from elsewhere in the body. Most commonly the long saphenous vein is used, although increasingly the internal mammary artery is being considered. Without antithrombotic therapy, a quarter of grafts will be occluded at one year, and mortality is closely related to graft patency. About 90% of vein grafts are occluded after 10 years and, thus, arterial grafts are now used routinely to promote long-term patency. Improved patient survival is evident in patients with left internal mammary artery grafts, either alone, or in association with saphenous vein grafts. Use of the bilateral internal mammary artery grafts appears to be safe, with less postoperative angina, fewer re-operations and better long-term results (Patil et al 2001).

CABG surgery is a palliative, not a curative intervention and is only feasible if the risk of the operation is less than continuing with medical therapy. Thus, age, diabetes and hypertension, as well as the general condition of the patient, in particular the efficiency of functional myocardium, need to be assessed. Bypass operations are costly and time consuming and they do not halt the progression of the underlying atherosclerotic process.

Bypass surgery is a potentially traumatic event, and patients who undergo this operation as a planned event will need careful and thoughtful preparation, assistance with recovery and preparation for discharge home. It is probable that the benefits of surgery could be substantially increased by provision of better facilities, including simple individually planned preparation and rehabilitation. Informed written consent will need to be obtained and the nurse should address any worries and misconceptions that the patient and family may have. A visit to the operating theatre and recovery room, including an inspection of relevant equipment and an introduction to the staff, may be helpful for some patients to cope with impending surgery.

Fulfilling informational needs is an important factor in assisting recovery and reducing anxiety. The provision of education that is tailored to individual needs and incorporates information and psychosocial support helps patients to cope with their illness and recovery. Such education should take account of beliefs, risk perception and emotional resistance. Patients seem to be mostly interested in short-term, practical information (van Weert et al 2003). A nurse-coordinated or interdisciplinary preoperative education programme is likely to be the best way of fulfilling the needs of this group of patients.

Patients are likely to remember their arrival in the intensive care unit and need to be prepared for the environment facing them on regaining consciousness. They need to know that they should expect initially to have an endotracheal tube, which will prevent them from talking, and they need to be prepared for the chest drains, intravenous infusions, arterial lines, urinary catheter, cardiac monitoring and possibly a nasogastric tube. The patients' family also need to be prepared for what to expect when they first see them after surgery. Patients need to be taught breathing exercises to ensure optimum lung expansion and oxygenation postoperatively, together with teaching about coughing and leg exercises.

Angiography will be performed on all prospective candidates for coronary artery bypass graft surgery in order to demonstrate the state of the vessels.

During surgery, the heart is exposed by median sternotomy, the aorta clamped off and extracorporeal cardiopulmonary bypass maintained via cannulae in the atria and ascending aorta. The body temperature is reduced to about 26°C and cardiac arrest induced with a cardioplegic solution. The heart can be stopped for up to 2 hours to allow anastomoses. The left internal mammary is mobilized from the chest wall and directly grafted onto the left anterior descending coronary artery. While this is happening, the long saphenous vein is stripped from the leg, flushed with heparinized blood and checked for leaks. The distal ends of the bypass vein grafts are sutured to as many vessels as require it. The aorta is then unclamped, the patient is rewarmed and normal cardiac rhythm re-established by defibrillation. The proximal ends of the grafts are sutured to the ascending aorta, cardiopulmonary bypass is stopped, the cannulae removed and the chest closed.

Patients are normally ventilated until haemodynamically stable. An arterial line and pulmonary artery flotation catheter will be used to monitor intracardiac pressures for the first 24h. Patients are mobilized quickly and are often fit for discharge within a week. The majority are able to return to work between 2 and 6 months after the operation. Aspirin must be started (preferably within 6 hours of surgery) because benefits of graft patency are lost when begun later. This should be continued indefinitely. Dressings on the chest and graft sites need to be checked regularly for excessive bleeding and haematoma formation. Elastic stockings are often used to reduce venous stasis and the risk of thromboembolic complications.

In most centres, the overall mortality is less than 3%. The most important complications are neurological caused by hypoxia, hypoperfusion, haemorrhage or metabolic problems. Perioperative stroke is a possible complication and the patient needs to be warned of this before surgery. Temporary impairment of concentration or memory is common, affecting up to half of patients in the first 6 weeks, but possibly persisting for many months afterwards (Newman et al 2001). The most common problem following bypass surgery is arrhythmias, most of a benign supraventricular nature. Perioperative myocardial infarction is a risk factor for premature death. Renal dysfunction is also a problem. Pain from the sternotomy can cause discomfort for a few weeks, as can pain around the long incision made for removing the saphenous vein. Mediastinitis from deep wound infections is more frequent where arterial grafts are used and can result in a high mortality.

Due to the increased trend for early discharge, planning for care at home becomes crucial in promoting optimum recovery. Patients need to know what to expect in terms of recovery at home, including expected symptoms and having realistic goals and expectations. Short-term anxiety and depression following bypass surgery can occur in as many as half of patients. Long-term psychological problems are less common, and patients with long-term psychiatric complications could possibly be identified prior to surgery and given extra support. There is some evidence that somatic factors lead to anxiety and depression in the preoperative period, whereas anxiety and depression lead to somatic factors in the postoperative period (Duits et al 2002).

Intra-aortic balloon counterpulsation

Although traditionally used for ventricular failure after cardiac surgery and cardiogenic shock after myocardial infarction, there have been limited clinical studies validating the benefits of intra-aortic balloon counterpulsation in the acute coronary patient. Prompt intervention may halt the progress of myocardial necrosis in the patient who is unresponsive to routine medical therapy.

Ventricular assist devices

These forms of mechanical intervention support systemic circulation, allow recovery of cardiac function, increase myocardial oxygen supply and reduce myocardial workload. Theoretically, they may be of use in limiting infarct size, but there is not sufficient evidence available to determine if their benefits outweigh their risks.

ANGIOTENSIN-CONVERTING ENZYME (ACE) INHIBITORS

Angiotensin II is a powerful vasoconstrictor that increases the afterload to the heart and stimulates aldosterone production. Angiotensin-converting enzyme (ACE) inhibitors prevent the production of angiotensin II thereby limiting vasoconstriction. A reduction in aldosterone decreases renal sodium reabsorption in the kidney and thus reduces the fluid load within the patient and the work of the heart.

ACE inhibitors have been shown to reduce mortality after acute myocardial infarction with residual impaired left ventricular function (Pfeffer et al 1992) and there is a case for administering ACE inhibitors to all patients with acute infarction on admission, providing there are no contraindications (Van de Werf et al 2003). There is evidence that the benefits of ACE administration in myocardial infarction are continued for at least 4–5 years, even in the absence of left ventricular dysfunction (Yusuf et al 2000).

A patient taking an ACE inhibitor needs to be started on a small dose and this dose then titrated. Patients will need monitoring for hepatic impairment as most ACE inhibitors (except captopril and lisinopril) are metabolized to more potent metabolites as they pass through the liver. Patients with renal failure may also need dose adjustments. Patients may complain of a dry cough and may benefit from a change in the ACE they are being prescribed.

MEETING BASIC NEEDS

Meeting basic needs of the patient, such as comfort, rest, sleep and elimination, is an essential and fundamental component of nursing intervention. Some of these needs will require immediate attention, whereas others may be postponed for a few days, although the nurse will need to anticipate them.

The acute coronary patient often feels stressed and anxious due to uncertainty and fear of outcome, loss of control, pain and lack of rest and sleep. The heart attack poses various threats for the patient and family which may be temporary or permanent in nature, including altered body image and self-image, as well as loss in terms of status in family, work and social circumstances, income and physical and psychological functioning. Patients also perceive a very real threat to their lives (Jaarsma et al 1995). The responses to these threats include a variety of crises, defences and coping behaviours. Personal beliefs, attitudes, values, responsibilities and experiences of the patient will influence how he perceives and responds to the heart attack. Cardiac patients have been shown to consider nursing competency, being taught about their illness and a human-centred approach to care as being most important to their care (Gay 1999). They have also been shown to feel reassured and secure when they perceive that the nurse caring for them is viligant and capable (Hunt 1999).

Nursing roles are becoming more complex and there is a real danger that basic patient needs such as comfort, dignity and psychological support get lost amidst technology and more medical aspects of care in the nursing role (Quinn and Thompson 1995).

PATIENT ADVOCACY

Patients who are unwell, anxious and away from their usual support networks are vulnerable. Medical culture, with its scientific expertise, technology and bureaucracy can make patients feel that they have surrendered their independence to the institutional care system resulting in a sense of loss of control. Nurses are ideally placed to be an advocate for the patient who may not understand the complexity of treatment options or be able to articulate their needs. This needs to be done in a manner that it is in the best interest of the patient who will be in an unfamiliar situation, and not just to give the nurse more power (Hewitt 2000). Nurses need to keep involved and up to date with their patients' care so that they can best contribute and expand upon the decision-making processes that occur, often briefly, on the ward round and at other times.

PATIENT INVOLVEMENT IN CARE

Patient advocacy is linked to patient involvement in care. Since the late 1980s patients have increasingly been invited to be involved in their care both at an individual and an organizational level (DoH 1989). The concept of patient participation has become widely accepted as a means of enhancing decision making, human dignity and enriching quality of life and patients are assuming more responsibility for the prevention, detection and treatment of health problems. Patient participation is an active process which involves the patient being involved in the decision-making process and goal setting.

The nurse needs to work with the patient to assess if, how and when they get involved in their own care. Some patients may not wish to be active in their care until the acute phase of their admission is over and it may not be appropriate for them to do so until then. Others may wish to remain passive recipients of care throughout their entire admission but may reluctantly comply with such an approach as they feel it is expected of them (Waterworth and Luker 1990).

SELF-CARE

Patients may be able to perform basic activities of living, including physical care, unaided if they are haemodynamically stable. They may also be involved in self-medication (Cahil 1998), although this may be inappropriate in the early stages when medication regimens are frequently changed and do not reflect what the patient will be prescribed long term, it may be appropriate towards the end of the patients' hospital stay. Self-medication has been shown to produce increased patient satisfaction and help enhance knowledge and compliance (Furlong 1996, Deeks and Byatt 2000).

Self-care forms one of the patient focused benchmarking frameworks designed to ensure quality patient care (DoH 2001). Important considerations for self-care include:

- patients being enabled to make choices about their self-care and these choices being respected
- continuous assessment of patients' self-care abilities
- risks for the patient undertaking self-care are assessed (e.g. risk of falling)
- patients have the knowledge to undertake self-care.

There is usually no reason why the haemodynamically stable patient cannot wash, eat and shave himself. In fact, it is likely that there is a danger of more stress resulting from not being allowed to do such activities than the actual performance of them. They may need some assistance if they are severely restricted by equipment such as short monitor cables, intravenous infusions and pacemakers, or if he is feeling weak or generally ill. The nurse should, in any case, offer to assist as the patient may feel unable to ask. If the patient is bedfast, then everything they need should be within easy reach.

PRIVACY AND DIGNITY

CCUs and ward areas are often areas where the patient may feel exposed and vulnerable. Having to use a bedside commode, having personal information broadcast on ward rounds and over the telephone and being unwell surrounded by strangers may cause distress. Bedside curtains offer less privacy than rooms with walls, particularly if they are not closed adequately.

Patient data are collected from many sources and widely disseminated both physically and electronically which has serious implications for patient confidentiality. While strategies are being implemented to limit the risks of breaches in confidentialty and each Trust now has a Caldicott Guardian (DoH 1997) to facilitate the process, it is the responsibility of the nurse to maintain individual patient confidentiality.

The Nursing and Midwifery Council (2002) states that nurses are professionally responsible for ensuring the promotion and protection of patient dignity, irrespective of the patient's gender, age, race, ability, sexuality, economic status, lifestyle, culture and religious and political beliefs. Dignity has been defined as ' being worthy of respect' and patients need to receive care that is focused upon respect for the individual, where they feel they matter all of the time (DoH 2001). A focus on emergency treatment and technological care is not an excuse for any patient to feel depersonalized or downgraded.

PATIENT ENVIRONMENT

The patient environment and immediate surroundings may influence the patient's sense of well-being and recovery. Patients who evaluate their environment as restful, clean, comfortable and quiet have been found to have a more positive outcome after a myocardial infarction than those who do not (Proctor et al 1996). A patient cared for in a side ward may have the benefit of privacy and quiet, but may suffer from social isolation. The patient out in an open ward lacks privacy and has to suffer in front of others but is able to talk to other patients, feel more involved in events and always knows the whereabouts of the nurse. Maintaining a safe environment depends on the nurse controlling lighting, noise, temperature, as well as less obvious but important considerations, such as asepsis during invasive procedures, ensuring adequate lengths of monitor cable and intravenous extension lines to allow safe patient movement and checking for and removing faulty electrical equipment.

COMMUNICATION

For nursing intervention to be effective, communication between the nurse, patient, family and other personnel has to be effective. The nurse is primarily involved in a caring role and an essential component of this is communication. Communication can take many forms: structured, informal, verbal or non-verbal, and tends to be a continuous process in situations where individuals are functioning within the same environment. Patient education, reduction of anxiety and contact at the bedside, while performing physical and technical activities, are all forms of communication between the nurse and patient.

The nurse is in a unique position where they have 24-hour patient contact, and the patient tends to look to them as a source of communication. It has been known for many years that the acute coronary patient often perceives the nurse to be the single most important factor in their care (Cassem et al 1970) and that the type of communication they receive can influence recovery and well-being (Garrity and Klein 1975). This is even more likely to be the case in an increasingly technological environment where patient stays are shorter and interventions more complex.

The nature of communication

The coronary patient is usually brought suddenly into an unfamiliar environment where they are no longer in control of their lives and events and have to accept a submissive role. One study examining the relationship between nurses and patients who had suffered a myocardial infarction concluded that the nurses sometimes found patients difficult to understand, particularly as patients often distanced themselves from what was happening to them (Svedlund et al 1999). However, other patients tended to appear to want to show their vulnerability to nurses and appeared to be actively seeking support. Effective communication should aim to retain the patient's individuality, and work with them to produce positive adaptation and coping mechanisms.

Communication has many components, including listening, reinforcing, encouraging, questioning, responding and giving information. This involves the nurse showing presence, perception, caring, acceptance, empathy, authenticity and respect.

The personality of both the nurse and the patient are ingredients contributing to the success or failure of communication. The nurse–patient relationship is an important factor in the ability of the nurse to contribute to patient well-being, and there needs to be a relationship of trust where the patient is valued as an individual. There is a real danger of patients becoming stereotyped, with individuals being attributed characteristics considered typical of their most prominent sociological feature. The Asian patient, the female patient and the middle-aged business executive all have individual needs. Patients who ask a lot of questions or do not conform with the stereotype image have

been shown to be considered unpopular by nurses (Stockwell 1972), yet it is sometimes those patients who are most likely to need the most support who are least likely to receive it. The 'model' patient is seen as being required to be uncritical, submissive and appreciative of his care. The patient who does not fit this mould may receive less nursing contact. Patients who are unable to communicate in English may also miss out on the social aspects of communication and have limited nurse contact only to carry out observations and interventions. This can mean that it is difficult to get to know the patient as an individual and this may have consequences for providing rehabilitation and support (Webster 1997).

Initially, the emphasis in communicating with the coronary patient and family is placed on conveying empathy and support and beginning to give information. More structured counselling and education should occur at a later stage. Patients are notoriously difficult at retaining information (Ley 1988) and the problem is compounded by the effects of high anxiety, pain and analgesia during the first hours following admission. The nurse needs to work with the patient and family to ensure that they are aware of the objectives of care, understand the procedures and management plan and develop a realistic outlook for the future. There is certainly a need to be clear and comprehensive, using language familiar to the patient and avoiding jargon.

Nursing skills

In order to participate in such communication, the coronary care nurse needs to possess a realistic outlook and the necessary knowledge and skills to convey information. Communication is a two-way process and the nurses need to be able to respond to feedback from the patient and adapt their approach to meet the patient's changing needs. Primary nursing is a way of maximizing this process. The nurse should be available to listen to the patient in a calm, unhurried, sympathetic and empathetic manner. The nurse needs to help the patient ventilate his fears and feelings and work to allay these feelings. Nursing intervention is recognizing the patients' manifestations of their reaction to their illness, particularly in relation to stress, and helping them to recognize their own responses and to cope with them.

Reassurance is a term often used in nursing, usually without clarification or evaluation. Broad promises such as 'Don't worry, everything will be all right' serve little purpose if patients lack a basic understanding of their condition, and may serve to lessen the credibility of the nurse in the eyes of the patient.

The nurse should respond to the patient's needs, not his overt behaviour (Ashworth, 1984). There is some evidence that working with the patient to work out an individual plan of daily activities can reduce anxiety (Zieman and Dracup 1990). However, the patient may not possess the necessary skills to be able to contribute. They may be too ill or anxious to represent themselves as they would wish; they may be physically or mentally handicapped; or may lack the knowledge and understanding to be able to make realistic decisions concerning the future. This may equally apply to the family, who may find the hospital imposing and may be influenced by the emotional impact of their loved one's illness.

In the highly clinical and technical environment there is sometimes a need for the nurse to stand back and carefully think about the care strategy best for the patient and whether it is realistic and appropriate. Allowing a critically ill patient to die with peace and dignity is not a failure and may be a better course of action than prolonging life with multiple therapy and technology which misleads the patient and family into thinking that there is a good deal of hope. Discussing such subjects openly in a constructive fashion with colleagues involves a sensitive and professional approach and will be a recurring problem.

Unstructured communication

As well as structured planned communication to convey specific information, there is also day-to-day conversation and non-verbal communication. Human contact is possibly more important in a technical environment such as a CCU than a general ward. The patient appreciates knowing that a nurse is always available and, if they are ill or bedridden, communication may be the only way they feel they can influence their environment and daily routine. There is a lot of time for patients to observe and react to what is going on around them,

and the atmosphere of the unit, whether it is relaxed, friendly, tense or chaotic, will convey certain impressions to and affect perception of the environment and the place they occupy in it. The way in which nurses communicate with each other and other patients will influence how readily they communicate with their fellow patients. Relatives will also take cues from the staff and patients when determining whether and how to approach the nurse to ask questions. Many staff communicate indirectly with the patient via the relatives.

In her review of staff–patient communication in the CCU, Ashworth (1984) sees its aims as being for the patient to perceive the nurse as friendly, helpful, competent and reliable, and for the nurse to recognize the patient as an individual and to be aware of his perceived needs and help him recognize other needs. Also, the nurse needs to provide factual information so that patients realistically knows what to expect and can help meet their own needs (Ashworth 1980).

Inadequate communication

There are various reasons why nurse–patient communication is often inadequate in the CCU, including the preoccupation with handling technology and the relegation of interpersonal skills. Other reasons may be the short duration of the patient's stay in the CCU, the severity of his heart attack, and anxiety or stress in the nurse. The nurse may be anxious about approaching patients, particularly if they are dying, and may be uncertain of the appropriate way to communicate with them. Specific issues, such as the occurrence of a cardiac arrest or death of a fellow patient, may pose communication difficulties. Personality differences and 'unpopular' characters are as likely to occur in the CCU as elsewhere.

Improving communication

Ashworth (1984) suggests three main approaches which might improve nurse–patient communication in the CCU:

1   planned education to develop communication knowlege and skills
2   discriminating reading and the use of relevant research-based nursing practice information

3 further research into staff–patient communication.

Fielding and Llewelyn (1987) advocate that there is a need for a careful assessment to identify precisely what form of communication training is needed, and to establish standards of communication competence.

PATIENT CONTACT

Nurse–patient contact is likely to be at its peak during the acute phase when the patient is subjected to observations and interventions designed to monitor and promote recovery. Thereafter, such contact often declines. The support given by physical presence should not be underestimated, although it is difficult to evaluate it formally (Routasalo 1999). Touch can be purely physical, carried out during procedures or therapeutic and carried out with the intention of bringing benefit. Touch can also occur spontaneously or be unintentional. Therapeutic touch can lead to a heightened sense of well-being and convey caring and support to patients and their families. It is a complex and ill defined concept (Williams 2001) that needs to be dealt with sensitively. Patients receiving caring touch and comforting emotional stimuli that is non-threatening are likely to experience a reduction in anxiety state (Glick 1986). Desire for touch often increases with the illness severity and massage has been shown to be effective in promoting rest and recovery in some critically ill patients (Richards 1998). The effects of massage and associated therapeutic touch have also been shown to reduce anxiety in patients in intensive care units (Cox and Hayes 1998). However, a number of studies have shown that changes in heart rate and rhythm can occur in response to human contact (Lynch et al 1974, Thomas et al 1975) which may not always be beneficial.

Nurses need to be alert for patients' negative attitudes and values towards touch (Davidhizar et al 1997). Touch can be perceived as intimate and an invasion of personal space that may not be appreciated by all patients and it may be used more appropriately in some instances than others. It may be used to convey hostility and anger, and may have sexual connotations. Patients may feel uncomfortable with close contact from relative strangers and may find it stressful, embarrassing and a barrier to effective communication.

COMFORT

The promotion of relaxation and comfort is an essential nursing skill which is sometimes overlooked when patients are perceived to have an acute cardiac problem and the focus of care is on doing things to the patient without necessarily considering the impact this might have. As Wilson-Barnett (1984) points out, careful positioning of the patient, reassurance with information, and the presence of a caring nurse, ensure that comfort assumes a high priority. Careful bed-making, regulation of light, temperature and noise, and the provision of hot milky drinks in the evening, may seem mundane and obvious, but are often delegated to the most junior nurse as they assume a low priority in the 'high-tech' environment of the CCU.

Patient discomfort is compounded by invasive techniques such as cannulation and catheterization, and the frequent disturbances that occur when routine observations and recordings are made. Invasive monitoring techniques often result in the general immobilization of the patient which carries with it attendant risks such as pressure sore development. Careful changing of the patient's position in bed and the use of fresh linen and pressure-relieving devices are important in reducing discomfort. Other considerations include the thoughtful siting of intravenous cannulae and the use of nasal cannulae instead of oxygen masks.

Music and relaxation therapy can be comforting and have been shown to reduce anxiety in patients with myocardial infarction (White 1999, Biley 2000).

ACTIVITY

Nursing intervention should reflect the current pattern of care for the acute coronary patient, which has been characterized by an increase in physical activity and a decrease in imposed invalidism and earlier discharge from hospital. A progressive reduction in the length of bed rest and stay in hospital for the coronary patient has occurred since the study by Levine and Lown (1952). A recent systematic review of bedrest after a heart attack concluded that longer periods of bedrest conferred no additional benefits over short periods, and recommended that unless there were compelling reasons patients should be mobilized early (Herkner et al 2003). Successful reperfusion therapies now mean that patients have less myocardial damage and will be able to resume activities relatively sooner than they could previously. The uncomplicated patient is now encouraged to sit out on the day of admission, provided that they are free of pain and significant arrhythmias.

If the patient is too unwell to get out of bed it is better if they sit upright in bed rather than lying flat, because the latter requires more myocardial work to pump blood through the excess pool of tissue fluid in the lungs.

Certainly, gradual but early mobilization should encourage the patient to walk around the ward by the end of a few days. It is important that an individualized approach takes preference over a standard regimen. Activity within the first day or so is likely to be sufficient to prevent the effects of immobility, and to maintain venous return, muscle tone and joint flexibility.

Inactivity is a major problem in that it is a source of frustration and boredom for the patient. The nurse should stress the need for temporary limitation. Enforced bed rest will only have an adverse effect on someone who is normally active. Relaxation, deep breathing and passive leg exercises on the CCU are useful in reducing boredom and mood changes and the physical consequences of immobility. Such activities will boost the patients' morale by making them feel they are playing an active part in their recovery. Activity allays depression and gives the patient a sense of active participation and control in their care and recovery, rather than merely being a passive recipient. A tentative plan needs to be formulated so that the patient has realistic guidelines to achieve certain levels of activity. Some patients may feel reluctant or hesitant to resume activity, whereas others are over-zealous. It is therefore important for the nurse to be optimistic and encouraging, but realistic and warn against undue fatigue and over-exertion. Activities should be interspersed with adequate rest periods. Although patients may be able to time their own activities, they may need

some advice from the nurse. For instance, it is advisable that the patient avoids undue exertion immediately after a meal: to digest a meal, blood flow to the gut has to increase and the heart will have a larger output demanded of it.

The ability to increase activity is a positive reinforcement for recovery. Patients able to participate in their own recovery experiences a restored confidence when it is shown that certain activities are once again possible. The family will also experience reassurance and relief to see them sitting comfortably in a chair.

Activity assessment

An ideal method of quantifying the energy spent undertaking various activities is the metabolic equivalents system (METs). One MET is equal to the resting oxygen uptake, or about 3.5 ml/kg per minute. The average man can attain a level of 12 METs, whereas an uncomplicated post-coronary patient can achieve a maximum capacity of 9 METs.

All activities can be assessed by observing heart rate and rhythm, respiratory rate and blood pressure. The nurse needs to monitor activities sensibly, in a manner that avoids unduly worrying the patient. The patient should be warned that the development of chest pain, shortness of breath, palpitations, faintness and dizziness are all indications to cease activity.

The immobile patient

Some patients will be too unwell to resume activity and will need to be cared for in the bed or chair. The complications of inactivity and bed rest include pressure ulcers, deep vein thrombosis and pulmonary embolism as well as psychological problems and difficulty carrying out activities of living. Bed- and chair-bound patients, or those with impaired ability to reposition need to be assessed for additional factors that increase the risk of developing pressure ulcers. These include incontinence, inadequate dietary intake and altered level of consciousness. Systematic assessment can be accomplished by using a validated risk assessment tool such as the Braden Scale or Norton Scale. Pressure ulcer risk needs to be assessed at periodic intervals. Skin care and early treatment needs to include (DoH 2001):

- inspection of the skin daily with particular attention to bony prominences
- skin cleansing at the time of soiling and at routine intervals – avoiding hot water and using a mild cleansing agent that minimizes irritation and skin dryness
- minimizing the force of friction when cleansing the skin
- avoiding massage over bony prominences
- minimizing exposure to moisture.

REST AND SLEEP

The purpose of rest is to decrease the myocardial demand for oxygen. The myocardium requires time, oxygen and nutrients to recover from the injury of infarction, and this recovery will be aided by reducing the amount of work, and therefore the oxygen demand, of the heart.

Although in theory the CCU should be the ideal environment for resting, in reality it rarely is and although patients may appear to sleep, it may not be refreshing or restorative (Reid 2001).

Physical and mental rest is achieved by a variety of factors, including adequate pain relief, the promotion of relaxation, comfort and sleep, and by ensuring that noise is kept to a minimum and that temperature and humidity are controlled. This requires that care be organized on a flexible and personalized basis.

Rest periods should be incorporated into the daily routine to guarantee the patient is free from unnecessary disturbance (Baker et al 1993). During these periods, peace and quiet should be encouraged, visitors to the unit (including health care professionals) discouraged and the lights dimmed and blinds drawn.

Disorientation, social isolation, sensory deprivation and unnecessary noise are not uncommon in the CCU. A warm stimulating environment should be encouraged, where patients feel they can relax and chat easily with fellow patients and staff. The provision of a suitable environment should include windows, calendars, clocks, radios and televisions equipped with headphones, newspapers, magazines and books, and personal items such as photographs. Visitors should be made welcome rather than viewed with suspicion by staff, and visiting times should be planned to fit the needs of the patient and family.

Sleep

The coronary patient will have individual sleep patterns and habits. The consequences of illness and its management and the unfamiliar environment may cause deprivation and fragmentation in sleep behaviour.

Traditionally, sleep is looked upon as a time of restoration and preparation for the next period of wakefulness. It has been suggested that sleep is a period of bodily and brain restitution, although there is much debate over its function (Horne 1988).

Sleep is not a steady state but a cyclic process characterized by different wave patterns in the brain. Sleep is conveniently divided into two distinct types defined by the presence or absence of rapid eye movements: REM (rapid eye movement or paradoxical) sleep and non-REM (orthodox) sleep. Human non-REM (NREM) sleep is further divided into four stages on the basis of specific EEG patterns. The individual becomes more deeply asleep as he passes through the stages. The periods of REM occurring at intervals during sleep have been linked to dreaming. REM sleep is characterized by an increase in blood pressure and heart and respiratory rates, whereas NREM sleep is characterized by a decrease in these parameters.

The sleep stages follow a fairly orderly cyclic pattern. In normal human adults, REM sleep begins about 90 min after sleep onset and recurs again at 90–100-min intervals. On average, the individual progresses through four to five cycles of sleep each night. Stage 4 sleep decreases and REM sleep increases in proportion progressively with each cycle, so that most stage 4 sleep occurs early in the night and most REM sleep occurs during the last few hours before arising. REM sleep periods usually account for 20–25% of the total sleep time throughout the night (Chokroverty 1999). On average, a person will awaken five times during the night and is twice as likely to wake from REM sleep as any other type. Bearing in mind that one complete sleep cycle lasts about 90 min it is possible that a patient being disturbed hourly will not progress through a full sleep cycle during his sleep. CCU patients have been found to feel that they had had a better nights sleep if they were not disturbed during the latter part of the night (Mitamura et al 1998). Patients with nocturnal angina are more likely to experience symptoms during periods of REM sleep and there is also an increase in ventricular activity in this sleep stage. The onset of symptoms of acute myocardial infarction are more frequent in bed, especially after just falling asleep and on waking (Thompson et al 1991).

Circadian rhythms

Sleep patterns follow an approximate 24-hour cycle known as a circadian rhythm. This innate pattern will continue to operate even when the typical external factors which influence behaviour, such as clocks, social and work routines, are removed. Humans are thought to have a natural free-running sleep cycle of 25 hours (Moore-Ede et al 1983), although there is much individual variation. People also differ in the time of day at which they function at their best. Horne and Ostberg (1976) identified two distinct groups of people, termed 'morning' and 'evening' types. The former prefer to go to bed early and get up early, performing best in the morning. The latter, conversely, prefer later nights and later arising, functioning best in the evening. In hospital, patients tend to be regarded uniformly with little thought given to individual preferences or attempts to adapt care to such variations. Circadian rhythms in hospital are likely to become desynchronized which results in poorer sleep quality (Taub and Berger 1976).

It is clear that coronary patients experience marked sleep disturbances in hospital, particularly in CCUs (Deamer et al 1972, Broughton and Baron 1973, 1978, Karacan et al 1973). Richards and Bairnsfather (1988) found that critical care unit patients spent more time in stage 1 sleep than did age- and sex-matched healthy subjects. There were also significant decreases in the percentage of time spent in any sleep stage during the night. It is possible that short naps taken in the morning and early afternoon could provide the extra REM sleep needed to approach normal values.

Studies in healthy volunteers and animal models have shown that sleep deprivation can cause increased oxygen consumption (Bonnet et al 1991), impaired cellular and humoral immunity (Benca et al 1997) and disrupted thermoregulation (Landis and Whitney 1997).

Promoting sleep

Sleep occurs when sleep-promoting factors outweigh arousal activity and sleep is affected by factors such as age, noise, temperature, light, pain and anxiety. Patients will be able to sleep better if they are comfortable, free from pain and in a quiet and peaceful environment. Hospital beds are often hard and narrow with plastic covered mattresses that limit effective sleep (Topf and Thompson 2001).

The average decibel rating for CCUs and other acute care areas has been reported as being 70 decibels (db) which is higher than those internationally recommended (30 db at night, 40 db during the evening, and 45 db during the daytime) (Topf 2000). Such units have equipment that produces sound levels near to 70 decibels which is close to that of heavy traffic or a noisy restaurant (Topf 2000). Equipment alarms, telephones, pagers, staff talking and visitors contribute to the noise (Hilton 1985). The nurse therefore needs to promote comfort and relaxation, and control the environment by reducing noise, regulating temperature and dimming lighting (Webster and Thompson 1986). Sleep will be disrupted by pain and therefore pain relief is essential. Often unnecessary nursing or medical observations and interventions disrupt the continuity and efficiency of patients' sleep. A large proportion of the noise that occurs will be amenable to behaviour modification (Kahn et al 1998). With the sophisticated technology available, such as multichannel monitoring facilities, many routine observations can be performed without waking the patient. Essential procedures should be organized so that the timing coincides with the patient being awake.

Hot milky drinks such as Ovaltine and Horlicks often form part of the night-time ritual and have been shown to improve sleep significantly (Brezinova and Oswald 1972).

Designing clinical areas to separate noisy admission areas away from other patient areas may help. It is also important to think about noise implications when purchasing new equipment.

Assessing sleep

Nursing assessment should incorporate information about the patient's usual sleeping behaviour, including data such as quality and quantity and the identification of any routines that may enhance his ability to sleep. Unfortunately, many nurses possess little knowledge about the assessment of sleep. The use of one of a variety of sleep measurement instruments that are available (Closs 1988), such as a sleep questionnaire, would be a useful adjunct in assessing the patient's normal sleeping habits and judging the efficacy of any intervention. Subjective reports tend to correlate significantly with objective assessments such as polygraphic recordings and are relatively easy and quick to perform.

DIET

The nurse should possess the knowledge and skills necessary to help assess and meet the nutritional requirements of the patient. Unfortunately, this fundamental aspect of nursing is often neglected and the patient is referred prematurely or inappropriately to the dietician. Patients need to be enabled to eat and drink so that (DoH 2001):

- they have a diet that meets their individual needs
- they are offered food and drink in an environment with acceptable sights, sounds and smells conducive to eating
- they are helped to eat and drink when required
- they are offered a replacement meal if one is missed
- diet and fluid intake is monitored
- all opportunities are taken to encourage healthy eating.

In the CCU, it may be appropriate for the patient, because they are generally inactive and may not feel hungry, to have nourishing drinks and small snacks. The Asian patient may require special consideration and relatives can offer valuable advice. Some patients may prefer to have meals brought in.

Fluid restriction may be warranted if the patient has developed heart failure. The patient may have been vomiting and will require thoughtful mouth care including mouthwashes and sips of cold or iced water.

A careful assessment of the patient's usual eating and drinking habits and lifestyle is important. Many patients will have preconceived ideas, usually obtained from relatives and the media, about diet. The nurse plays a key role in nutrition education and in performing the difficult task of changing inappropriate habits. A major problem is not in the giving of advice but in achieving appropriate long-term behavioural responses which are in the patient's best interests.

Many misconceptions regarding diet litter the popular press and even the scientific literature. The problem is compounded by conflicting and unsubstantiated information and advice given by friends, relatives and health professionals. This is particularly true regarding coronary heart disease. If the nurse is to be successful in achieving compliance, it is vital that factual information is presented objectively, consistently and in a way that can easily be understood by the patient and his family. Unfortunately, many health professionals seem to forget that eating and drinking are pleasurable experiences as well as providing the essential nutrients to the body. Any dietary modification often requires a major change in the patient's habits. Gradual change is likely to be more successful in achieving compliance. The involvement of the family is usually necessary, as eating and drinking are often a family or communal activity and the women of the household are the ones normally expected to do the shopping and cooking.

ELIMINATION

Prolonged bed rest should be avoided because this decreases gastrointestinal activity and the faeces may become hardened because of water reabsorption, leading to constipation. Constipation may lead to straining which should be avoided because it may result in excessive isometric work which serves as a vagal stimulant and can produce bradycardia and other arrhythmias. Similar effects may result with the use of a bedpan which patients often find uncomfortable and stressful to use. Using a bedside commode is easier and places the patient in a more familiar position for defecation (Winslow et al 1984). There appears to be little evidence for promoting the use of the bedpan in preference to the commode.

Laxatives may be required to prevent excessive straining during bowel movements, but, more importantly, careful attention should be paid to the diet, particularly fluid and fibre content. The patient should be reassured that it is not unusual for patients to have altered bowel habits on admission to hospital. Certain drugs will alter the patient's normal bowel movement pattern. For instance, opioids cause constipation and antibiotics may cause diarrhoea.

The patient is likely to feel embarrassed about using a commode or urinal in the vicinity of fellow patients and staff, and this can be minimized by ensuring that the curtains are drawn to provide at least some privacy. Patients are likely to feel more at ease in a private room or cubicle than in an open-plan area and some units encourage the patient to be taken to a toilet in a wheelchair and to walk to the toilet at an early stage.

Careful monitoring of the patient's fluid balance is necessary to monitor cardiac function and the effects of treatment. Daily weighing of the patient may be more accurate than a fluid balance chart for assessment of congestive cardiac failure. The male patient may find it easier to use a urinal while standing at the bedside rather than lying supine in bed. Patients who are prescribed diuretics need to be warned that urine output is likely to increase in amount and frequency. Careful timing of the administration of diuretics is necessary to minimize disturbing the patient during the night.

BATHING AND HYGIENE

Many patients admitted to hospital with a suspected cardiac problem will be unprepared because of the sudden onset of symptoms and the urgency of the admission. Patients may feel embarrassed and uncomfortable particularly if they have vomited, are sweating and are partly naked. Those that have suffered a cardiac arrest may have been incontinent of urine. Single use toiletries should be provided if the patient has not brought any in with him (DoH 2001). Patients may be too unwell initially to care for themselves and appreciate help. The psychological aspects of bathing and hygiene are

important. Patients may feel better after a shower or bath, and appreciate simple things such as the provision of hand-washing facilities after using a commode and before a meal, being able to soak their feet in a bowl of water and having their hair washed.

Mouth care

Mouth care needs to be offered to all patients, especially those who wear dentures, have fluid intake restricted or have been vomiting. Patients with dentures may be embarrassed about cleaning them in the presence or others and should be offered the necessary privacy and facilities.

Bathing

The patient may move more slowly and deliberately when bathing in order to conserve energy (Winslow et al 1985). They may, however, prefer to shower, in accordance with their normal domestic routine, particularly during the later stages of stay in the CCU. The mean oxygen consumption during showering is higher than during bathing (Johnston et al 1981).

The isometric activity required by some patients to climb out of the bath may cause a steep rise in arterial pressure which increases myocardial work. Therefore, before the patient first bathes the nurse needs to evaluate the patient for potential difficulty in getting out of the bath. For instance, if the patient is weak or obese or is generally likely to experience difficulties, then assistance in the form of handrails, rubber non-slip mats and an extra nurse may be required.

SUPPORTING THE PATIENT

Coping

A heart attack is perceived as a life crisis by most patients. It is seen as a threat to the individual and it interferes with normal coping responses. The patient may need help in coming to terms with his heart attack and without which ineffective coping mechanisms may have a negative impact and delay adaptation.

Coping involves the use of innate or acquired mechanisms or ways of responding to a stimulus in order to adapt to change. Coping is initiated once a situation is perceived as threatening (Lazarus 1966). Adaptation is a positive response to changes in the individual's internal or external environment.

Moving from being a healthy individual to becoming sick and admitted to hospital necessitates some form of coping. The style of adjustment to the myocardial infarction will be determined by the premorbid personality of the patient and will be influenced by a variety of factors.

Patients may already be coping with other disruptive events in their lives, such as changing or losing their job, moving house, or divorcing (Holmes and Rahe 1967). The heart attack may be seen as a natural consequence of 'having too much on their plate'. A recent event may be selected as being the cause for the heart attack in an effort to apportion some blame. The success or failure of coping with previous or ongoing life events may shape the way the patient responds to the heart attack. An individual's response does not seem to be related to the severity of the heart attack (Cay 1982).

Coping involves involuntary physiological responses or emotional behavioural responses with varying degrees of cognitive control. The sick role may or may not be accepted easily. Admission to hospital is often unexpected and usually not initiated by the patient. Being obliged to accept help from others, being exempt from normal social responsibilities and being obliged to get well and go about seeking competent help (Parsons 1964), may not coincide with the patient's response to the heart attack.

The way in which the person perceives a heart attack is likely to influence coping behaviour. Burgess and Hartman (1986) found that 94% of the patients they studied regarded their heart attack as a serious illness, although 74% saw it as something that was controllable. Treatment for a heart attack tends to assume that the disorder is controllable, which is likely to colour the patient, family and health professionals' understanding of the illness and the possible coping options available.

The extent to which an individual believes they can actually influence their own health can be linked to the concept of locus of control (Rotter 1966), whereby health (or illness) is seen either as being a product of one's own behaviour (internal locus of control) or a result of apparently unchangeable and often unpredictable outside circumstances (external locus of control).

Table 6.3   Factors influencing coping style

Culture and associated health beliefs
Previous experience of illness (either of self or others)
Attitude and perceived support of family
Perceived implications of having a heart attack
Level of acceptance
Level of knowledge and understanding
Usual coping style
Personality
Self-motivation, self-esteem and self-image
Presumed benefits of hospital treatment
Belief that all actions are relevant to recovery
Tolerance for unwelcome situations
Need and desire to return to premorbid lifestyle
Recognition and desire for any benefits of being treated
    as sick
Support and resources available

Admission to hospital in itself necessitates adaptation. Wilson-Barnett (1980) lists some of the factors that the patient has to cope with:

- unexpected events
- unpleasant symptoms
- loss of function
- loneliness
- unfamiliar surroundings and relationships
- altered status and role.

Stress

Stress may be viewed as either a stimulus or a response. Selye (1976) defines stress as the nonspecific response of the body to any demand made upon it. According to Selye's concept, stress is divided into various stages (Selye 1976). First, the individual experiences loss or threat, such as loss of health and threat to previous lifestyle; secondly, the individual tries to adjust to or cope with the situation by taking active measures, such as seeking help and complying with advice; and, finally, if the stress persists a stress reaction may follow resulting in physiological and psychological changes in behaviour. Illness and fatigue will ensue if the situation continues.

Physical producers of stress (stressors) include pain, altered tissue perfusion, hypoxia and electrolyte imbalance. Psychological stressors include changes in lifestyle, loss, frustration and confusion.

Response to stress

Both the nervous and endocrine systems play a major part in the response to stress. Reasoning and thought processes will affect the interpretation of stimuli.

Increased catecholamine (adrenaline and noradrenaline) release in response to autonomic nerve action can lead to alterations in heart rate, external work performed by the heart, energy required to activate cardiac contraction, and metabolic state of the myocardium. All of these factors mean that myocardial oxygen demand is increased and both electrical and mechanical instability may follow.

A combination of the action of the adrenocortical and autonomic responses to stress are thought to include increased levels of free fatty acids, serum cholesterol and plasma glucose, together with alterations in blood viscosity and platelet stickiness, and a decreased resistance to infection.

A cluster of certain social events, all of which require life adjustment, appears to be significantly associated with the time of onset of illness. The Social Readjustment Rating Scale (Holmes and Rahe 1967) was developed to measure the magnitude of such events. Significant events include a death of a partner, divorce or separation and moving house.

Fear

The patient's immediate reaction is fear, not only of death, but, more commonly, of the threat the infarct poses to his lifestyle (Thompson 1995). This fear can be reduced by emphasizing the nature of the CCU, explaining about the monitoring equipment, the possibility of artefacts, the routine observations of heart rate and blood pressure, investigative procedures, and administration of drugs. The CCU environment, including staff and technology, is generally more reassuring than frightening to the patient and partner.

Dependency

This can be reduced by encouraging the resumption of normal activities as soon as possible in an attempt to minimize the sense of damage and helplessness. Involving the patient in decision making about his own care helps to increase feelings of self-worth and independence. Involving the partner and other family members may also help.

Disorientation

This and social isolation can be reduced by the provision of a suitable environment which includes calendars, clocks, radios, televisions, newspapers, windows and personal items such as photographs.

Threats posed by myocardial infarction

Myocardial infarction poses threats such as death, altered body image and self-image, helplessness and loss, with the result that the patient feels damaged, incompetent and dependent upon others.

Death

This is perhaps the most immediate perceived threat to the acute coronary patient. They will have gathered information, often based on folklore, from the media, relatives and colleagues about a heart attack and will have formed ideas about his condition and the likelihood of death. The death of another patient on the unit will increase such fear. Relatives, especially the partner, may experience this threat to a greater extent than the patient, who may feel too ill or fatigued to contemplate any future event.

Altered body image

Body image evolves throughout the person's life, gradually adapting to his changing structure and function. Illness or injury to a part of one's body requires a more sudden change in this process so that the person can perceive it realistically and then adapt to it. A heart attack may pose particular problems in terms of perception of the body image by the patient and others, as the damage is not externally visible.

Altered self-image

The perceived threat to self-image is related to the interruption of usual roles and function and will be influenced by previous priorities and lifestyle.

Helplessness

This tends to occur when events are perceived as being uncontrollable (Seligman 1975), and often results in embarrassment about needing help with micturition and defecation, and worry about the use of technology and feelings of being trapped or restricted.

Loss

The patient may experience losses, both real and imagined, for example, loss of income, status and role within the family and local community, and leisure and work activities.

The patient responds to such threats by using defence mechanisms and coping behaviours. Anxiety, denial and depression are the most common emotional responses.

Anxiety

Anxiety is a normal but enormously complex human phenomenon which is notoriously difficult to define. In a mild or moderate degree, anxiety is part of normal experience. In excess it impairs effectiveness. Empirically, anxiety is used to describe an unpleasant emotional state or condition. Anxiety is also used to describe relatively stable differences in anxiety-proneness as a personality trait. Spielberger (1966) suggests that ambiguity in the term arises from the indiscriminate use of it in referring to two different concepts: a transitory *state* which fluctuates over time, and a personality *trait* that remains relatively stable over time. A person who perceives a situation as threatening experiences a transitory rise in state anxiety. Trait anxiety, however, is an acquired behavioural disposition based primarily on experiences and reflected in behaviour by relatively stable individual differences in anxiety-proneness in response to stress. Persons high in trait anxiety are more disposed than those low in trait anxiety to perceive situations as threatening.

Raised anxiety levels in coronary patients admitted to hospital have been well documented, with serial measurements generally showing that anxiety is highest on admission to the CCU and immediately after transfer to the ward, falling rapidly over the following week, and rising just prior to discharge (Thompson et al 1987). The degree of anxiety often bears little relation to the severity of the infarct, and women are often more anxious than men (Kim et al 2000).

Anxiety is certainly the most common initial response to myocardial infarction. The main source of anxiety is probably the prospect of sudden death, and the signs of anxiety are more likely to be noticed during the initial phase of the illness, when recurrent symptoms, such as chest pain, develop, or when special procedures, such as the insertion of a temporary pacing wire, are required. A less obvious problem that evokes anxiety is the sensation of weakness. Anxiety about transfer to the ward or discharge home is likely to be high if the patient is suddenly transferred without prior warning and preparation.

The patient with mild anxiety is usually alert and able to absorb information and solve problems, although they may be restless and irritable. The patient who has very high level of anxiety is often too distressed to absorb or remember information. They may be unable to concentrate and find it difficult to sleep.

A significant reduction in anxiety can often be achieved by a considerate, attentive and competent nurse using simple measures. Close and consistent nurse–patient contact increases the patient's feeling of security (Thompson 1990). Feelings of strangeness and isolation can be reduced by simple but careful and effective information and support. Relaxation techniques involving progressive muscle relaxation may be effective in minimizing undue stress.

Depression

Depression is common in coronary patients particularly if anxiety is unrelieved and may persist for some time (Lane et al 2002). It is an understandable response when one considers the implications of a myocardial infarction, such as loss of earning capacity, activities and general status within the family and society.

The moderate to severely depressed patient may experience sadness, disinterest, sleep disturbances and loss of appetite. They may be irritable, oversensitive or prone to bouts of tearfulness.

However, depression may be difficult to recognize, since the patient may appear quiet and pleasant, and complies with treatment and advice. It is important that depression is recognized and dealt with promptly because it may interfere with the process of recovery.

In the acute phase, depression usually appears on the third to fifth day, when the patient is less able to maintain denial. However, it is often accompanied and may be masked by anxiety.

The patient is likely to experience feelings of hopelessness and helplessness which results in a generally pessimistic outlook. Certainly, a depressed patient is likely to make a poor long-term recovery as measured by the ability to return to work and resume sexual functioning. It may be helpful for the nurse to sit down with patients and attempt to find out what is making them depressed. Many of their fears may be realistic, which are likely to prove difficult to resolve or alleviate, for there is nothing that the nurse can do to reassure them that all will be well. Some concerns may be unfounded, and once these are identified the nurse can help correct any misconceptions that he may have. Often, having someone to sit down and talk with, or hold and cry with, may enable them to reorganize their thinking and help him positively reassess their future. The nurse should avoid overprotection or the encouragement of patient dependency. The patient should be given an optimistic, but realistic, outlook which conveys hope and gives the patient energy and enthusiasm. Probably the best antidote is early and progressive mobilization to counter the physical and psychological problems associated with immobility. The sooner the patient is mobilized, the sooner will feelings of self-worth and self-esteem return.

Denial

Denial, the commonest coping mechanism in coronary patients, is usually temporary and may serve to protect them from emotional disturbances such as anxiety, which could aggravate or prolong the illness. Gradual acceptance of the illness and active participation in recovery usually follow. However, denial is dangerous to the patient when its presence allows engagement in some form of behaviour that threatens their welfare.

Denial can often be recognized by statements the patient makes: denial of fact (e.g. refusing to acknowledge that one has suffered a heart attack) and denial of meaning (e.g. refusing to admit one is anxious or depressed). Four levels of denial are often apparent:

1   Major denial: no fear is expressed at any time during the course of the illness.
2   Moderate denial: initial denial is eventually followed by the admission of at least some degree of fear.
3   Mild denial: the verbal stance against fear is not consistent, and some fear is admitted from the beginning.
4   Minimal denial: complaints of fear are spontaneously made or easily elicited.

Anger and hostility

Once patients are aware that they have suffered a heart attack and what it may imply, it is not uncommon for their reaction to be one of anger or hostility or both. There is much emphasis and media coverage today on healthy living, and patients who consider that they have taken special care of their own health may feel cheated. Anger occurs in response to frustration, threat or injury. It may be expressed actively or passively or may be self-directed. Active expressions of anger include sarcasm, criticism, irritability and arguing. Passively, anger may be expressed through non-compliance, boredom, sudden withdrawal or forgetfulness. Self-directed anger is manifested as depression, self-deprecation, accident proneness, and somatic symptoms such as headaches.

It is often difficult for the nurse to remain objective, especially when the patient is critical. Staff may feel powerless or become angry themselves. They need to try to help patients clarify and describe their ideas and feelings through focusing on their anger and deciding upon a constructive way of dealing with it. The behaviour needs to be explained to relatives and the nurse should avoid being judgemental and taking the patient's actions personally.

Guilt

In seeking a reason or justification for an event that is often sudden and unexpected, the patient and his relatives may feel guilty that things they have or have not done may be responsible for the present illness. The patient may blame himself for letting his family down and being absent from work. If he feels relatively well shortly after admission, he may feel guilty at occupying a hospital bed.

Resolution and restitution

This is the time when patients begin to cope constructively with their heart attack and its consequences. They begin to talk rationally and realistically about their future hopes and plans. They may reassess their self-image, priorities and goals and have some sense of pride at having survived the crisis. They may even begin to see positive aspects of having suffered a heart attack. This can be termed secondary gain, and includes components such as a welcomed opportunity to reassess priorities and lifestyle, a chance to spend more time with the family, a justifiable reason for taking early retirement, appreciation that loved ones have shown concern and feelings for them, and the feeling of increased self-worth that comes with being the centre of attention for a while.

Unfortunately, some patients may never fully adapt to the fact that they have suffered a heart attack.

Religion and culture

Religious and cultural beliefs may influence attitudes to health and health care and play an important role in the outcome of the patient's illness.

The social institution of religion often plays a key role in determining attitudes and customs associated with life and death, even if the religion is not actively practised. Thus, it is often an important source of comfort and support during illness, especially the crisis stage, for the patient and family.

The cultural response to sickness needs to be considered when planning care and respect given to individual customs and beliefs (Webster 1997).

RESPONSE OF THE FAMILY

The sudden onset of acute myocardial infarction, with little or no warning, and the perception of the illness as a devastating threat to physical, emotional and social well-being, often create a crisis state for the family as well as the patient. Family members often feel that their loved one has been removed and isolated from them, making them feel helpless, frightened and unnecessarily excluded from intimate involvement. They, in particular the spouse, have the potential death of the patient uppermost in their mind, and experience guilt over the illness, feeling that they have possibly caused or contributed to it in some way, for instance, through recent friction or tension within the family unit. They often experience intense feelings of loss; for instance, they no longer have certain needs such as economic and emotional security consistently and reliably being met. Although they require information, reassurance, support, and especially to feel that there is hope (Leske 1986), they may feel reluctant to seek out staff and indicate their concerns. In fact, many are likely to feel that if they do so they may be in the way or upset staff, possibly resulting in patient care being adversely affected. Therefore, the nurse must often take the initiative in approaching the family. If the family members are ineffectively using coping mechanisms, they may seek support rather than provide it, thereby placing additional stress on the already compromised patient (Chavez and Faber 1987).

Nursing intervention aims to assess and support the family's coping mechanisms, providing information and reassurance, and referring the patient and family to other appropriate agencies for expert consultation.

If the crisis is not relieved by mobilizing adequate and necessary resources to deal with the threat, or by altering the perception of the situation, the patient is likely to suffer.

Continuous interaction with the patient and family places the nurse in an ideal position to help them cope with the crisis in a positive and adaptive manner (Leske 1986). The ability of the spouse in particular to deal in an optimal manner with the patient's illness has a significant impact on the health and functioning of the family (Runions 1985) and on the physical and psychological adaptation of the patient.

The partner

The partner is often more anxious than the patient, at least during the initial phase and there is evidence that professional support is inadequate or inappropriate (Thompson and Cordle 1988). Support is often provided by family, friends and relations.

Early after admission to hospital, the family, especially the partner, is likely to be in a state of shock and, once the crisis is over, relieved that the patient has survived. They are likely to be faced with crushing anxiety and overwhelming emotional turmoil (Theobold 1997). The partner frequently initiates direct coping strategies in response to the threats associated with the patient's heart attack (Nyamathi 1987). This may involve taking action to strengthen their resources to deal with the threat, for example by telephoning relatives for company or asking the nurse for information about the patient. Alternatively, the partner may attempt to cope by attacking the threat, for example by verbally abusing staff or friends. This is usually associated with anger and some feelings of guilt (Nyamathi 1987). The partner may use cognitive, indirect coping and palliative coping strategies in an attempt to deal with the threat; for example, denial, rationalization or fantasy are commonly used.

The partner's main need is to feel that there is hope (Norris and Grove 1986), although other needs include support from the family and health professionals, and the need for information and relief from anxiety.

Early after the patient's admission is unlikely to be the most appropriate time to provide detailed advice and information. What is perhaps needed at this time is a simple explanation of what has happened and what to expect, together with ample opportunity to express feelings and concerns (Thompson and Cordle 1988). Essentially, the spouse and family need to:

- feel helpful
- be kept informed
- express feelings
- receive support.

The partner can provide a unique service to the patient, staff and others by providing or relaying information, highlighting the patient's preferences and dislikes, and supporting their recovery in general. Unnecessary distress can be prevented by including them in all aspects of care decision making, including discharge planning and preparation for the usual homecoming difficulties, thereby facilitating a more smooth and continuous transition (Thompson 2002).

The partner needs to be provided with information about the emotional and physical responses they are likely to experience in response to the patient's heart attack, including:

- anxiety
- depression
- guilt
- tearfulness
- sleep disturbance
- anorexia
- fatigue
- weight loss
- headache
- faintness
- stomach pain
- sickness
- chest pain
- dizziness
- shortness of breath
- sexual difficulties.

All of these are common characteristics of the stress response The partner often experiences a dilemma about how to care for the patient. They often feel, perhaps justifiably, that if they appear to show concern they may be accused of being overprotective or smothering, whereas if they appear calm and composed they may be regarded as callous or unsympathetic. Their reactions to the patient will be influenced by a variety of factors, not least of which will be the state of their relationship prior to the illness.

Nurse-directed in-hospital groups for spouses may produce significant reductions in self-reported anxiety and depression, and significant increases in self-reported satisfaction and in knowledge (Thompson 1990). Such a programme needs to be structured sufficiently to provide guidelines for the nurse and yet be flexible enough to accommodate the individual needs of the patient and partner. Careful thought needs to be given to the timing and place where the intervention is carried out. The use of side rooms allows privacy for the couple, although time should be set aside for each partner to talk privately with the nurse.

Once the patient returns home, the family is often afraid to express true feelings in case they induce adverse physical or emotional reactions. Such cautious suppression of feelings often inhibits frank and easy communication and often results in a general atmosphere of tension, which in the long term is deleterious for the patient. These problems can be controlled if the family is encouraged to be open to frank discussions, provided that feelings and concerns are expressed sensitively and constructively.

The family often needs to be reassured that its responses are normal, and encouraged to develop existing relationships to cope with the period of inevitable change. The family should be reassured that it is not isolated, and maintaining a link with the hospital without promoting dependence needs to be fostered. Although the patient and family may want advice and support, they may feel their needs are too trivial to concern their family doctor. Other sources of support need to be explored. Telephone links with the CCU, and outpatient rehabilitation involving the spouse, may be beneficial. Groups for partners may be helpful in offering support, providing information and encouraging changes in lifestyle. Such groups can be organized from the hospital or exist independently, and rely on varying degrees of professional input.

It seems likely that there is a need for close professional involvement with the family after the patient has been discharged home. Ideally, the family should be included in follow-up visits to continue the information process and to provide a more reliable indication of progress.

Grief and bereavement

People who fear the death of a close one often begin the process of grieving before any loss actually occurs, a phenomenon known as anticipatory grief (Lindemann 1944). Although the majority of patients in hospital do return home following a heart attack, spouses may experience intense feelings of loss due to the perceived threat of their partner's death. Hampe (1975) has identified eight needs that are acutely felt by the partner going through the stages of anticipatory grief:

1 The need to be with the person.
2 The need to be helpful to the person.

3 The need for assurance of the comfort of the person.
4 The need to be informed of the person's condition.
5 The need to be informed of impending death.
6 The need to ventilate one's emotions.
7 The need for comfort and support for family members.
8 The need for acceptance, support and comfort from the health professionals.

If the patient's condition does become terminal, then support prior to the death is likely to help the family work through guilt and grief afterwards (Kubler-Ross 1970). The death, or impending death, of a family member usually increases the emotional dependency of other members upon each other. The family is usually a source of comfort, support and sympathy for all of its members.

While family members are experiencing grief through the process of mourning, they are likely to pass through several stages of shock and disbelief, developing awareness, and restitution. These stages may begin before the patient's actual death and will be experienced differently by each family member. They may fear their loved one is dying when this is actually an unlikely event. If, however, the patient's condition does become grave, then the need for sensitive support for the family is paramount. This often requires that nurses come to terms with their own feelings about death and dying, and that they receive support and guidance from their peers and seniors. The conflict between professional distance and emotional involvement has been identified as a central problem for nurses in their care of dying patients (Field 1989). Talking frankly to the relatives of a dying patient is a stressful situation for many nurses. News of death or impending death is best communicated to the family group rather than to an individual member, and should be done in a setting of privacy where the family can behave naturally without restraint of public display (Engel 1964).

If the death is expected there is time for preparation and support and for the family to begin its grieving process. If the death is unexpected, for instance following a cardiac arrest, the situation is more complex with relatives likely to display grieving reactions such as shock, anger, disbelief and bargaining, as they try to come to terms with the sudden loss.

Relatives who have been presented with an optimistic outlook will need extra support, and feelings of guilt may need to be worked through by relatives and the nurse together.

Ideally, the bereaved individual should feel that someone has a personal interest in their welfare and that there is someone available to whom they can talk with freely and who will not consider it an imposition. All too often, nurses use 'distancing tactics' to remove themselves from patients' and relatives' emotional suffering as a way of coping with the stress of the situation (Maguire 1985).

The bereaved should be encouraged to express their emotions through talking, crying and venting their hostility and feelings of guilt. Their responses need to be accepted without criticism or shock.

In the CCU, where the organization of nursing work is centred around a primary nursing style, this facilitates close and continuing contact between nurses and their patients, thereby increasing the chance that emotional involvement will develop. This presents increased difficulties in the handling of death and dying in the unit, for which most nurses are ill-prepared. A good and easily available system of social and psychological support for nurses is required (Field 1989). Bereavement support services have been implemented successfully in some areas (Wilson et al 2000).

Visitors

Visitors may be viewed as potential sources of noise, disturbance and stress. As relatives of coronary patients they are likely to be highly anxious and find the CCU an alien place, with unfamiliar sights and sounds which provoke stress. Although there is no doubt that they are in need of support (Daley 1984), this tends to be ignored because nurses have difficulty in identifying and meeting their needs (Davis 1987). However, planned education and orientation of relatives to the environment seems to reduce their stress levels (Chavez and Faber 1987).

Visiting helps relatives to come to terms with what has happened to the patient, and some relatives use 'being there' as a way of coping with the impact of their loved one's crisis. Nyamathi (1987) found that 90% of spouses expressed intense satisfaction at visiting their partners.

Although the relatives may benefit from visiting, it is ultimately what is best for the patient that matters. Some patients benefit from having members of their family sitting quietly around the bedside, whereas others may be stressed and easily tired at feeling obliged to engage in conversation. Brown (1976) found that CCU patients being visited for a period of up to 10 min each hour responded with significant rises in blood pressure and heart rate – the increased blood pressure being sustained for 5 min after the visit. Increasing the frequency of the visits produces a sustained elevation of systolic blood pressure, and ectopic beats have been found to be provoked by the onset of interactions (Thomas et al 1975) suggesting that it is perhaps best for some patients to have one longer visit than several short ones.

The patient may feel unable to ask relatives to leave or not to visit, and so it falls to the nurse to assess the situation and ask the relatives to comply with the patient's needs and wishes. Other patients' relatives may be a disruptive influence. The sound of someone else's child crying, for instance, may be upsetting. Thought needs to be given to whether it is appropriate to permit children to visit, and there needs to be an awareness of the customs and practices of different cultures. Respect for the wishes of individual patients and their relatives has to be weighed against the needs of fellow patients. In some instances, knowing that the visit can only last half an hour may cause increased strain and stress on both patient and relatives. Allowing open visiting may prevent a mass influx of people for a concentrated period of time. Setting aside a period during the day when visiting is discouraged provides an opportunity for the patient to rest, including a daytime nap.

There does appear to be a need for individualized visiting times, with the needs of both partners and other close relatives being taken into account. Visiting policies need to be monitored and evaluated for their effectiveness (Simpson et al 1996).

The nurse should set aside time to spend with relatives early after the patient's admission, so that support and information can be offered before misconceptions, uncertainty and worries set in. Involving the partner in the admission, for example, to provide certain demographic data, helps them to feel useful, involved and less lonely and anxious. Providing information booklets giving details of the CCU, staff, routines, visiting times, a telephone number and the name of the primary nurse, keeps close relatives informed and involved. Giving written information ensures that it is available for reference after leaving the hospital. Encouraging relatives to telephone at any time fosters links between the patient, relatives and nurse.

TRANSFER FROM THE CORONARY CARE UNIT TO THE WARD

Although transfer to the ward may be interpreted by the patient as evidence of improvement, it can also be construed as loss and rejection. The CCU is often seen as a place that is secure, safe and familiar (Coyle 2001) and anxiety, and even fear, about impending transfer is not uncommon. This is likely to be increased if the patient is transferred abruptly, with little planning, especially if this is during the middle of the night. Such negative reactions can be reduced by thoughtful preparation by the nurse who appreciates that a sudden change in the patient's environment is likely to cause both the patient and relatives concern about safety and comfort (Jenkins and Rogers 1995).

Klein et al (1968) found that the incidence of cardiovascular complications was reduced in patients prepared for transfer and cared for by the same nurse and doctor throughout their stay in hospital. There is also evidence that family support during the transfer phase appears to reduce associated cardiovascular problems and patient stress (Schwartz and Brenner 1979). Toth (1980) found that anxiety levels of patients who had received structured pre-transfer teaching were significantly lower on the day and time of transfer than those patients who had not received such intervention. Therefore, it would seem that such a programme would be appropriate on a routine basis. This would prepare the patient for an, often marked, alteration in routine and environment, such as a significant reduction in nursing and medical attention, and changes in medication, diet and activity. Such an intervention is likely to be best accomplished if the primary nurse on the CCU follows the patient through and liaises with the ward nurse.

With the virtual revolution that has occurred due to the advent of thrombolytic therapy and latterly PCI, it seems likely that the length of stay in hospital, including the CCU, will become much shorter. In fact, it is likely that patients will be discharged home directly from the CCU. This will mean that the nursing role will be very much geared towards the provision of education and support to the patient and family. It will also mean that nurses will need to assess carefully the patient's psychological and physical viability for transfer or discharge.

Surprisingly, perhaps, most coronary patients are not concerned about being disconnected from an ECG monitor (Thompson et al 1986), possibly viewing this as a sign of progress. In addition, they generally appear physically well, and the ward nurses may believe that they require minimal care and contact because the coronary care nurse will have dealt with the important things. Because of these factors, there is a real danger that they may be left alone to care for themselves. It is therefore important that when the coronary care nurse hands over to the ward nurse a full explanation of what has happened to the patient in terms of care is given and a proposed tentative plan of activities is outlined. The patient should be included in these discussions, so that they can clarify issues and make useful suggestions.

Preparing the patient for transfer from the CCU to the ward, or direct discharge to home, is an important nursing activity that needs further evaluation.

References

ACC/AHA (2000). Guidelines for the management of patients with unstable angina and non-ST elevation myocardial infarction. Executive summary and recommendations. *Circulation*, 102: 1193–1209.

Anderson DJ, Jenkins C, McInally C (1999). Using spinal cord stimulation to manage angina pain. *Dimensions of Critical Care Nursing*, 18 (3): 12–13.

Antithrombotic Trialists' Collaboration (2002). Collaborative meta-analysis of randomised trials of antiplatelet therapy for prevention of death, myocardial infarction, stroke and high risk patients. *British Medical Journal*, 324: 103–105.

Antman EM, Cohen M, Radley D et al (1999). For the TIMI 11B (Thrombolysis in Myocardial Infarction) and ESSENCE (Efficacy and Safety of Subcutaneous

Enoxiparin in non-Q wave coronary myocardial infarction. *Circulation*, 100: 1602–1608.

Ashworth P (1980). *Care to Communicate. An Investigation into Problems of Communication between Patients and Nurses in Intensive Therapy Units*. Royal College of Nursing, London.

Ashworth P (1984). Staff–patient communication in coronary care units. *Journal of Advanced Nursing*, 9: 35–42.

ASSENT-2 (1999). Single-bolus tenecteplase compared with front-loaded alteplase in acute myocardial infarction: the ASSENT-2 double blind randomised trial. *Lancet*, 354: 716–722.

Attree M (2001). Patients' and relatives' experiences and perspectives of 'good' and 'not so good' quality care. *Journal of Advanced Nursing*, 33: 456–466.

Baker CF, Garvin BJ, Kennedy CW et al (1993). The effect of enviromental sound and communication on CCU patients' heart rates and blood pressure. *Research in Nursing Health*, 16: 415–421.

Beeby JP (2000). Intensive care nurses experiences of caring. Part one, Consideration of the concept of caring. *Intensive and Critical Care Nursing*, 16: 76–83.

Benca RM, Quintans J (1997). Sleep and host defences: a review. *Sleep*, 20: 1027–1037.

Bertrand ME, Simoons ML, Fox KAA (2000). Management of acute coronary syndromes without persistent ST elevation. Recommendations of the Task Force of the European Society of Cardiology. *European Heart Journal*, 21: 1406–1432.

Biley FC (2000). The effects on patient well being of music listening as a nursing intervention: a review of the literature. *Journal of Clinical Nursing*, 9: 668–677.

Birkhead JS (1992). Time delays in the provision of thrombolytic treatment in six district hospitals. *British Medical Journal*, 305: 445–448.

Birkhead JS (2000). Responding to the requirements of the national service framework for coronary disease: a core data set for myocardial infarction. *Heart*, 84: 116–117.

Boden WE, Van Gilst WH, Scheldewaert RG et al (2000). Diltiazem in acute infarction treated with thrombolytic drugs: a randomised placebo-controlled trial. INTERCEPT. *Lancet*, 355: 1751–1756.

Boersma E, Maas ACP, Deckers JW et al (1996). Early thrombolytic treatment in acute myocardial infarction: reappraisal of the golden hour. *Lancet*, 348: 771–775.

Bondestam E, Havgren K, Gaston-Johansson F, Jern S, Herlitz J, Holmberg S (1987). Pain assessment by patients and nurses in the early phase of acute myocardial infarction. *Journal of Advanced Nursing*, 12: 677–682.

Bonnet MH, Berry RB, Arand DL (1991). Metabolism during normal, fragmented and recovery sleep. *Journal of Applied Physiology*, 71: 1112–1118.

Bowles KH (2000). Patient problems and nurse-led interventions during acute care and discharge planning. *Journal of Cardiovascular Nursing*, 14: 29–41.

Brezinova V, Oswald I (1972). Sleep after a bedtime beverage. *British Medical Journal*, 2: 431–433.

British Cardiac Society (2001). Guidelines for the management of patients with acute coronary syndromes without ST segment elevation. *Heart*, 85: 133–142.

British Heart Foundation (2003). *Coronary Heart Disease Statistics*. British Heart Foundation, London.

Broughton R, Baron R (1973). Sleep of acute coronary patients in an open ward ITU. *Sleep Research*, 2: 144–149.

Broughton R, Baron R (1978). Sleep patterns in the ICU and on the ward after acute myocardial infarction. *Electroencephalography and Clinical Neurophysiology*, 45: 348–360.

Brown AJ (1976). Effect of family visits on the blood pressure and heart rate of patients in the coronary care unit. *Heart and Lung*, 5: 291–296.

Burgess AW, Hariman CR (1986). Patients' perceptions – key to recovery. *American Journal of Nursing*, 86: 568–571.

Cahil J (1998). Patient participation – a review of the literature. *Journal of Advanced Nursing*, 7: 119–128.

CAPRIE Steering Committee (1996). A randomised double blind trial of clopidogrel versus aspirin in patients at risk of ischaemic events. *Lancet*, 1329–1339.

Cassem NH, Hackett TP, Bosom C, Wishnie H (1970). Reactions of coronary patients to the CCU nurse. *American Journal of Nursing*, 70: 319–325.

Caunt J (1995). The advanced nurse practitioner in CCU. *Care of the Critically Ill*, 12: 136–139.

Cay EL (1982). Psychological problems in patients after a myocardial infarction. *Advances in Cardiology*, 29: 108–112.

Chavez CW, Faber L (1987). Effect of an education-orientation program on family members who visit their significant other in the intensive care unit. *Heart and Lung*, 16: 92–99.

Chilcott J, Hunt A (2001). Nurse-friendly integrated care pathways (development of cardiology pathways based on the Roper, Logan and Tierney model of nursing). *Nursing Times*, 97: 32–34.

Chokroverty S (1999). *Sleep Disorders Medicine: Basic Science, Technical Considerations, and Clinical Aspects*. Butterworth-Heinemann, Boston.

Closs SJ (1988). Assessment of sleep in hospital patients: a review of methods. *Journal of Advanced Nursing*, 13: 501–510.

Cohen M, Demers C, Gurtinkel EP et al (1997). A comparison of low molecular weight heparin with unfractionated heparin for unstable coronary artery disease. Efficacy and safety of subcutaneous Enoxiparin in non-Q wave coronary events study group. *New England Journal of Medicine*, 337: 447–452.

Collinson J, Flather M, Fox KA et al (2000). Clinical outcomes, risk stratification and practice patterns of unstable angina and myocardial infarction without ST elevation. *European Heart Journal*, 21: 1450–1457.

Coyle MA (2001). Transfer anxiety: preparing to leave intensive care. *Intensive and Critical Care Nursing*, 17: 138–143.

Cox C, Hayes J (1998). Experiences of administering and receiving therapeutic touch in intensive care. *Complementary Therapies in Nursing and Midwifery*, 4: 128–133.

Cucherat M, Bonnefoy E, Tremeau G (2004). Primary angioplasty versus intravenous thrombolysis for acute myocardial infarction. (Cochrane Review). In: *The Cochrane Library* Issue 1. Wiley, Chichester.

CURE Investigators (2001). Effects of clopidogrel in addition to aspirin in patients with acute coronary syndromes without ST segment elevation. *New England Journal of Medicine*, 345: 494–502.

Currell R, Wainwright P, Urquhart C (2002). Nursing record systems: effects on nursing practice. *Cochrane Database of Systematic Reviews. Issue 4.*

Dalby M, Montalescot G (2002). Transfer for primary angioplasty: who and how? *Heart*, 88: 570–572.

Daley M (1984). Families in critical care. *Heart and Lung*, 13: 231–237.

Davidhizar R, Giger JN (1997). When touch is not the best approach. *Journal of Clinical Nursing*, 6: 203–206.

Davis JM (1987). Visiting acutely ill patients: a literature review. *Intensive Care Nursing*, 2: 16–165.

Day W (2000). Relaxation: a nursing therapy to help relieve cardiac chest pain. *Australian Journal of Advanced Nursing*, 18: 40–44.

Deamer RM, Scharf MB, Kales A (1972). Sleep patterns in the CCU. *US Navy Medicine*, 59: 19–23.

de Belder MA (2001). Acute myocardial infarction: failed thrombolysis. *Heart*, 85: 104–112.

deBono D, Simoons ML, Tijssen L et al (1992). Effect of early intravenous heparin on coronary patency, infarct size, and bleeding complications after alteplase thrombolysis: a randomised double blind European Cooperative Study Group Trial. *British Heart Journal*, 67: 122–128.

Deeks P, Byatt K (2000). Are patients who self-administer their medicines in hospital more satisfied with their care? *Journal of Advanced Nursing*, 31: 395–400.

de Luc K (2000). Care pathways: an evaluation of their effectiveness. *Journal of Advanced Nursing*, 32: 485–496.

Department of Health (1989). *Working for Patients: The Health Service Caring for the 1990s*. HMSO, London.

Department of Health (1997). *The Caldicott Committee: Report on the Review of Patient-Identifiable Information*. Department of Medicine, London.

Department of Health (2000). *National Service Framework for Coronary Heart Disease*. Department of Health, London.

Department of Health (2001). *The Essence of Care – Patient Focused Benchmarking for Health Care Professionals*. Department of Health, London.

DeWood M, Berg R (1987). The role of surgical reperfusion in myocardial infarction. *Cardiology Clinics*, 2: 113–117.

Duits AA, Duivenvoorden HJ, Boeke S, Mochtar B, Passchier J, Erdman RAM (2002). Psychological and somatic factors in patients undergoing coronary artery bypass graft surgery: towards building a psychological framework. *Psychology and Health*, 17: 159–171.

Ellis SG, da Silva ER, Heyndrickx G et al (1994). Randomised comparison of rescue angioplasty with conservative management of patients with early failure of thrombolysis for acute myocardial infarction. *Circulation*, 90: 2280–2284.

EMIP Study (1993). Pre-hospital thrombolytic therapy in patients with suspected acute myocardial infarction. *New England Journal of Medicine*, 329: 383–389.

Engel GL (1964). Grief and grieving. *American Journal of Nursing*, 64: 93–98.

Erhardt L, Herlitz J, Bossaert L et al (2002). Task force on the management of chest pain. *European Heart Journal*, 23: 1153–1176,

Every N, Hochman J, Becker R et al (2000). Critical pathways: a review. *Circulation*, 101: 461–469.

Fibrinolytic Therapy Trialists' (FTT) Collaborative Group (1994). Indications for fibrinolytic therapy in suspected myocardial infarction: collaborative overview of early mortality and major morbidity results from all randomised trials of more than 1000 patients. *Lancet*, 343: 311–322.

Field D (1989). Emotional involvement with the dying in a coronary care unit. *Nursing Times* (Occasional Paper), 85 (13): 46–48.

Fielding RG, Llewelyn SP (1987). Communication training in nursing may damage your health and enthusiasm: some warnings. *Journal of Advanced Nursing*, 12: 281–290.

Fox KAA (2000). Acute coronary syndromes: presentation, clinical spectrum and management. *Heart*, 84: 93–100.

Freemantle N, Cleland J, Young P et al (1999). Beta-blockade after myocardial infarction: a systematic review and meta-regression analysis. *British Medical Journal*, 318: 1730–1737.

Fredrikson L (1999). Modes of relating in a caring conversation: a research synthesis on presence, touch and listening. *Journal of Advanced Nursing*, 30: 1167–1176.

Furlong S (1996). Do programmes of medicine self administration enhance patient knowledge, compliance and satisfaction? *Journal of Advanced Nursing*, 23: 1254–1262.

Garrity TF, Klein RF (1975). Emotional responses and clinical severity as early determinants of six-month mortality after myocardial infarction. *Heart and Lung*, 4: 730–737.

Gay S (1999). Research dimension. Meeting cardiac patients expectations of caring. *Dimensions of Critical Care Nursing*, 18: 46–50.

Glick MS (1986). Caring touch and anxiety in myocardial infarction patients in the intermediate cardiac care unit. *Intensive Care Nursing*, 2: 61–66.

Goodacre S, Mason S, Arnold J et al (2001). Psychologic morbidity and health related quality of life of patients assessed in a chest pain observation unit. *Annals of Emergency Medicine*, 38: 369–376.

Great Britain (2003). *The Misuse of Drugs* (Amendment) (No 3) Stat. Inst. No 2429. HMSO, London.

GREAT Study Group (1992). Feasibility, safety and efficacy of domiciliary thrombolysis by general practitioners: the Grampian Regional Early Anistreplase Trial. *British Medical Journal*, 305: 548–553.

GUSTO-1. Global utilisation of streptokinase and t = PA for occluded coronary arteries (1993). An international randomised trial comparing four thrombolytic strategies for acute myocardial infarction. *New England Journal of Medicine*, 329: 673–682.

Hampe SO (1975). Needs of the grieving spouse in a hospital setting. *Nursing Research*, 24: 113–120.

Hautvast RWM, Blanksma PK, Dejonqste MJL et al (1999). Effect of spinal cord stimulation on myocardial blood flow assessed by positron emission tomography in patients with refractory angina. *American Journal of Cardiology*, 77: 462–467.

Herkner H, Thoenissen J, Nikfardjam M et al (2003). Short versus prolonged bed rest after uncomplicated acute myocardial infarction: a systematic review and meta-analysis. *Journal of Clinical Epidemiology*, 56: 775–781.

Hewitt J (2000). A critical view of the arguments debating the role of the nurse advocate. *Journal of Advanced Nursing*, 439–445.

Hilton B (1985). Noise in hospitals: its effects on the patient. *Research in Nursing Health*, 8: 283–291.

Holmes TH, Rahe RH (1967). The social readjustment rating scale. *Journal of Psychosomatic Research*, 11: 213–218.

Holter NJ (1961). New methods for heart studies. *Science*, 134: 1214–1217.

Holub N, Eklund P, Keenan P (1975). Family conferences as an adjunct to total coronary care. *Heart and Lung*, 4: 767–769.

Horne JA (1988). *Why We Sleep: The Functions of Sleep in Humans and Other Mammals*. Oxford University Press, Oxford.

Horne JA, Ostberg O (1976). A self assessment questionnaire to determine morningness–eveningness in human circadian rhythms. *International Journal of Chronobiology*, 4: 97–110.

Hudson GR (1993). Empathy and technology in the coronary care unit. *Intensive and Critical Care Nursing*, 9: 55–61.

Hughes C, Scott K, Saltissi S et al (1997). The effect of an acute chest pain nurse (ACPN) on door to needle time at an inner city teaching hospital. *Heart* 77 (Suppl 1): 49–54.

Hunt JM (1999). The cardiac surgical patient's expectations and experiences of nursing care in the intensive care unit. *Australian Critical Care*, 12: 47–53.

INJECT International Joint Efficacy Comparison of Thrombolytics (1995). Randomised double blind comparison of retaplase double bolus administration with streptokinase in acute myocardial infarction. (INJECT) trial to investigate equivalence. *Lancet*, 366: 336–339.

ISIS-2 (Second International Study of Infarct Survival) Collaborative Group (1988). Randomised trial of intravenous streptokinase, oral aspirin, both, or neither among 17187 cases of suspected acute myocardial infarction. *Lancet*, 2: 349–360.

Jaarsma T, Kastermans M, Dasen T et al (1995). Problems of cardiac patients in early recovery. *Journal of Advanced Nursing*, 21: 21–27.

Jenkins D, Rogers H (1995). Transfer anxiety in patients with myocardial infarction. Pre-transfer teaching programme to prepare patients for move from coronary care unit to general ward. *British Journal of Nursing*, 4: 1248–1252.

Johnson JE (1973). Effects of accurate expectations about sensations on the sensory and distress components of pain. *Journal of Personality and Social Psychology*, 27: 261–275.

Johnston BL, Watt EW, Fletcher GF (1981). Oxygen consumption and hemodynamic and electrocardiographic responses to bathing in recent post-myocardial infarction patients. *Heart and Lung*, 10: 666–671.

Joint European Society of Cardiology/American College of Cardiology Committee (2000). Myocardial infarction redefined: a consensus document for the redefinition of myocardial infarction. *European Heart Journal*, 21: 1502–1513.

Kahn D, Cook T, Carlisle C et al (1998). Identification and modification of environmental noise in an ICU setting. *Chest*, 114: 535–540.

Karacan I, Green JR, Taylor WJ et al (1973). Sleep characteristics of acute myocardial infarction patients in an ICU. *Sleep Research*, 2: 159.

Kim KA, Moser DK, Garin BJ et al (2000). Differences between men and women in anxiety after acute myocardial infarction. *American Journal of Critical Care*, 9: 245–253.

Klein RF, Kliner VA, Zipes DP, Troyer WG, Wallace AG (1968). Transfer from a coronary care unit. *Archives of Internal Medicine*, 122: 104–108.

Kubler-Ross E (1970). *On Death and Dying*. Tavistock, London.

Landis CA, Whitney JD (1997). Effects of 72 hours sleep deprivation on wound healing in the rat. *Research in Nursing and Health*, 20: 259–267.

Lane D, Carroll D, Ring C et al (2002). The prevalence and persistence of depression and anxiety following myocardial infarction. *British Journal of Health Psychology*, 7: 11–21.

Lazarus RS (1966). *Psychological Stress and the Coping Process*. McGraw-Hill, New York.

Leske JS (1986). Needs of relatives of critically ill patients: a follow-up. *Heart and Lung*, 15: 189–193.

Levine SA, Lown B (1952). Armchair treatment of acute coronary thrombosis. *Journal of the American Medical Association*, 148: 1365–1369.

Ley P (1988). *Communicating with Patients*. Croom Helm, London.

Lindemann E (1944). Symptomatology and management of acute grief. *American Journal of Psychiatry*, 101: 141–148.

Lynch J, Thomas S, Mills M, Malinow K, Katcher A (1974). The effects of human contact on cardiac arrhythmias in coronary care patients. *Journal of Nervous and Mental Disease*, 158: 88–99.

Maguire P (1985). Barriers to psychological care of the dying. *British Medical Journal*, 291: 1711–1713.

McFarlane J (1980). *Essays on Nursing*. King's Fund, London.

McKenna CJ, Forfar JC (2002). Was it a heart attack? *British Medical Journal*, 324: 377–378.

Meurier CE (1998). The quality of assessment of patients with chest pain: the development of a questionnaire to audit the nursing assessment records of patients with chest pain. *Journal of Advanced Nursing*, 27: 140–146.

Meurier CE, Vincent CA, Palmer DG (1998). Perception of causes of omissions in the assessment of patients with chest pain. *Journal of Advanced Nursing*, 28: 1012–1019.

Mickley H (1994). Ambulatory ST segment monitoring after myocardial infarction. *British Heart Journal*, 71: 113–114.

Miller-Craig MW, Joy AV, Adamowicz M et al (1997). Reduction in treatment delay by paramedic ECG diagnosis of myocardial infarction with direct CCU admission. *Heart*, 78: 456–461.

Mitamura S, Nakamura M, Yamamoto T et al (1998). Observational assessment of patients' sleep complaints in the coronary care unit. *Psychiatry and Clinical Neurosciences*, 52: 164–165.

Moore-Ede MC, Czeisler CA, Richardson GS (1983). Circadian time keeping in health and disease. Part 1. Basic properties of circadian pacemakers. *New England Journal of Medicine*, 309: 469–476.

Morris MC, Serruys P, Sousa J for the RAVEL study group (2002). A randomised comparison of a sirolimus-eluting stent with a standard stent for coronary revascularisation. *New England Journal of Medicine*, 366: 1773–1780.

Morrison LJ, Verbeek PR, McDonald AC et al (2000). Mortality and prehospital thrombolysis for acute myocardial infarction: a meta-analysis. *Journal of the American Medical Association*, 283: 2686–2692.

Murphy R, Mackway-Jones K, Sammy I et al (2001). Emergency oxygen therapy for the breathless patient. Guidelines prepared by North West Oxygen Group. *Emergency Medicine Journal*, 18: 421–423.

National Institute of Clinical Excellence (2002a). *Thrombolysis*. Technology Appraisal Guidance, NICE, London.

National Institute of Clinical Excellence (2002b). *Guidance on the Use of Glycoprotein IIb/IIIa Inhibitors in the Treatment of Acute Coronary Syndromes*. Technology Appraisal Guidance No 47, NICE, London.

Newman MF, Kirchner JL, Phillips-Bute B et al (2001). Longitudinal assessment of neurocognitive function after coronary artery bypass. *New England Journal of Medicine*, 334: 395–402.

NHS Executive (1996). *Review of Ambulance Performance Standards*. Final Report of steering group. NHS Executive, London.

Norris LO, Grove SK (1986). Investigation of selected psychosocial needs of family members of critically ill adult patients. *Heart and Lung*, 15: 194–199.

Norris RM (1998). Fatality outside hospital from acute coronary events in three British health districts, 1994–5. United Kingdom Heart Attack Study Collaborative Group. *British Medical Journal*, 316: 1065–1070.

Nursing and Midwifery Council (2002). *Code of Professional Conduct*. NMC, London.

Nyamathi AM (1987). The coping responses of female spouses of patients with myocardial infarction. *Heart and Lung*, 16: 86–99.

O'Connor L (1995). Pain assessment by patients and nurses, and nurses notes on it, in early myocardial infarction. Part 1. *Intensive and Critical Care Nursing*, 11: 183–191.

Parsons T (1964). *The Social System*. Free Press, New York.

Patil CV, Nicolsky E, Boulos M et al (2001). Multivessel coronary artery disease: current revascularisation strategies. *European Heart Journal*, 22: 1183–1197.

Pearson SD, Goulart-Fisher D, Lee TH (1995). Critical pathways for improving care: problems and potential. *Annals of Internal Medicine*, 123: 941–948.

Pell JP, Simpson E, Rodger C (2003). Impact of changing diagnostic criteria on incidence, management and outcome of acute myocardial infarction: retrospective cohort study. *British Medical Journal*, 326: 134–135.

Pepine CJ (1989). New concepts in the pathophysiology of acute myocardial infarction. *American Journal of Cardiology*, 64: 2B–8B.

Peric-Knowlton W (1984). The understanding and management of acute pain in adults. The nursing contribution. *International Journal of Nursing Studies*, 21: 131–143.

Pfeffer MA, Braunwald E, Moye LA et al (1992). Effect of captopril on mortality and morbidity in patients with left ventricular dysfunction after myocardial infarction. Results of the survival and ventricular enlargement trial. The SAVE investigators. *New England Journal of Medicine*, 327: 669–677.

Pontin D (1999). Primary nursing: a mode of care or a philosophy of nursing? *Journal of Advanced Nursing*, 29: 584–591.

Potts SG, Lewin R, Fox KA et al (1999). Group psychological treatment for chest pain with normal coronary arteries. *Quarterly Journal of Medicine*, 92: 81–86.

Prasad N, Wright A, Hogg M, et al (1997). Direct admission to the coronary care unit by the ambulance service for patients with suspected myocardial infarction. *Heart*, 78: 462–464.

Proctor TF, Yarcheski A, Orscello R (1996). The relationship of hospital process variables to patient outcome post-myocardial infarction. *International Journal of Nursing Studies*, 33: 121–130.

Quinn T (1995). Can nurses safely assess suitability for thrombolytic therapy? A pilot study. *Intensive and Critical Care Nursing*, 11: 126–129.

Quinn T, Morse T (2003). The interdisciplinary interface in managing patients with suspected cardiac pain. *Emergency Nurse*, 11: 22–24.

Quinn T, Thompson DR (1995). The changing role of the nurse. *Care of the Critically Ill*, 73: 48–49.

Quinn T, Butters A, Todd L (2002). Implementing paramedic thrombolysis – an overview. *Accident and Emergency Nursing*, 10: 189–196.

Quinn T, MacDermott A, Caunt J (1998). Determining patient suitability for thrombolysis: coronary care nurses' agreement with expert cardiological 'gold standard' as assessed by clinical and electrocardiological vignettes. *Intensive and Critical Care Nursing*, 14: 219–224.

Rawles J (1997). Pre-hospital coronary care. *Pre-hospital Immediate Care*, 1: 12–18.

Reid E (2001). Factors affecting how patients sleep in the hospital environment. *British Journal of Nursing*, 10: 912–915.

Rhodes MA (1998). What is the evidence to support nurse led thrombolysis? *Clinical Effectiveness in Nursing*, 2: 69–77.

Richards KC, Bairnsfather L (1988). A description of night sleep patterns in the critical care unit. *Heart and Lung*, 17: 35–42.

Richards K (1998). Effect of back massage and relaxation intervention on sleep in critically ill patients. *American Journal of Critical Care*, 7: 288–299.

Rotter JB (1966). Generalized expectations for internal versus external control of reinforcement. *Psychological Monographs*, 80: 1–28.

Routasalo P (1999). Physical touch in nursing studies: a literature review. *Journal of Advanced Nursing*, 30: 843–850.

Royal College of Nursing (1999). *Guidance for Nurses Giving Intravenous Therapy*. Royal College of Nursing, London.

Royal College of Nursing (2000). *Patient Group Directions. Guidance and Information*. Royal College of Nursing, London.

Runions J (1985). A program for psychological and social enhancement during rehabilitation after myocardial infarction. *Heart and Lung*, 14: 117–125.

Savage MW, Channer KS (2002). Improving the management of myocardial infarction. *British Medical Journal*, 325: 1185–1186.

Schwartz LP, Brenner ZR (1979). Critical care unit transfers. Reducing patient stress through nursing interventions. *Heart and Lung*, 8: 540–546.

Seligman ME (1975). *Helplessness*. W.H. Freeman, San Francisco.

Selye H (1976). *The Stress of Life*. McGraw-Hill, New York.

Simpson T, Wilson D, Mucken N, Martin S, et al (1996). Implementation and evaluation of a liberalized visiting policy. *American Journal of Critical Care*, 6: 255–256.

Spielberger CD (1966). *Anxiety and Behaviour*. Academic Press, New York.

Stockwell F (1972). *The Unpopular Patient*. Royal College of Nursing, London.

Sutton AG, Campbell PG, Price DJ et al (2000). Failure of thrombolysis by streptokinase: detection with a simple electrocardiographic method. *Heart*, 84: 113–115.

Svedlund M, Danielson E, Norberg A (1999). Nurses' narrations about caring for in-patients with acute myocardial infarction. *Intensive and Critical Care Nursing*, 15: 34–43.

Taub JM, Berger RJ (1976). The effects of changing the phase and duration of sleep. *Journal of Experimental Psychology: Human Perception and Performance*, 2: 30.

Theobold K (1997). The experiences of spouses whose partners have suffered a myocardial infarction: a phenomenological study. *Journal of Advanced Nursing*, 26: 595–601.

Thieman DR, Coresh J, Schulman SP et al (2000). Lack of benefit for intravenous thrombolysis in patients with myocardial infarction who are older than 75 years. *Circulation*, 101: 2239–2246.

Thomas SA, Lynch JJ, Mills ME (1975). Psychological influences on heart rhythm in the coronary care unit. *Heart and Lung*, 4: 746–750.

Thompson DR (1990). *Counselling the Coronary Patient and Partner*. Scutari, London.

Thompson DR (1995). Fear of death. In *The Cardiac Patient: Nursing Interventions* (S O'Connor ed). Mosby, London. pp. 117–126.

Thompson DR (2002). Involvement of the partner in rehabilitation. In *Advancing the Frontiers of Cardiopulmonary Rehabilitation*. (J Jobin, F Maltais, P Poirier, P LeBlanc, C Simard eds). Human kinetics, Champaign, IL. pp. 211–215.

Thompson DR, Bailey SW, Webster RA (1986). Patient's views on cardiac monitoring. *Nursing Times* (Occasional Paper), 82 (9): 54–55.

Thompson DR, Cordle CJ (1988). Support of wives of myocardial infarction patients. *Journal of Advanced Nursing*, 13: 223–228.

Thompson DR, Sutton TW, Jowett NI, Pohl JEF (1991). Circadian variation in the frequency of onset of chest pain in acute myocardial infarction. *British Heart Journal*, 65: 177–178.

Thompson DR, Webster RA, Cordle CJ, Sutton TW (1987). Specific sources and patterns of anxiety in male patients with first myocardial infarction. *British Journal of Medical Psychology*, 60: 343–348.

Thompson DR, Webster RA, Sutton TW (1994). Coronary care unit patients' and nurses' ratings of the intensity of ischaemic chest pain. *Intensive and Critical Care Nursing*, 10: 83–88.

Tiefenbrunn AJ, Sobel BE (1991). Thrombolysis and myocardial infarction. *Fibrinolysis*, 5: 1–15.

Topf M (2000). Hospital noise pollution: an environmental stress model to guide research and clinical interventions. *Journal of Advanced Nursing*, 31: 520–528.

Topf M, Thompson S (2001). Interactive relationships between hospital patients' noise-induced stress and other stress with sleep. *Heart and Lung*, 30: 237–243.

Toth JC (1980). Effect of structured preparation for transfer on patient anxiety. *Nursing Research*, 29: 28–34.

United Kingdom Central Council for Nursing, Midwifery and Health Visiting (1998). *Guidelines for Records and Record Keeping*. UKCC, London.

Van de Werf F, Ardissino D, Betriu A, et al (2003). The Task Force on the Management of Acute Myocardial Infarction of the European Society of Cardiology: Management of acute myocardial infarction with ST-segment elevation. *European Heart Journal*, 24: 28–66.

van Weert J, van Dulmen S, Bar P, Venus E (2003). Interdisciplinary preoperative patient education in cardiac surgery. *Patient Education and Counseling*, 49: 105–114.

Vermeer F, Oude OAJ, vd Berg EJ et al (1999). Prospective randomised comparison between thrombolysis, rescue PTCA and primary PTCA in patients with extensive myocardial infarction admitted to a hospital with extensive myocardial infarction admitted to hospital without PTCA facilities: a safety and feasibility study. *Circulation*, 101: 101–108.

Wallentin L, Lagerqvist B, Husted S et al (2000). Outcome at one year after an invasive compared with a non-invasive strategy in coronary artery disease: the FRISC 11 invasive randomised trial. *Lancet*, 356: 9–16.

Waterworth S, Luker K (1990). Reluctant collaborators in care: do patients want to be involved in decisions concerning care. *Journal of Advanced Nursing*, 15: 971–976.

Weaver WD, Cerqueira M, Hallstrom AP et al for the Myocardial Infarction Triage and Intervention (MITI) Project Group (1993). Pre-hospital initiated versus hospital initiated thrombolytic therapy. *Journal of the American Medical Association*, 270: 1211–1216.

Webster R (1997). The experience and health care needs of Asian coronary patients and their partners: methodological issues and preliminary findings. *Nursing in Critical Care*, 2: 215–223.

Webster RA, Thompson DR (1986). Sleep in hospital. *Journal of Advanced Nursing*, 11: 447–457.

Wells N (1984). Responses to acute pain – the nursing implications. *Journal of Advanced Nursing*, 9: 51–58.

White JM (1999). Effects of relaxing music on cardiac autonomic balance and anxiety after acute myocardial infarction. *American Journal of Critical Care*, 8: 220–230.

Williams A (2001). A literature review on the concept of intimacy in nursing. *Journal of Advanced Nursing*, 33: 660–667.

Wilmhurst P (1999). What is meant by 'thrombolysis nurse'? *Journal of the Royal College of Physicians of London*, 33: 284–285.

Wilson A, Norbury E, Richardson K (2000). Caring for broken hearts: patients and relatives: three years of bereavement support in CCU. Account of follow-up support service in a coronary care unit. *Nursing in Critical Care*, 5: 288–293.

Wilson-Barnett J (1984). *Key Functions in Nursing* (Winifred Raphael Memorial Lecture). Royal College of Nursing, London.

Winslow EH, Lane LD, Gaffney FA (1984). Oxygen consumption and cardiovascular response in patients and normal adults during in-bed and out of bed toileting. *Journal of Cardiac Rehabilitation*, 4: 348–354.

Winslow EH, Lane LD, Gaffney FA (1985). Oxygen uptake and cardiovascular responses in control adults and acute myocardial infarction patients during bathing. *Nursing Research*, 34: 164–169.

Woodward V (1997). Professional caring: a contraindication in terms? *Journal of Advanced Nursing*, 26: 999–1004.

World Health Organisation Expert Committee (1959). *Hypertension and Coronary Heart Disease: Classification and Criteria for Epidemiological Studies*. World Health Organisation, Geneva. (Technical Support Series 168).

Yusuf S, Wittes J, Freidman L (1988). Overview of results of randomised clinical trials in heart disease. 11. Unstable angina and heart failure. Primary prevention with aspirin and risk factor modification. *Journal of the American Medical Association*, 260: 2259–2263.

Yusuf S, Sleight P, Pogue J et al (2000). Effects of an angiotensin converting enzyme inhibitor, ramapril on cardiovascular events in high risk patients. The Heart Outcomes Prevention Study Investigators. *New England Journal of Medicine*, 324: 145–155.

Zieman KM, Dracup K (1990). Patient-nurse contracts in critical care: a controlled trial. *Progress in Cardiovascular Nursing*, 5: 98–103.

Further reading

Hatchett R, Thompson DR (eds) (2002) *Cardiac Nursing: A Comprehensive Guide*. Harcourt, London.

Jowett NI, Thompson DR (2003) *Comprehensive Coronary Care*. 3rd edn. Baillière Tindall, London.

Stewart S, Moser DK, Thompson DR (2004) *Caring for the Heart Failure Patient*. Martin Dunitz, London.

Chapter **7**

Dealing with complications

CHAPTER CONTENTS

INTRODUCTION

Complications that follow acute myocardial infarction tend to be dependent on:

- the cumulative loss of functional myocardium as a result of current and previous ischaemic damage
- the extent of coronary artery disease
- other disease processes (e.g. diabetes, renal disorder).

DISORDERS OF HEART RATE AND RHYTHM

The term *arrhythmia* is used to imply an abnormality either in:

- electrical impulse *formation*
- electrical impulse *conduction* within the heart.

About 90% of coronary patients will experience some sort of arrhythmia, particularly in the first 24 hours following infarction. The detection and treatment of arrhythmias is one of the main primary purposes of the coronary care unit. Arrhythmias producing circulatory impairment or compromising ischaemic myocardium, or which predispose to more serious arrhythmias, require prompt and effective therapy. Therefore, the nurse needs to be able to recognize arrhythmias, interpret their significance and take appropriate action to minimize their potential deleterious effects on the patient.

It is likely that both the extent and location of the infarction will play an important part in the cause of the arrhythmia. While many (usually pre-hospital) deaths occur in the setting of minimal myocardial damage, the more extensive the myocardial damage, the more likely the patient will experience arrhythmias particularly late in the hospital course. Patients admitted with extensive (particularly anterior) infarcts, heart failure, obesity and a history of anxiety are more prone to arrhythmias post-infarction. Arrhythmias may also be precipitated by certain endocrine disorders, electrolyte imbalance, hypoxia, drug toxicity and free radicals released following reperfusion.

Clinically, arrhythmias may be considered either as primary electrical disorders or as secondary disturbances reflecting impaired pump action.

An arrhythmia may cause its effects by any of the following changes:

1   change in heart rate
2   loss of atrial transport
3   increase in myocardial oxygen requirement
4   decrease in myocardial blood flow
5   loss of synchronicity of ventricular contraction
6   any combination of the above.

Consequences of arrhythmias arise because of impaired circulation or myocardial oxygenation. Although the healthy heart is able to withstand many rhythm disturbances, the diseased heart cannot. Any circulatory embarrassment is serious following acute myocardial infarction, since it may compromise perfusion in areas of marginally ischaemic myocardium and cause further infarction.

As heart rate is a major determinant of myocardial oxygen requirements, tachycardia consistently increases demand. Most patients (particularly those with anterior infarction) have enhanced activity of the autonomic nervous system which predisposes to transient hypertension and to tachycardias. Increases in heart rate are associated with a reduction in diastolic timing. Ventricular filling may therefore be critically reduced with a dramatic fall in cardiac output. Since coronary flow occurs mainly during diastole, especially to the left ventricular myocardium, but the duration of diastole is reduced during tachycardia, coronary perfusion is decreased. Thus, tachyarrhythmias increase myocardial oxygen requirements and decrease myocardial oxygen supply. A tachycardia has been found to be a factor favouring extension of the infarct and is associated with a worse outcome.

With any tachyarrhythmia, the patient may experience palpitations, shortness of breath, feelings of dizziness, faintness, sweating and a reduced exercise tolerance.

Parasympathetic (vagal) overactivity is particularly common following inferior and posterior myocardial infarction and predisposes to a reduced heart rate and hypotension. Bradycardias, occurring either as a result of disorder of impulse formation or of a conduction disturbance, can also produce symptoms of decreased cardiac output. Initially, cardiac output is maintained by an increase in stroke volume achieved by an increased end-diastolic volume and/or an increased ejection fraction. Thus, bradycardia can optimize the chance of myocardial preservation during acute infarction by reducing myocardial oxygen requirements while maintaining cardiac output. The effectiveness of such compensatory mechanisms is, however, limited, especially in the patient with myocardial disease. Cardiac output may become critically low with associated heart failure at rates that the normal heart could withstand, i.e. at rates below 40 beats/min. The duration of the bradycardia influences the haemodynamic effect. Thus, trained athletes and individuals with chronic heart block can maintain a near normal cardiac output at rates that would compromise the patient with acute heart block.

In the healthy heart, the atrial component of cardiac output maintenance is of little haemodynamic consequence, except at fast rates or during exercise. However, following acute myocardial infarction with resultant impaired left ventricular function, atrial transport may assume prime importance in maintaining cardiac output.

Effective ventricular function depends upon synchrony of left ventricular contraction. Intraventricular conduction disturbances, such as left bundle branch block, which produce only slightly less synchronous activation of the ventricle, can have a significant haemodynamic effect on the infarcted ventricle.

MANAGEMENT OF ACUTE CARDIAC ARRHYTHMIAS

Medical management of arrhythmias aims to restore sinus rhythm and to prevent recurrences.

If it is not possible to restore sinus rhythm, then the aim is to 'normalize' the ventricular rate and increase cardiac output. Therapy on the coronary care unit is usually initiated for arrhythmias which (a) are producing, or are likely to produce, haemodynamic decompensation, or (b) may be a precursor of cardiac arrest. Attention needs to be directed towards the precipitating cause, for instance pain, fear, hypoxia, acidosis or electrolyte imbalance, otherwise if they persist restoration of sinus rhythm may prove difficult.

Management of cardiac arrhythmias usually takes the form of drugs or electrical (defibrillation or pacing) intervention.

PRINCIPLES OF CARE OF THE PATIENT WITH A CARDIAC ARRHYTHMIA

The clinical manifestation of an arrhythmia depends on the ventricular rate, the conduction of the myocardium and the physiological and psychological response of the patient.

Arrhythmias may produce a variety of problems for the patient:

- palpitations
- dizziness
- fainting
- shortness of breath
- chest pain
- headache
- reduced activity tolerance
- anxiety.

Patient assessment should include:

- the apparent effect of the arrhythmia on the patient
- a history of any past experiences with arrhythmias
- a knowledge of any relevent medications or other treatments
- the identification of any possible precipitating factors.

The deviation of the heart rate and rhythm from the normal is not in itself a reason for intervention. Whether treatment is warranted depends on the occurrence, or possibility, of a reduction in cardiac output, a progression to more sinister arrhythmias, the psychological effect on the patient and the likely success and safety of treatment.

The nurse seeks to care for the patient rather than solely focusing on the arrhythmia, and this involves the alleviation of any associated symptoms, providing explanations of problems together with any treatment, and continued monitoring for adverse effects resulting from reduced cardiac output.

Regular recordings of the patient's blood pressure and careful observation for cyanosis, pallor, sweating, and alterations in urine output, mental alertness and activity tolerance, will give an indication of cardiac output. The patient may be the best judge of the effects of the arrhythmia, and their involvement in aspects of decision making about care planning and evaluation is crucial.

The patient who is aware of the arrhythmia, whether through its effects or because of perceived increased medical and nursing attention, is likely to be anxious, perceiving the, often sudden, change in his condition as a life-threatening event and a major setback to the recovery process. The obvious change in the bedside electrocardiogram (ECG) monitor tracing may be a cause of alarm for both the patient and his relatives. If ischaemic chest pain occurs with the arrhythmia, the patient may worry that they are suffering another heart attack.

Decreased activity tolerance may mean increased dependency on the nurse, with associated feelings of helplessness and frustration. The patient may need help to carry out desired and necessary activities while maintaining optimum independence and control. Poor tissue perfusion, coupled with decreased mobility, will increase the likelihood of skin breakdown at pressure point sites. Many arrhythmias increase the likelihood of systemic emboli. Thus, patients may require encouragement regarding changes of body position and the performance of passive exercises.

ANTI-ARRHYTHMIC DRUG THERAPY

Anti-arrhythmic drugs tend to exert their effect by blocking the underlying stimulus which originally initiated the arrhythmia, blocking the formation of the impulse, or blocking impulse conduction. There are many ways of classifying anti-arrhythmic drugs, including the type of arrhythmia, the site of action and how the drug works electrophysiologically.

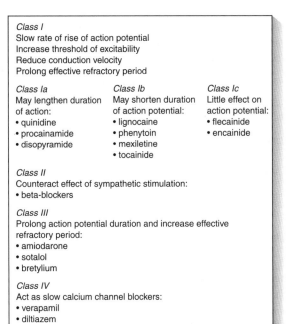

Class I
Slow rate of rise of action potential
Increase threshold of excitability
Reduce conduction velocity
Prolong effective refractory period

Class Ia	Class Ib	Class Ic
May lengthen duration of action:	May shorten duration of action potential:	Little effect on action potential:
• quinidine	• lignocaine	• flecainide
• procainamide	• phenytoin	• encainide
• disopyramide	• mexiletine	
	• tocainide	

Class II
Counteract effect of sympathetic stimulation:
• beta-blockers

Class III
Prolong action potential duration and increase effective refractory period:
• amiodarone
• sotalol
• bretylium

Class IV
Act as slow calcium channel blockers:
• verapamil
• diltiazem

Figure 7.1 Summary of action potential classification of anti-arrhythmic drugs.

Most of these drugs may also be classified according to their effects, either directly or indirectly, on the action potentials of normal cardiac cells. A classification system described by Vaughan-Williams (1984) is often used (Figure 7.1).

Action potential classification

Class I. Membrane stabilizing agents

This class of drugs impedes the transport of sodium across the cell membrane during the initiation of cellular activation and thereby reduces the rate of rise of the action potential (phase 0). The many drugs that fall into this group are subdivided into classes A, B and C according to their effect on the action potential (manifested in the ECG by the Q-T interval).

Class Ia drugs prolong the action potential duration and inhibit the fast sodium current and the upstroke of the action potential. They are more cardiodepressant than other drugs in this class. Examples of this class of drugs include quinidine, procainamide and disopyramide.

Class Ib drugs decrease ventricular conduction cell automaticity, possibly by shortening the refractory

period. These drugs have an increased effect on diseased myocardial tissue and they shorten the action potential duration. Examples of this class of drugs include lidocain, mexiletine and phenytoin.

Class Ic drugs have a membrane stabilizing capacity on the atria and ventricles. They slow intraventricular conduction but have little, if any, effect on the action potential. Examples of this class of drugs include flecainide and propafenone.

Class II. Beta-adrenergic receptor blocking agents – beta-blockers

This class of drugs interferes with the effects of the sympathetic nervous system by reducing the effects of circulating catecholamines on the adrenergic receptor cells known as beta-receptors. Ahlqvist (1948) proposed the term alpha- and beta-receptors for sites on smooth muscle where catecholamines produce excitatory and inhibitory responses, respectively. Subsequently, Lands et al (1967) categorized beta-adrenergic receptors into a subclassification: beta-1 receptors (chiefly at cardiac sites) and beta-2 receptors (elsewhere). However, different tissues may possess both types in varying proportions. Beta-adrenergic receptor blocking agents (beta-blockers) have received major attention because of their utility in the management of cardiovascular disorders, including angina pectoris, hypertension and cardiac arrhythmias. However, because of the ability of certain drugs, such as propranolol and timolol, to block beta-receptors in bronchial smooth muscle and skeletal muscle, they have to be used with caution, particularly in those with asthma. As a consequence, selective beta-1 blockers have been introduced, e.g. metoprolol and atenolol. However, it is important to remember that the selectivity of beta-1 blockers is not absolute: larger doses of these compounds will inhibit all beta-receptors.

This class of drugs reduces the slope of spontaneous depolarization (phase 4) of cells with pacemaker activity and therefore the rate of pacemaker discharge.

Class III. Agents prolonging action potential duration

This class of drugs prolongs the duration of the action potential, consequently increasing the effective refractory period. The conduction time, contractility and rate of rise of the action potential are not affected. They suppress ventricular ectopic activity, ventricular tachycardia (VT) and ventricular fibrillation (VF). Examples of this class of drugs include amiodarone, sotalol and bretylium.

Class IV. Slow calcium channel blockers

This class of drugs antagonizes the transport of calcium across the cell membrane which follows the inward flux of sodium during cellular activation and depresses the plateau phase of the action potential. Cells in the sinus and atrio-ventricular (AV) nodes are particularly susceptible. Examples include verapamil and diltiazem. Their action is particularly significant in the upper part of the AV node as they block circus movements during re-entry tachycardias. Some calcium antagonists, such as nifedipine, do not appear to have any anti-arrhythmic action.

Clinical classification

Anti-arrhythmic drugs may also be divided into three groups according to their principal site(s) of action. This classification is generally used for practical therapeutic purposes. The first group consists of drugs whose predominant action is to slow conduction in the AV node, and are thus used in the management of supraventricular arrhythmias. The second group includes drugs that mainly affect ventricular arrhythmias. The third group comprises drugs that act mainly on the atria and ventricles and may thus prove useful in the management of both supraventricular and ventricular arrhythmias (Table 7.1).

Drug administration

In the coronary patient, the absorption of drugs from the gastrointestinal tract may be unpredictable. Decreased blood flow produced by reduced cardiac output or by vasoconstrictor agents may slow drug absorption at this site.

Drugs are frequently given by the intravenous route, as the desired concentration of a drug in the blood is obtained with an accuracy and immediacy not possible by any other route.

Table 7.1 Summary of clinical classification of anti-arrhythmic drugs according to their principal site(s) of action

Site of action	Anti-arrhythmic drug
AV node	Verapamil, diltiazem, digoxin, beta-blocker, adenosine
Ventricles	Lignocaine, mexiletine, tocainide, phenytoin
Atria and ventricles	Amiodarone, quinidine, disopyramide, flecainide, procainamide

Loading dose

If a rapid effect is required, a bolus loading dose is often given to achieve a therapeutic blood level at the onset of therapy. A loading dose may be desired if the time required to attain a steady state by the administration of drug at a constant rate is long relative to the demands of the condition being treated. Loading doses tend to be large and are often administered parenterally and rapidly. This can have significant disadvantages. For example, the particularly sensitive individual may be exposed abruptly to a toxic concentration of a drug. Moreover, if the drug used has a long half-life (denoted by $t_{1/2}$; the time it takes for the plasma concentration or the amount of drug in the body to be reduced by 50%), it will take a long time for the concentration to fall if the level initially achieved was excessive.

Maintenance dose

In most clinical situations the drug will be administered in a series of repetitive doses or as a continuous infusion, in order to maintain a steady-state concentration of drug in plasma within a given therapeutic range. The timing of drug administration is usually most effective if there is no pronounced fluctuation in drug concentration between doses.

Limitations of drug therapy

Despite advances in the knowledge of the pharmacological management of arrhythmias, management is still often unsatisfactory, with many patients being treated empirically. Although drugs tend to be used as a first option for anti-arrhythmic therapy, their limitations need to be appreciated.

Most drugs have the potential for initiating arrhythmias, in other words they are arrhythmogenic. They tend to be negative inotropes and hence reduce coronary perfusion which predispose to pre-existing or new cardiac arrhythmias.

Arrhythmias are more likely to occur if more than one agent is being prescribed at the same time. Therefore, careful selection of an appropriate drug as first choice is important. Anti-arrhythmic drugs may also produce other unwanted or deleterious effects, such as gastrointestinal and central nervous system symptoms, hypotension, heart failure and impairment of the cardiac conducting system.

It is often difficult to maintain therapeutic drug levels, and frequently the process of selecting the most appropriate drug that is both effective and well tolerated for a given patient becomes a method of educated trial and error for the physician. In some cases, it is often advantageous to use alternative and more appropriate approaches, such as cardioversion, vagal stimulation or artificial cardiac pacing.

DISTURBANCES OF IMPULSE FORMATION

The common arrhythmias, due to some abnormality of impulse formation, seen in the acute coronary patient include the following.

Sinus bradycardia

This is arbitrarily defined as a sinus rhythm at 60 beats per minute or lower. It is common in healthy individuals during sleep and will be apparent in patients receiving beta-blockers or digoxin. It is a particularly common physiological phenomenon in athletes. It is also seen in about a third of all coronary patients, particularly in the first hour after inferior infarction. It is usually benign and may have advantages for compromised myocardial perfusion by limiting the myocardial work of an acutely injured heart. It may, however, result in hypotension secondary to a low cardiac output and a reduction in coronary perfusion. There is also a theoretical likelihood of increased risk of VF, as

escape rhythm and ventricular ectopic activity is more likely with a slow heart rate.

Sinus bradycardia tends to occur most frequently with an inferior infarction because the right coronary artery supplies the inferior aspects of the heart and, in most cases, the sinus and AV nodes. Following infarction, increased acetylcholine release from the autonomic fibres of these nodes makes bradycardia more likely. Sinus bradycardia may sometimes occur following reperfusion of the right coronary artery. Occurrence later in the course of myocardial infarction is usually a favourable sign and requires no treatment.

Treatment is warranted if the bradycardia is associated with signs and symptoms of hypoperfusion, for instance chest pain, dizziness, faintness, frequent ectopic beats, low blood pressure or signs of reduced cerebral or renal perfusion.

In general, patients with acute inferior infarction do well without any active intervention. Atropine (0.5 mg) is effective if a slow heart rate develops due to increased vagal stimulation. Further doses may be given at 2–3 minute intervals, up to a total dose of 2.0 mg. Sinus bradycardia in patients with an anterior infarction is indicative of extensive myocardial damage and therefore a worse prognosis.

On the occasions that drugs prove ineffective, temporary pacing is used to increase the ventricular rate. Pacing is preferred to the use of positive chronotropic agents, which increase oxygen demand, myocardial work and possibly the size of the infarct.

The ECG shows normal P waves followed by QRST complexes at a regular rate less than 60 per minute (Figure 7.2).

Sinus tachycardia

This is arbitrarily defined as a sinus rhythm greater than 100 per minute. Sinus tachycardia is normal during exercise, but if it occurs at rest it may be as a result of a primary electrical disturbance or secondary to pain, anxiety, pericarditis, heart failure, hypovolaemia and high output states.

Sinus tachycardia is thought to occur in about a third of acute myocardial infarction patients probably as a result of enhanced catecholamine activity. The mortality of patients with sinus tachycardia is

Figure 7.2   Sinus bradycardia.

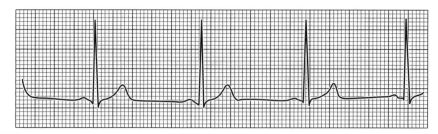

usually higher in those with sinus bradycardia, usually as a result of left ventricular failure. Reflex tachycardia occurs as a compensatory mechanism in an attempt to maintain cardiac output in the face of a reduced stroke volume. Sinus tachycardia usually occurs in the patient with previously relatively good left ventricular function, whereas other supraventricular tachycardias predominate in the older and more debilitated patient.

As myocardial oxygen consumption is related to heart rate and infarct size, sinus tachycardia can carry an ominous prognosis for the coronary patient. As sinus tachycardia is usually a physiological response to other disease or stimuli, treatment of the arrhythmia usually means treatment of the cause such as chest pain, anxiety, heart failure or even the discomfort associated with faecal impaction.

Although sinus tachycardia is a physiological response to myocardial damage, it may benefit from beta-blockade, particularly if there is associated hypertension. Intravenous beta-blockade has been shown to improve prognosis after acute myocardial infarction (Freemantle et al 2001). Metoprolol and atenolol are safe to use intravenously, providing there is no asthma or advanced heart failure. The short-acting esmolol can be used if there is any doubt about cardiac decompensation. Intravenous beta-blockers need to be given by slow intravenous injection while monitoring for any significant fall in heart rate and blood pressure. The pulse rate should be maintained at around 60 beats per minute.

The ECG shows normal P waves followed by QRST complexes at a regular rate exceeding 100 per minute. Often the rate is about 120 per minute and very rarely may reach 180 per minute. The PR and QT intervals decrease as the heart rate increases, so that the P wave merges with the preceding T wave. The rate varies with inspiration.

Atrial ectopic beats (synonyms: atrial extrasystoles; atrial premature beats; premature atrial contractions)

An *ectopic* impulse is one that arises at any site other than the sinus node. A *premature* impulse is one that arises earlier than is anticipated. Most ectopic impulses are premature.

Atrial ectopic beats are common in the acute coronary patient. They occur when the atrial ectopic focus discharges before the sinus node and can indicate sympathetic overactivity, hypoxia or anxiety. They are usually asymptomatic and of no haemodynamic significance, although they may reflect progressive atrial dilatation, in which case, treatment of heart failure is necessary. Atrial ectopics are often precursors to sustained supraventricular re-entry tachycardia by initiation of the re-entry circuit.

The ECG usually shows a premature P wave, often of abnormal configuration, followed usually by a QRST complex which is usually normal but may occasionally be slightly widened and deformed in shape (aberrant). The further the ectopic focus is from the sinus node, the greater the abnormality in the shape of the P wave. The P-R interval varies with each ectopic site, but with most atrial ectopic beats it is about 0.12 s. An incomplete compensatory pause usually follows the ectopic beat and thus the P-P interval will be slightly longer than the normal P-P interval (Figure 7.3).

Narrow complex tachycardias

The main tachycardias with a narrow QRS complex are:

- atrial fibrillation
- atrial flutter
- AV nodal re-entry tachycardia, AV re-entry tachycardia, and paroxysmal tachycardia.

Figure 7.3   Atrial ectopic beat (indicated by arrow).

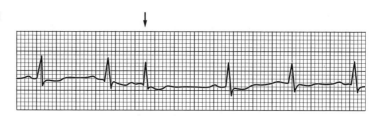

With the exception of atrial fibrillation (AF), most narrow complex tachycardias are regular and the P wave, if seen, may be a different shape from the P wave of sinus rhythm.

The term supraventricular tachycardia is often used to refer to any tachycardia originating above the ventricles, but this term is anatomically incorrect as most narrow complex tachycardias incorporate both ventricular and atrial myocardium within the circuit. Narrow complex tachycardias may be short lived (paroxysmal) or sustained. The aim of treatment is to restore sinus rhythm, or if this is not likely to be successful (as in chronic or unstable rhythms) to reduce the ventricular rate.

Atrial fibrillation

AF is the most common arrhythmia encountered in clinical practice and complicates 15–20% of myocardial infarctions. It is frequently associated with severe left ventricular damage and heart failure. Atrial ischaemia, right ventricular infarction and hypoxia may also be contributory factors. It is usually self-terminating and episodes may last from minutes to hours and are often repetitive (Van de Werf et al 2003). It is often preceded by frequent and multifocal atrial ectopic beats or atrial flutter. The incidence of AF after acute myocardial infarction has decreased since the introduction of thrombolysis, but it still indicates a poor prognosis. (Pizzetti et al 2001).

AF is thought to occur as a result of either enhanced automacity in one or more rapidly depolarizing foci or re-entry involving one or more circuits. Normal atrial contraction is replaced by a continuous series of irregular fibrillation waves which are ineffective for atrial emptying and so functionally the atria remain in diastole. Sustained AF usually indicates extensive myocardial damage and hence a poor long-term prognosis (Davies 2001). The loss of the atrial transport mechanism that occurs with AF means that there is a loss of atrial contribution to the ventricular stroke volume. The atrial component is usually some 10–20% of total cardiac output and without this there is a decreased ventricular filling time and diastolic coronary perfusion time.

Thromboembolism, especially resulting in a stroke or pulmonary embolus, is an important consequence arising from stasis in the right or left atrial appendage. It is particularly likely to occur when AF reverts to sinus rhythm. AF is the single most important cause of ischaemic stroke in those over 75 years of age (Hart and Halpern 2001).

Treatment depends on the ventricular rate, haemodynamic state and the risk of thromboembolism. It is acknowledged that there is a lack of good evidence to support clinical management decisions that take into account the different mechanisms and duration of the arrhythmia (ACC/AHA/ESC 2001). If the ventricular rate is not fast and the arrhythmia is well tolerated then no treatment is required. Symptomatic AF complicating myocardial infarction is probably best treated with amiodarone or by electrical cardioversion. Digoxin will tend to slow the ventricular response rather than produce sinus rhythm and also increase myocardial workload and oxygen consumption. The heart rate can be slowed with a small dose of beta-blocker if required.

If AF persists for more than 2 or 3 days and the patient is asymptomatic, the risk of systemic emboli following cardioversion is 3–5% and so it is prudent to anticoagulate the patient for at least 4 weeks prior to elective DC cardioversion.

Non-pharmacological treatment of persistent AF includes:

- AV node ablation, in order to prevent conduction from the atria to the ventricles, with the insertion of a permanent pacemaker

Figure 7.4 Atrial fibrillation.

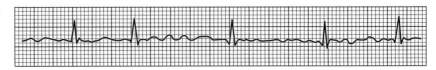

Figure 7.5 Atrial flutter.

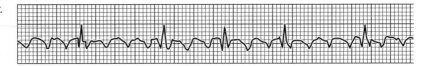

- surgical techniques involving the atrial myocardium to redirect the flow of atrial impulses.

The ECG shows absent P waves, irregular ventricular response (R-R interval) and chaotic fibrillatory waves indicative of rapid atrial depolarization at a rate of 400–600 per minute (Figure 7.4). The atrial rate greatly exceeds the ventricular rate because the majority of impulses are not conducted through the AV junction. The QRS complexes are usually of normal configuration. The rhythm may appear regular if the rate is very rapid.

Atrial flutter

Atrial flutter is seen in about 5% of acute coronary patients. Atrial flutter is thought to originate from a re-entry mechanism in the right atrium that spreads to the left atrium. There is rapid regular atrial activity, usually at a rate of between 220 and 350 per minute. This is characterized on the ECG by a 'saw-tooth' appearance due to the very rapid, wide and bizarre flutter waves. These flutter waves can be best revealed when the AV block, which inevitably occurs and may be variable (e.g. 2:1, 3:1), is increased by carotid sinus massage.

The ventricular rate depends upon the degree of block of the atrial impulses at the AV node, which depends upon its state of refractiveness. In the healthy AV node, the block will usually be 2:1, resulting in a heart rate of about 150 beats per minute. If there is damage to the conduction system, this block tends to increase. Varying AV conduction ratios mean that the pulse may feel irregular and there will be variable R-R intervals

on the ECG. Exercise decreases AV blockade and it is possible therefore for the pulse rate to increase with exercise.

Atrial flutter may be transient but may degenerate to AF, cause the patient to be haemodynamically compromised and be a precursor of heart failure. Spontaneous reversion to sinus rhythm is, however, quite common.

As atrial flutter is unstable, it should always be converted to sinus rhythm unless it is known that the patient has been in the rhythm for many months or years. Verapamil increases the AV block and reverts to sinus rhythm in about 20% of cases. Low dose direct current (DC) cardioversion is particularly useful for converting as is rapid atrial pacing.

The ECG shows that there is no isoelectric interval between adjacent flutter waves giving rise to the characteristic 'saw-tooth' appearance. The flutter waves range from about 220 to 350 per minute. AV block is present, i.e. 2:1, 3:1, 4:1 or higher. This may be variable, thus the ventricular (QRS) response is correspondingly variable: a regular irregularity (Figure 7.5).

The atrial flutter rate is calculated by measuring the interval between flutter waves in seconds, and dividing this into 60 gives the rate per minute. For example, an interval of 0.20 s represents a flutter rate of 60/0.20 or 300 per minute. It is largely the differences in atrial rate which differentiate between atrial tachycardia, AF and atrial flutter.

It is not unusual when the atrial rate speeds up to around 350–400 per minute on the ECG that there seems to be a combination of flutter waves and fibrillation waves. This is referred to as *coarse fibrillation* or *flutter/fibrillation* and often progresses to overt AF.

AV nodal re-entry tachycardia

AV nodal re-entry tachycardia originates from a focus within, or immediately next to the AV node. There is a re-entry circuit consisting of a slow antegrade pathway and a fast retrograde pathway, resulting in almost simultaneous atrial and ventricular activation.

The ECG shows rapid normal QRS complexes at a rate of 160–220 beats per minute. The P wave is buried in the QRS complex.

AV re-entry tachycardia

AV re-entry tachycardia occurs when there is an accessory AV pathway such as the bundle of Kent in Wolff–Parkinson–White syndrome. This occurs in about 2 in 1000 people. The rate of the tachycardia is usually about 150–250 beats per minute. During the tachycardia, slow antegrade conduction occurs through the AV node and fast retrograde conduction occurs through the additional pathway. There a pause between atrial and ventricular activation so that P waves may be seen between the QRS complexes. The P waves can be seen more easily if the rate is temporarily reduced with carotid sinus massage (CSM) or adenosine.

Paroxysmal atrial tachycardia

Paroxysmal atrial tachycardia is uncommon and occurs when there is a rapid discharge of an atrial pacemaker from one or more foci in the atria at a rate of 150–250 beats per minute. It is a true supraventricular tachycardia. There may be an intra-atrial re-entry circuit or occasionally an enhanced automaticity of an atrial focus. There is often second or third degree AV block so that the ventricular response is not unduly fast and haemodynamic stability is not compromised (Figure 7.6).

Treatment of tachycardias originating in the atria depends on the symptoms they produce. A loss of synchronized atrial activity and resulting fall in cardiac output may lead to the patient becoming haemodynamically compromised. There is then a danger of infarct extension and electrical cardioversion becomes the treatment of choice.

CSM, which increases vagal tone and inhibits sinus node firing and slows AV conduction, may slow or terminate the rhythm. It is also useful to differentiate between arrhythmias. For example, CSM will slow down but not terminate atrial flutter, whereas it will break the cycle of re-entry in AV re-entry tachycardias by blocking the AV node and therefore terminate the arrhythmia. CSM is performed by digital pressure, using the first and second fingers, over the carotid artery at the level of the upper border of the thyroid cartilage. It is massaged against the transverse process of the sixth cervical vertebra for about 15 s. It is not without risk and may produce cerebral hypotension. The Valsalva manoeuvre will also produce vagal stimulation and can be achieved by splashing the face with cold water or stimulating the gag reflex.

Various drugs may be used to restore sinus rhythm. Adenosine is particularly useful if there is left ventricular dysfunction or hypotension. Verapamil is not recommended in the setting of acute

Figure 7.6   ECG: atrial tachycardia with 2:1 AV blocks (leads aVF and V1). The atrial rate is 175 beats per minute.

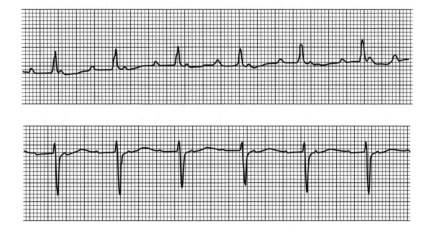

myocardial infarction (Van de Werf et al 2003). Beta-blockers may be successful but should be avoided in uncontrolled cardiac failure or if patients have been pre-treated with verapamil. Refractory tachycardias usually respond to amiodarone.

Cardioversion

The term cardioversion generally refers to external transthoracic electrical cardioversion. Electrical treatment has the advantage of being free from pharmacological side effects which often involve depression of myocardial contractility. Electrical cardioversion involves the use of a predetermined energy current. The current is timed (synchronized) with the intrinsic activity of the heart. This is to avoid electrical stimulation in the vulnerable part of cardiac repolarization, which is the downward slope of the T wave precipitating VF. Successful cardioversion relies on jolting the majority of cardiac cells, including fibrillating cells, into a transient state of simultaneous excitation. Then, once the cells collectively repolarize, the sinus node resumes its role as dominant pacemaker. Energy levels are titrated upwards if an initial shock is unsuccessful. Typical initial monophasic energy levels are at least 200 J, and possibly 360 J for AF (Joglar et al 2000) and at least 100 J for atrial flutter and other non-VTs.

Increasingly, biphasic defibrillators are used. With biphasic waveform, current is delivered in one direction, stops and is then reversed to travel in the opposite direction. There are different types of biphasic waveform produced by different defibrillators and there is much debate over which form is most effective and what energy levels to use (Achleitner et al 2001). The biphasic waveform is said to induce depolarization in the mid-refractory period and produce a graduated depolarization response which makes it more effective than monophasic depolarization. Biphasic waveforms appear to achieve cardioversion at lower energy levels than monophasic waveforms. On average, two-thirds less current is required for the equivalent effect (Tang et al 2001). Biphasic wave form has been shown to be more effective than monophasic wave form for cardioverting AF to sinus rhythm, with patients having a higher success rate and requiring lower energy levels (Mittal et al 2000).

Success of cardioversion depends on a variety of factors including:

- the nature of the underlying heart disease
- length of time in the arrhythmia
- energy levels and type of wave form used
- transthoracic impedance – influenced by size of patient, bone density, skin contact, position, size and pressure of paddles, interval between shocks, number of shocks delivered and phase in respiratory cycle.

Some biphasic defibrillators are able to adjust the amount and duration of the current delivered based on a measurement of transthoracic impedance. Reported initial success rates for cardioverting AF range from 20% to 90%, although patient characteristics and definition of success vary between studies (ACC/AHA/ESC 2001).

Electrical cardioversion is usually performed electively, with the patient lightly anaesthetized or sedated.

Metabolic and drug considerations

Patients with hypoxia and acidosis are difficult to cardiovert. Abnormal potassium levels may also render the procedure less successful. Digoxin reduces the energy threshold required, and digoxin toxicity can result in an increased risk of ventricular arrhythmias after cardioversion. Quinidine, lignocaine and phenytoin increase the energy threshold and higher amounts of energy will therefore be required to restore sinus rhythm. Ideally the patient should be fully anticoagulated with warfarin and have an International Normalised Ratio (INR) of greater than 2.0 for more than a month. However, this will not be possible early post-infarction, and intravenous heparin should be given prior to the procedure.

Procedure

The procedure should be fully explained to the patient so that they are aware of what to expect. This should include a description of the procedure, including the length of time it will take, the personnel involved, where it will take place, the expected outcome and aftercare. Since the procedure is elective, a consent form is required to be signed by the patient. A light general anaesthetic is usually given, although intravenous diazepam or midazolam can be used to achieve conscious sedation (Mitchell et al 2003). Patients need to be informed of whether they will be aware of what is going on around them. If an anaesthetic is used the patient should have fasted for 4–6 hours beforehand.

The procedure is often performed at the bedside or in theatre recovery, with the patient lying flat and their head supported by a pillow. The patient should have been asked to remove any dentures, jewellery and restrictive clothing. A 12-lead ECG is usually obtained prior to and following cardioversion to assess the efficacy of the procedure. Oxygen is usually administered before the procedure and during recovery. Resuscitation equipment, including suction, should be readily available.

The actual procedure is similar to that used in defibrillation, but the defibrillator will need to be set to synchronized mode so that the shock is delivered just after the R wave to avoid the shock being delivered on the vulnerable 30 ms preceding the apex of the T wave. Unsynchronized shocks could potentially precipitate VF. Ideally, the ECG should be set to display the most upright R wave to aid the process of synchronization. If a first shock is unsuccessful an attempt needs to be made at a higher energy level.

Electrolyte impregnated pads should be used to minimize electrical resistance. Large pads result in lower impedance than smaller ones, but if pads are too large the current density through the cardiac tissue will be insufficient to achieve cardioversion. A size of between 8 and 12 cm is usually used. Shocks delivered during expiration deliver higher energy levels to the heart. Traditionally hand-held paddles are used to deliver the shocks, although increasingly hand-free systems are being used.

One pad is placed below the right clavicle and the other paddle over the apex of the heart in the fifth intercostal space on the left side of the thorax in order to depolarize an optimum mass of myocardial cells. Pads need to be placed directly against the chest wall rather than over breast tissue. It is also possible to cardiovert from chest to back with one paddle placed on the left of the base of the sternum and the other between the shoulder blades slightly to the left of the spine. This alternative method is particularly useful for obese patients who will have increased transthoracic impedence. It is also useful for patients where the underlying pathology affects both the right and left atrium, such as atrial septal defect or cardiomyopathy. Careful positioning of gel pads and firm pressure if applying the paddles will minimize the risk of chest wall burning.

Although it usually is a medical responsibility to perform cardioversion, it presents a good opportunity for the nurse to become acquainted with the procedure in a more controlled non-emergency situation. Nurses are increasingly taking on the responsibility for leading and coordinating cardioversion, particularly in the outpatient and day case setting (Quinn 1998).

Aftercare

After the procedure the nurse should be present, while the patient recovers, to monitor physical parameters, including any adverse reactions to the anaesthetic, and to provide emotional support and information.

If a general anaesthetic has been given, the patient may remain unconscious for 10–15 min depending on the number of shocks required and the amount of anaesthetic given. Attempts at cardioversion are usually abandoned after four or five shocks to avoid excessive trauma to the patient.

Post-cardioversion recovery is as for any procedure involving a general anaesthetic, with the patient lying on his side until regaining consciousness. Blood pressure, pulse oximetry and heart rate require regular monitoring. It is likely that the patient will feel weak and lethargic for several hours. Nausea and vomiting are not uncommon and appropriate measures should be taken to provide relief. Paddle burns are uncommon if careful attention is paid to application of the gel pads. Any inflammation should respond to topical steroid cream such as 1% hydrocortisone.

The patient should be given a clear and simple explanation of the outcome of the procedure and given ample opportunity to ask questions and discuss concerns.

Possible complications

Complications resulting from cardioversion are rare and tend to be related to the amount of energy used, the efficiency of the procedure and underlying electrolyte and metabolic abnormalities. Arrhythmias, especially sinus bradycardia, wandering pacemakers and junctional rhythm, can occur up to 8 h after cardioversion. Ventricular ectopics are not uncommon. These arrhythmias are more likely if anti-arrhythmic drugs have been taken or if the patient is hypokalaemic. Whether raised cardiac markers after cardioversion are a result of the procedure or underlying pathology is a meet point (Lund et al 2000). Thromboembolic complications are rare, but can occur up to 10 days after the procedure (Berger and Schweitzer 1998) and anticoagulation therefore needs to continue for at least 4 weeks after the procedure especially if sinus rhythm returns.

Junctional bradycardia

The AV junction has an intrinsic discharge rate of about 50 per minute, and may assume the role of dominant pacemaker if it is discharging at a faster rate than the sinus node. Junctional bradycardia may follow, particularly after inferior infarction, where action of the sinus node has been depressed. Vasotonic agents such as diamorphine can also produce junctional rhythms.

The atria and ventricles are stimulated simultaneously; the stimulus spreading normally to the ventricle but retrogradely into the atria. As a result the P wave may appear slightly before, after or buried in the QRS complex. Because the atria and ventricles beat simultaneously, the atria have to contract against a closed mitral and tricuspid valve. Blood is pumped retrogradely, thus producing palpable waves in the venous pulses of the neck.

Junctional bradycardia is usually short-lived and self-terminating, thus requiring no treatment. However, if the bradycardia is associated with signs of a low cardiac output, atropine should be given. Occasionally temporary pacing may be required in preference to frequent doses of atropine.

The ECG shows a rate of about 30–60 per minute. The P waves (if present) are usually inverted and may precede, coincide with, or follow, the normal QRS complexes. The P-R interval is variable.

Ventricular ectopic beats (synonyms: ventricular extrasystoles; ventricular premature beats; premature ventricular contractions)

During the early phase of myocardial cell damage there is a high degree of electrical instability in the ventricular myocardium. Factors predisposing to ventricular arrhythmias include:

- myocardial ischaemia
- hypoxia
- electrolyte and acid base imbalance – particularly hypokalaemia
- effect of drugs.

Cells have differing action potentials and refractory periods which can produce bursts of complex re-entry arrhythmias anywhere within the AV bundle or the ventricular conducting system. The incidence of ventricular ectopic beats in acute coronary patients is probably near 100%. Scarred or ischaemic areas of the myocardium can act as a focus for arrhythmias and extensive infarctions are generally associated with a higher frequency of ventricular ectopy.

Infrequent ventricular ectopic beats do not cause significant haemodynamic deterioration but frequent, or bigeminal activity produces a bradycardia requiring treatment.

Certain types of ventricular ectopic beats are thought to be precursors of ventricular tachycardia or fibrillation. These ventricular ectopic beats are those that:

- occur at a rate of more than 5 per minute
- are of the 'R-on-T' type: the ectopic occurs on the apex of the preceding T wave
- are multifocal
- occur in runs of two or more
- are bigeminal.

However, the concept of these 'warning arrhythmias' is questionable, as they are only associated with about half the patients who develop VF. It is no longer policy to consider routine prophylaxis against ventricular arrhythmias in the post-myocardial infarction patient. However, ventricular ectopic beats exhibiting the R-on-T phenomenon, occurring in salvos or with multifocal origins, may be considered for treatment. The choice of treatment remains controversial although lignocaine is still probably the most frequently used prophylactic agent. Care is needed in the elderly and those with hypotension or conduction defects. With the high doses needed to reduce the incidence of primary VF, there is a high incidence of side effects, which include fatal episodes of bradycardia and asystole.

The ECG shows a broad (>0.12 s) and bizarre-shaped QRS complex reflecting abnormal conduction through the ventricles. The T wave points in an opposite direction from the main QRS deflection. The ectopic beat often occurs prematurely, is not preceded by a P wave, and is followed by a compensatory pause (Figure 7.7).

Significant ventricular arrhythmias can occur after patients go home from hospital. Patients who are susceptible to these can be identified by an early exercise test, 24-hour ECG monitoring or electrophysiological testing.

Ventricular tachycardia

VT is defined as four or more ventricular ectopic beats in rapid succession. The rate is usually between 120 and 250 per minute. It may be self-limiting (non-sustained) or prolonged (sustained), and may be preceded by either R-on-T or late

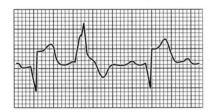

Figure 7.7 An isolated ectopic beat occurring in a patient with acute myocardial infarction.

ventricular ectopic beats. VT is potentially a serious arrhythmia as it can produce shock, cardiac arrest, or lead to VF. It is most likely to occur post-infarction in the first 48 hours following the onset of muscle damage and is often a one-off event. Short bursts of VT are particularly common in the first 24 hours. This does not necessarily require treatment and has no bearing on prognosis. This is in contrast to VT occurring beyond 48 hours after infarction. This is often a feature of larger infarcts and associated scar tissue.

The choice of treatment depends on the degree of haemodynamic embarrassment caused by the tachycardia. VT is sometimes difficult to distinguish from paroxysmal supraventricular tachycardia, with aberrant conduction, as both will have broad QRS complexes, although a regular tachycardia with broad ventricular complexes, post-infarction, is usually ventricular in origin.

The ECG shows widened (>0.12 s) QRS complexes occurring regularly at a rate usually between 120 and 250 per minute (Figure 7.8). In about half of the cases of VT, atrial activity continues to be initiated by the sinus node and therefore proceeds independently of, and at a slower rate than, ventricular activity. In other cases of VT, the ventricular impulses are conducted via the AV junction to the atria (retrograde conduction) producing inverted P waves after the QRS complex. Sometimes atrial impulses may be conducted through to the ventricles in the normal way, producing a 'captured' beat which produces a QRS of normal sinus rhythm. Fusion beats may be observed when a normal atrial stimulus travelling down the conducting system meets and combines with a ventricular stimulus being conducted retrogradely. This produces a QRS complex that has some characteristics of a normal QRS complex, and some of a ventricular ectopic beat.

Figure 7.8 Ventricular tachycardia.

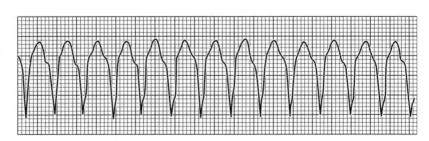

VT is distinguished from other tachycardias if the ECG shows AV dissociation, capture or fusion beats, and a QRS axis more negative than −30°. Uniformly negative or positive deflections (referred to as monomorphic) in the chest leads are almost certain to be evidence of VT (Table 7.2).

Variants of ventricular tachycardia

There are four main variants of VT, as given below.

Accelerated idioventricular tachycardia

Accelerated idioventricular tachycardia or 'slow' VT, is usually benign and requires no treatment. It is often associated with successful thrombolysis and is the result of an escape rhythm initiated in the ventricles.

The ECG shows a regular rhythm at a rate usually between 60 and 100 per minute. P waves, if apparent, tend to be abnormal in shape, and the QRS complexes are wide and bizarre in configuration. Sinus rhythm usually takes over after about 30 beats (Figure 7.9).

Torsade de pointes tachycardia

Torsade de pointes, or twisting of points, occurs when the polarity of the VT appears to spiral around the isoelectric line, i.e. there are frequent and marked changes in the direction of the QRS axis (also referred to as polymorphic VT). This rhythm is found most frequently in patients with a prolonged Q-T interval and can be precipitated by severe left ventricular function following infarction, and is presumably initiated by ventricular ectopic beats occurring during the vulnerable repolarization period. It often reverts spontaneously to sinus rhythm, but may degenerate to VF.

The recognition of this arrhythmia is important because it may be aggravated by anti-arrhythmic agents and because correction of the underlying cause usually prevents it. Causes include bradycardia and AV block, and drugs such as disopyramide, or disorders such as hypokalaemia, that lead to abnormal ventricular repolarization. Although it is usually self-terminating it may need to be abolished by overdrive pacing, correcting electrolyte imbalance or withdrawing responsible drugs.

The Q-T interval normally shortens with increasing heart rate, thus necessitating correction when measuring it with the following formula:

$$\text{Corrected Q-Tc interval} = \frac{\text{Q-T interval}}{\sqrt{\text{R-R interval}}}$$

The normal Q-Tc should not exceed 0.42 s.

Table 7.2 Features that help in the differentiation of ventricular tachycardia from an aberrantly conducted supraventricular tachycardia (SVT)

	Ventricular tachycardia	SVT
Rate	140–180	150–240
Rhythm	Regular or irregular	Regular or irregular
RBBB pattern	Rare	Common
P waves	AV dissociation	Usually 1:1
Morphology of preceding ectopics	Same	Different
Capture/fusion beats	Present	Absent
Vagal stimulation	No effect	May help
QRS in V leads	Concordant	Discordant
QRS axis	<−30°	Normal

Figure 7.9   Idioventricular tachycardia.

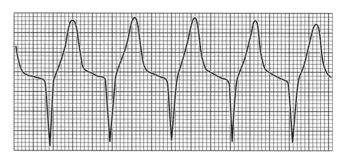

The ECG shows progressive changes in the direction of the QRS axis every 5–30 beats. The rate is usually 200–240 per minute.

Extrasystolic ventricular tachycardia

This arrhythmia occurs only occasionally in the acute coronary patient and does not necessarily deteriorate to sustained VT. Treatment may not be necessary, although lidocaine is often administered.

The ECG shows the occurrence of episodes of VT following a ventricular ectopic beat which originates at a fixed interval from the QRS complex of a sinus beat. After a short burst of tachycardia, there is often a long pause before sinus rhythm recommences.

Parasystole

This phenomenon may occasionally occur in the acute coronary patient. It is particularly common in patients taking digoxin. A ventricular ectopic focus discharges regularly, independent of the dominant rhythm which is usually sinus rhythm. Depolarization from the ventricular focus captures the ventricles, provided that they are not refractory as a result of activation by the dominant rhythm. Fusion beats will occur if the two pacemakers discharge simultaneously.

The ECG shows characteristic coupling intervals, interectopic intervals which are multiples of a common factor, and fusion beats (complexes which in configuration are a fusion between normal and ectopic beats) because the ventricles may by chance be simultaneously activated by both ectopic and normal pacemakers.

Treatment of ventricular tachycardia

Treatment of VT depends on the haemodynamic consequences for the patient. Some patients will tolerate VT very well. However, most sustained episodes will require treatment as they have deleterious effects on cardiac output leading to hypotension and heart failure. Beta-blockers, unless contraindicated, are the first line of therapy. If the risk of VF is thought to be high then lidocaine is usually the drug of choice. However, intravenous amiodarone may be more effective, especially in

patients with recurrent, sustained VT requiring cardioversion (Van de Werf et al 2003). Raising the legs to promote venous return may terminate the arrhythmia as may getting the patient to cough forcefully. Some patients can maintain cerebral circulation as a result of the pressure changes in the chest brought about by repeated coughing. Defibrillation is indicated if the patient loses consciousness. If there is not a defibrillator immediately available, then a precordial thump is worth trying while equipment is brought to the patient.

Ventricular fibrillation

A significant proportion of deaths caused by myocardial infarction are due to VF (primary VF). VF is the rapid, totally uncoordinated contraction of ventricular myocardial fibres, reflected in the ECG by irregular, chaotic electrical activity. VF causes circulatory arrest, and unconsciousness develops within 10–20 s of the onset of the arrhythmia.

The only reliable management for VF is immediate defibrillation. Occasionally, a precordial thump is effective and takes little time to perform. However, a defibrillator should be readily available so that little or no time need be spent on cardiopulmonary resuscitation (CPR).

VF is most likely to occur in the first few hours after acute infarction, although it may also occur during convalescence. It is sometimes divided into four categories:

1. Reperfusional VF – occurring following thrombolysis and reflecting a good prognosis as it probably indicates opening of the infarct-related artery.
2. Primary VF – occurring in the early hours of infarction and not associated with severe myocardial damage.
3. Secondary VF – occurring in the context of heart failure or cardiogenic shock. The prognosis is poor.
4. Late onset VF – occurring 3–4 or more days after acute infarction.

The final category comprises between 10% and 30% of all hospital deaths. Immediate defibrillation is the only effective treatment and is discussed in the section on resuscitation. The long-term survival is relatively good for patients with primary VF. VF (or VT) occurring within the first 24 hours after acute infarction is unlikely to recur after discharge from the coronary care unit and there is usually no need for oral anti-arrhythmic therapy. However, problems occurring after 48 hours are usually indicative of extensive myocardial damage and recurrence is likely. Oral anti-arrhythmic therapy is therefore often given for several months following later onset of a ventricular arrhythmia or if there are recurrent episodes of VT or VF. Patients with heart failure, prolonged ST segment elevation and persistent third heart sound have an increased likelihood of VF during convalescence and should be evaluated for insertion of an implantable cardioverter defibrillator (ICD).

The ECG shows fine or coarse, irregular, chaotic waves at a rate of between 300 and 500 per minute. Fine VF may mimic asystole and produce what appears to be a flat line on the ECG.

DISTURBANCES OF IMPULSE CONDUCTION

The conducting system of the heart, responsible for the formation and conduction of electrical impulses, is prone to disruption following acute myocardial infarction, either transiently through oedema and ischaemia, or permanently through necrosis. It is estimated that up to a quarter of acute coronary patients demonstrate conduction disturbances. The significance of the problem depends on the extent and location of myocardial damage.

Injury to the reflexes acting on the sinus node may produce sinus arrhythmias. However, the most clinically relevant disruptions to conduction occur in the location of the AV junction and bundle branches.

The term AV block is applied when the atrial impulse is delayed or completely fails to reach the ventricle. It is customary and convenient to classify impaired AV conduction into:

- first-degree AV block
- second-degree AV block
- third-degree AV block – complete AV block.

Conduction disturbances of the intraventricular conducting system (bundle branches) occur in about one-fifth of coronary patients. They are more likely to occur with anterior infarcts and have more serious consequences than blocks occurring higher in the cardiac conducting system. Haemodynamic instability is more likely because subsidiary pacemakers below the level of the block are slower and less reliable. Also, the area of myocardial damage is likely to be greater when the bundle branches are affected.

Sinus arrest

This occurs when the sinus node fails to deactivate the atria. In the absence of sinus node activity, subsidiary pacemakers in the atria, AV junction or ventricles normally give rise to an escape rhythm until sinus rhythm recommences. Both sinus arrest and sinoatrial block produce an absence of P waves. However, it is possible to distinguish between them. In sinus arrest, no P waves are generated for varying periods of time, so that whatever P-P intervals there are vary in length. In sinoatrial block, impulses are being generated regularly, although some of them do not reach the surrounding myocardium, so the longer P-P intervals will be an exact multiple of the basic P-P cycle.

The ECG shows periods where there are absences of P waves and therefore no ensuing QRS-T complexes. When P-P intervals do occur they are irregular.

Sinoatrial block

This occurs when there is a block of transmission of the impulse into the atria from the sinus node (Figure 7.10). In theory, SA block can be classified, like AV block, into first, second or third degree. However, only second-degree SA block can be

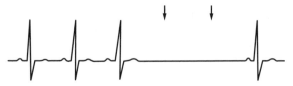

Figure 7.10 Sinotrial block showing two omitted PQRST complexes.

confidently diagnosed from the ECG. SA block is particularly common with inferior infarction because, in most cases, the right coronary artery supplies the sinus node as well as the inferior myocardium.

First-degree SA block

This implies a slowing of conduction through the SA junction. It cannot be diagnosed from an ECG because all P waves will be equally late in reaching the surrounding myocardium and so the P-P intervals will be normal.

Second-degree SA block

This occurs when, intermittently, conduction into the atrial myocardium slows to such an extent that it is interrupted. If the impulse is not conducted, then there is no atrial or ventricular activation and hence no corresponding P wave or QRS complex visible on the ECG. This degree of SA block may be regular, producing conduction ratios of 2:1 or 3:2, or it may be irregular when the sinus impulses are blocked intermittently. It can occur with Wenckebach conduction or in a manner analogous to Mobitz type II AV block.

Type I conduction produces progressive slowing of SA conduction until finally conduction is completely blocked and there is a long pause between complexes on the EGG. The 'dropped' beat gives the SA junction the opportunity to recover in order that the next sinus impulse can be conducted, and the whole sequence starts again. It is usually associated with inferior infarction and seldom causes adverse haemodynamic effects.

Type II second degree SA block produces a constant P-P interval, but P waves are periodically dropped every three to four beats. No treatment is required if the patient is asymptomatic. Atropine, adrenaline and pacing may be required, as for sinus bradycardia.

Third degree SA block

This occurs when the sinus node fails to deactivate the atria. As no impulses reach the atrial myocardium, P waves are not recorded on the ECG even though they are being initiated by the sinus node. In the absence of sinus node activity,

subsidiary pacemakers in the atria, AV junction or ventricles normally give rise to an escape rhythm. Dropped beats may be felt on palpation of the pulse and the patient may complain of palpitations. The patient with SA block is usually asymptomatic and requires no treatment although atropine, adrenaline and pacing may be necessary, as for sinus bradycardia.

The ECG shows periods where there are absences of P waves and therefore no ensuing QRS-T complexes. When P-P intervals do occur they are an exact multiple of the basic P-P cycle.

Atrioventricular block

AV heart block may be short lived, transient or permanent. It has been classified as first, second or third degree AV block.

First-degree AV block

Each impulse passing through the AV node is delayed, resulting in an increase in the P-R interval on the ECG. Each atrial complex is followed by a ventricular complex. The patient is usually unaffected by this partial block and so no immediate action is necessary, although cardiosuppressant agents should be avoided. First degree heart block complicates about 15% of acute myocardial infarctions and is more common with inferior infarcts. It can also follow the administration of digoxin, diltiazem and beta-blockers which affect the AV node. If the AV block becomes progressively more severe, the conduction time is further prolonged. First-degree AV block may be the forerunner of more serious disturbances and careful observation is warranted. Approximately 40% of those with first degree block post-infarction will go on to develop more serious heart block problems.

The ECG shows a prolonged (>0.2 s) P-R interval, a normal P wave and a normal QRS complex (Figure 7.11).

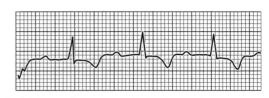

Figure 7.11   First-degree AV block.

Second-degree AV block

There are two types of second-degree AV block.

Wenckebach type (Mobitz type I) AV block
The Wenckebach phenomenon is characterized by a progressive prolongation of the P-R interval until a ventricular complex fails to follow an atrial complex. Following a pause, the same cycle is then repeated. It is usually due to a lesion involving the AV junction and accounts for about nine out of ten cases of second degree heart block. The patient will not usually be aware of this disturbance, although they may experience palpitations. The arrhythmia often complicates inferior myocardial infarctions and may occasionally progress to complete AV block. There is usually no need for active treatment, although drugs, such as verapamil and digoxin, that may exacerbate the functioning of the AV node should be avoided. On the rare occasion that the patient does become haemodynamically compromised, atropine should be tried before initiating temporary pacing.

The ECG shows a progressive lengthening of the P-R interval until a point is reached at which no QRS complex follows the P wave. Then the cycle repeats itself. The ratio of the number of P waves to the number of QRS complexes may be fixed or variable (Figure 7.12).

Mobitz type II AV block   This is a less common type of AV block, characterized by the sudden failure of a P wave to elicit a QRS complex without a previous warning prolongation of the P-R interval. It is a more serious partial block and can progress to complete AV block or ventricular asystole.

In its mildest form with intermittent 'dropped' beats, there is no previous prolongation of the P-R interval, which remains normal up to the blocked beat. In more severe forms, an AV ratio of 2:1, 3:1 or even 6:1 is obtained, the P-R interval of the conducted beat being normal. The patient may be unaffected by this. Any effect depends on the ventricular rate and the efficiency of the ventricles. Bradycardia is often present and may have serious effects on the circulation, for example, heart failure and cardiogenic shock. Temporary pacing should be considered.

The ECG shows a fixed P-R interval (which may exceed 0.2 s). At intervals, one or more QRS complexes are dropped. Widening of the QRS complexes may occur (Figure 7.13).

Third-degree AV block

Complete AV block can be one of the most serious complications the acute coronary patient can develop. It is characterized by a failure of atrial impulses being transmitted to the ventricles (Figure 7.14) and a continued circulation then depends on the ventricles being activated by a subsidiary pacemaker. The atrial rate is faster than the ventricular rate.

Complete AV block is commonly due to fibrosis of the conducting system, either alone or in association with diffuse myocardial fibrosis. It is most commonly a complication of occlusion of the right coronary artery which usually supplies blood to the AV junction. This artery is also responsible for supplying the inferior aspects of the heart, and a

Figure 7.12   Second-degree AV block (Mobitz type I).

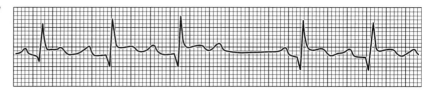

Figure 7.13   Second-degree AV block (Mobitz type II).

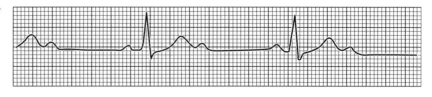

combination of complete AV block and inferior infarction is common.

In complete AV block complicating an inferior myocardial infarction, the subsidiary pacemaker usually discharges at a rate above 40 beats per minute with a narrow QRS complex. Complications of asystole and symptoms resulting from a low ventricular rate are uncommon and treatment is usually not required. Recovery of the AV node usually occurs within a few hours or days, although it may take up to 3 weeks and any decisions around permanent pacing need to take this into account.

In patients with an anterior infarction, complete AV block usually indicates extensive myocardial damage, often affecting bundle branch tissue, the AV node and extensive septal infarction. In this situation, complete heart block often occurs suddenly without any evidence of pre-existing conduction disturbance. The heart rate is often about 30 per

minute and the QRS complex broad. The patient is likely to feel weak, lethargic, faint and dizzy. Ventricular asystole or VF may develop, or extreme bradycardia, resulting in heart failure or shock. The mortality rate is as high as 75%. Treatment requires the insertion of a temporary pacemaker, although whether this has any impact on long-term survival is debatable. The heart block is likely to be permanent and those patients who survive may subsequently require permanent pacing.

The ECG shows P waves at a regular rate which bear no relationship to the QRS complexes (Figure 7.15).

Atrioventricular dissociation

Confusion often exists in distinguishing between complete AV block and AV dissociation. In the latter there is no organic block between the atria and the ventricles, but two separate pacemakers discharge almost simultaneously, one (usually the sinus node) controlling the atria and the other (either from a junctional or ventricular focus) controlling the ventricles. When these two pacemakers become out of synchronization, the impulse from the atria may descend into the AV junction before the pacemaker from this area is ready to discharge again and the atria then 'capture' the ventricles. There is, therefore, no organic block but only a physiological block due to the two pacemakers competing with each other. AV dissociation is always secondary to some other abnormality, with either slowing of the sinus node or acceleration of a lower pacemaker, or a combination of the two. This explains why the rate of the QRS complexes is usually faster than that of the P waves and this is one way of distinguishing this rhythm from complete heart block on the ECG.

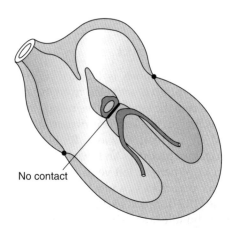

No contact

Figure 7.14   Representation of complete heart block.

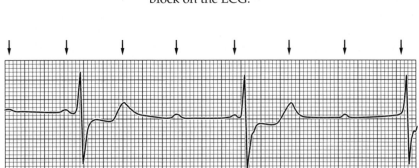

Figure 7.15   Complete heart block. Some of the P waves are hidden in the T waves; arrows indicate position of P waves.

No specific treatment is required unless drugs are the contributing cause, in which case they should be withdrawn.

The ECG shows P waves 'marching through' the QRS complexes (i.e. they are dissociated). At some time, P waves are followed by a QRS complex at the normal interval (capture beats).

Bundle branch block

In this condition either the right or the left branch of the AV bundle fails to conduct impulses. Bundle branch block often appears as a complication of ventricular hypertrophy, although a local lesion of the conducting system may be responsible for this condition.

The pathological significance of the two types of bundle branch block differs. The prognosis for right bundle branch block is generally good, whereas that of left bundle branch block is much more serious. The acute coronary patient who has left bundle branch block is at increased risk of developing ventricular arrhythmias and AV block.

Right bundle branch block

In this condition there is a defect of the right bundle which gives rise to a characteristic electrocardiographic appearance. Although the right bundle is blocked, the interventricular septum is activated from left to right, as in the normal heart. The left ventricle is depolarized before the right. This produces a further R wave (R') in the right chest leads: an M pattern is seen in leads such as V_1.

Right bundle branch block may be partial (QRS width <0.12 s) or complete (QRS width >0.12 s). It is of little clinical significance, except as an indication of possible heart disease.

On the ECG the right chest leads show a delayed positive deflection as depolarization spreads in a right anterior direction. Lead V_1 shows an M pattern with a normal initial small R wave, a normal S wave and a further R wave (R') as the impulse bypasses the block and spreads from the left ventricle to the right ventricle. Leads I, V_5 and V_6 record a normal Q wave, a normal R wave, but a wide deep S wave due to the delayed right ventricular depolarization away from these leads (Figure 7.16).

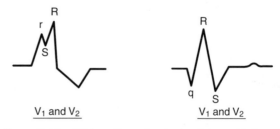

Figure 7.16   QRS configuration in the right and left chest leads in a right bundle branch block.

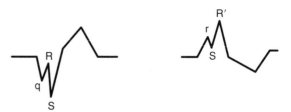

Figure 7.17   QRS configuration in the right and left chest leads in left bundle branch block.

Left bundle branch block

The left bundle branch is blocked so the interventricular septum is activated from the right side instead of from the left side. This results in the normal Q wave in the left ventricular leads being replaced by a small R wave. Right ventricular depolarization produces an R wave in V_1 and an S wave in V_6. When the left ventricle is depolarized an R wave occurs in V_6 and a broad S wave in V_1. Thus, the QRS duration exceeds 0.12 s.

The left bundle branch block pattern often masks the ECG changes of myocardial infarction. Left bundle branch block is rare in the otherwise normal individual and is most commonly seen in ischaemic heart disease. Treatment, if warranted, depends on the cause of the block. The acute coronary patient with this type of block has a tendency to develop ventricular arrhythmias and AV block.

On the ECG small R waves are seen in leads I, aVL and V_4–V_6. As the right ventricule is activated before the left, there is also a wide, sometimes notched, QRS complex in these leads, and a wide QS wave in V_1–V_3 (Figure 7.17).

'New' left bundle branch block is an indication for thrombolytic therapy if the history suggests myocardial infarction and there are no contra-indications.

Hemiblock

This is the term used for describing a block in one of the two main divisions of the left bundle branch: anterior and posterior fascicles.

Usually the wave of depolarization spreads through both fascicles simultaneously. If one fascicle is blocked, the impulse passes through the other at the usual rate. The direction of the QRS vector is altered depending on which fascicle is affected. Blockage shifts the portion of the QRS complex in the direction of the blocked division and produces corresponding axis deviation.

Left anterior hemiblock

Left anterior hemiblock is common because this fascicle is very thin and susceptible to damage. Interruption of this fascicle due to infarction results in activation occurring predominantly through the fibres of the left posterior fascicle. Activation is directed upwards and to the left, resulting in left axis deviation. This is manifested on the ECG with deep terminal S waves in leads II, III and aVF and a tall R wave in lead aVL. The mean frontal plane QRS axis is commonly in the region of $-30°$ to $-60°$.

Left posterior hemiblock

Left posterior hemiblock occurs less frequently because this fascicle is thick, short and fan-shaped and has a double blood supply. Left posterior hemiblock indicates extensive left ventricular damage. Activation occurs predominantly through the fibres of the anterior superior division, downwards and to the right, resulting in right axis deviation. This results in prominent S waves in leads I and aVL and tall R waves in leads II, III and aVF. The mean frontal plane QRS axis is directed in the region of $±90°$ to $+120°$.

Bifascicular block

Bifascicular block occurs when two of the three fascicles are blocked. This means that ventricular conduction depends on the remaining unblocked fascicle. Pre-existing right bundle branch block complicated by blockage of either of the left fascicles

as a result of infarction will develop into complete AV block if the remaining clear fascicle also becomes blocked.

Treatment for bifascicular block remains controversial, with arguments both for and against prophylactic temporary, or even permanent, pacing.

Trifascicular block

Trifascicular block occurs when there is right bundle branch block and a block in both the anterior and posterior fascicles of the left bundle branch. Trifascicular block is a term used to describe the situation whereby at least one of the three fascicles is only partially blocked, to distinguish it from complete AV block where all three fascicles are completely blocked.

Complete AV block is likely to develop if alternating right and left bundle branch block patterns are observed on the ECG.

Ventricular asystole

Asystole may affect about 10% of coronary patients and the prognosis is very poor: mortality exceeds 90%. Asystole is characterized by ventricular standstill caused by suppression of pacemaker activity; thus, ventricular activity is absent on the ECG. Strong cholinergic activity may suddenly depress sinus or AV node function, especially when sympathetic stimulation is decreased by ischaemia, infarction or beta-blockade. Asystole may also follow AV block, bi- or trifascicular block, or electrical countershock and is a final common pathway for untreated VF.

In ventricular asystole there is no cardiac output and therefore the patient will be unconscious. CPR is therefore initiated and adrenaline and atropine may prove effective but prognosis is poor. Cardiac pacing may be attempted if there is some evidence of P wave activity. Cardiac pacing is often unsuccessful, particularly when asystolic arrest occurs because of extensive myocardial damage or is a sequelae of prolonged arrest.

Pulseless electrical activity (PEA)

Previously known as electromechanical dissociation, PEA is profound myocardial pump failure despite near or near to normal electrical excitation. It usually occurs secondary to drugs, hypoxia, hypovolaemia or mechanical embarrassment such as cardiac tamponade, trauma, pulmonary embolism and tension pneumothorax. It may also occur as the end point of VF. The occurrence of PEA following myocardial infarction usually indicates a terminal event such as rupture of the heart or cardiac tamponade. The patient's best chance of survival is the prompt identification and treatment of the underlying problem.

CPR will need to be initated as there is no cardiac output. Adrenaline, and other pressor agents, are useful adjuncts. Calcium may be considered if there is accompanying hyperkalaemia, hypocalcaemia or if calcium antagonists have been taken.

CARDIAC PACING

Control over the electrical activity of the heart is frequently made by means of an artificial pacemaker. Pacemakers have several basic components:

- a *pulse generator,* containing a chemical battery power source, an output circuit, a timing circuit and a sensing circuit
- an *electrode* which is able to make direct contact with the heart
- *connecting cable leads* for temporary pacing systems.

Pacemakers may be either *temporary* or *permanent,* depending on whether the pulse generator is located externally or implanted. If pacing is planned for a short duration only, an external power source is used to deliver electricity to the heart either transvenously to the endocardium, via the skin or via the oesophagus. When long-term control is required, a permanent pacemaker is implanted. Thus, there are four main ways of cardiac pacing:

1 temporary transvenous pacing
2 temporary transcutaneous pacing
3 temporary oesophageal pacing (rare)
4 permanent pacing.

Recommendations for when pacing should be carried out vary and tend to be based on clinical experience rather than clinical trials. The two main indications for pacing are:

- failure of impulse generation
- failure of AV conduction.

The American College of Cardiology, American Heart Association and North American Society for Pacing and Electrophysiology (ACC/AHA/NASPE 2002) have produced pacing guidelines (ACC/AHA 1998) and some of the indications for temporary and permanent pacing are summarized in Tables 7.3 and 7.4.

The two most common modes of pacing are *demand* and *fixed rate.* The former senses intrinsic cardiac rhythm and stimulates myocardial depolarization and contraction as necessary; the latter fires at a predetermined rate, irrespective of intrinsic cardiac activity.

Temporary cardiac pacing

Temporary endocardial cardiac pacing has been used since the early 1960s to maintain cardiac output

---

Table 7.3   Some indications for temporary pacing

Acute myocardial infarction
1 Anterior myocardial infarction accompanied by:
    Complete heart block
    Second-degree heart block
    First-degree heart block with bifascicular block
    Newly acquired left bundle branch block (rare)
2 Inferior myocardial infarction accompanied by:
    Any of the above, accompanied by actual or
    threatened haemodynamic decompensation

Prior to permanent pacing
When patients are symptomatic and immediate permanent pacing facilities are not available

Prophylactic perioperatively
1 During general anaesthesia or cardiac catheterization in patients with:
    Intermittent heart block
    Bifascicular block with first-degree heart block
2 During cardiac surgery
    Especially for aortic and tricuspid surgery
    Septal defect closure

Treatment of tachycardias
Overdrive pacing (rare)

during episodes of extreme bradycardia, heart block and asystole. Thrombolysis and other acute reperfusion strategies have resulted in a decline in the number of patients requiring temporary pacing post-infarction (Petch 1999). It is usually only performed when the patient is haemodynamically compromised. Other indications include diagnostic uses, as in stress testing, and the prevention and suppression of tachyarrhythmias which are resistant to drug therapy, by means of overdriving an ectopic focus or by breaking a re-entry circuit with a critically timed impulse.

Although there is little doubt that temporary cardiac pacing may save life acutely, its long-term value is more difficult to assess. Prognosis is influenced not only by complications of the procedure, such as arrhythmias, cardiac perforation and septicaemia, but also by the degree of underlying myocardial damage which originally led to the conduction defect. The principal determinant of prognosis is the site of the infarct. Anterior myocardial infarction is caused by the occlusion of the left anterior descending coronary artery, which also provides the major blood supply to the AV bundle and bundle branches. Proximal occlusion of the left

coronary artery leads to extensive myocardial damage, often resulting in heart failure and cardiogenic shock. Heart block is a sinister and sudden complication and is due to ischaemic destruction of the conducting tissue below the AV node. Inferior myocardial infarction, on the other hand, does not usually involve so much critical myocardium and normally only results in reversible ischaemia and oedema in the region of the AV node. Inferior infarction is usually caused by occlusion of the right coronary artery, which supplies the inferior wall of the heart. The AV node receives its blood supply by the right coronary artery in 90% of cases, or by the left circumflex artery in the rest. As a result, conduction disturbances commonly occur following acute inferior infarction. Fortunately, for unknown reasons, unless there is pre-existing damage to the conducting tissues, ischaemic injury to the AV node following inferior infarction is rarely permanent. Thus, for the majority of patients with an inferior infarction associated with heart block, normal AV conduction recurs within a few days, whereas, for the patient with an anterior infarction with heart block, the prognosis is poor, and the indications for pacing are controversial. Certainly acute complete heart block requires pacing, and permanent pacing may be required for anterior infarction complicated by high-grade AV block.

Technique

It is usual for a special lead-insulated room to be set aside for temporary cardiac pacing, with facilities for ECG monitoring, fluoroscopy and resuscitation being readily available.

The procedure should, ideally, be fully explained to the patient who should sign a consent form if possible. However, in many instances the patient will obviously have a compromised cardiac output and will thus not be fully conscious.

Transvenous pacing

Although transvenous pacing is the most common method of temporary pacing, medical experience of performing the procedure is less widespread than previously, and it has been estimated that on average, a doctor will see two temporary pacings and perform two under supervision before being

---

Table 7.4   Some indications for permanent pacing

General agreement
Acquired symptomatic complete heart block
Symptomatic second-degree heart block
Symptomatic sinus bradycardia
Sinus node dysfunction
Carotid sinus syndrome

Frequent indications
Asymptomatic complete heart block
Asymptomatic second-degree heart block
Transient Mobitz type II heart block following acute
    myocardial infarction
Bifascicular block in patients with syncope
Overdrive pacing for recurrent ventricular tachycardia

Generally not indicated
Syncope of unknown cause
Asymptomatic bradycardia
Sinus bradycardia with non-specific symptoms
Asymptomatic sinus arrest
Nocturnal bradycardia

left unsupervised (Murphy et al 1995). The use of fluoroscopy is governed by a European Economic Community Directive (EEC 1988) which requires that those operating such equipment be assessed and certified as competent to use it.

The procedure involves two components:

- the insertion, under local anaesthetic, of a bipolar catheter into the subclavian, internal jugular, femoral or brachial vein. The British Cardiac Society recommends the right internal jugular route (Parker and Cleland 1993), this route being the most direct to the left ventricle. The subclavian route is more risky and may lead to arterial puncture and pneumothorax. The femoral and brachial routes can cause problems with electrode stability but may be more appropriate choices for those patients in whom thrombolytic therapy has been recently received or is imminent. The method of choice for catheter insertion is the Seldinger technique using a guide-wire as the use of a long cannula helps the passage of the pacing wire into the heart, limits the risk of catheter displacement and can be used for infusing drugs and other intravenous fluids. Alternative techniques are the percutaneous needle and sheath approach and the cut down technique which is more suitable for venous access via the arm veins.

- the passage, usually under the guidance of fluoroscopy, of the catheter into the superior vena cava, and thence the right atrium, through the tricuspid valve and into the apex of the right ventricle. Position of the tip in the ventricle should be slightly downward pointing and lateral.

The catheter electrodes sense spontaneous electrical activity. Two types of electrodes are seen. The most common are bipolar electrodes where both the negative electrode (cathode) and the positive electrode (anode) are contained in a plastic coating and rest endocardially a few millimetres apart. Unipolar electrodes have one negative cathode on the endocardium and the positive anode on the skin surface.

The various pacing options for temporary pacing are:

- atrial pacing – the electrode is in the right atrial appendage and paces and senses the atria only (AAI pacing)

- ventricular pacing – the electrode is in the right ventricular apex and paces and senses the ventricle only (VVI pacing). This is the most common form of temporary pacing
- dual chamber pacing – there is an electrode in both the atrial and ventricular position and these electrodes pace and sense both chambers (DDD pacing).

Verification of pacing is judged from the appearance of a pacing spike (a vertical line) preceding the QRS complex on the ECG. Each spike should 'capture' a QRS complex. Pacing 'threshold' is obtained by determining the lowest pacing voltage needed to elicit a paced beat: ideally the threshold should be less than 1 V and preferably below 0.5 V.

Temporary transvenous pacing is not without problems, with some form of complication reported to occur in a third to a half of cases (Murphy 2001). Complications include arrhythmias (especially VT and VF) probably produced by mechanical irritation of the endocardium; perforation of the heart or septum; and failure to pace, sense and capture (Table 7.5). Other complications include the following:

1 *Ventricular irritability* at the site of the endocardial catheter tip is common following initial catheter insertion. The ECG usually shows ventricular ectopic beats and the patient may complain of 'dropped beats'. The irritability from the catheter as a foreign body usually disappears after a couple of days.

2 *Abdominal muscle twitching or hiccoughs* occur occasionally as a result of electrode stimulation of the phrenic nerve, myocardial perforation or excessive pacemaker voltage. They are usually very uncomfortable for the patient and should be corrected as soon as possible either by repositioning, replacement or decreasing the voltage.

3 *Infection* is more common if the wire is left in for several days. One study has reported that almost a fifth of patients with a pacing wire left *in situ* for over 48 hours developed septicaemia (Murphy 1996). Infection is more likely if the temporary wire is introduced by the femoral vein, when antibiotic prophylaxis should be considered. Because of the problems with infection, temporary pacing should be avoided

Table 7.5 Some common problems with pacemakers

Problem	Features	Common causes	Interventions
Failure to capture	ECG: absence of QRS complexes immediately following pacing spike (if ventricular paced) Bradycardia Hypotension Fatigue	Electrode displaced Pacemaker voltage too low Lead wire fracture Battery failure Oedema or scar tissue formation at electrode tip	Reposition electrode Increase voltage (mA)* Replace lead Replace battery Reposition or replace electrode
Failure to pace	ECG: absence of pacing activity Hypotension Bradycardia	Battery failure Circuitry failure Lead wire fracture Broken or loose lead – generator connection	Replace battery Replace generator Replace lead Repair connection
Failure to sense	ECG: inappropriately placed pacing spikes Palpitations Dropped beats Ventricular Tachycardia	Battery failure Electrode displaced Lead wire fracture Increased sensing threshold due to oedema or fibrosis at electrode tip	Replace battery Reposition electrode Replace lead Adjust sensitivity setting

* mA, milliamperes.

if at all possible in those patients who are going to need permanent pacing.

4 *Pacemaker dependence* occurs when the pre-existing rhythm is abolished after pacing for a while, leaving complete asystole as the underlying 'rhythm' (seen if the pacing box is momentarily switched off). Transient rises in the threshold or movement of the wire may then be associated with Stokes-Adams attacks as a result of the heart becoming pacemaker dependent. This problem can be rectified by the insertion of a second wire to take over while the first is relocated or removed.

Care of the patient with a temporary transvenous pacemaker

Care of the patient essentially includes:

- assessing pacemaker function
- maintaining system integrity
- ensuring patient comfort and safety

- preventing and dealing with complications
- teaching the patient about his condition and management.

The patient who has had a pacemaker inserted usually shows a marked improvement in mental state, blood pressure, skin colour and general well-being. They should be carefully monitored until either a permanent unit is implanted or pacing is discontinued.

Initially the patient is usually nursed in bed. Mobility will necessarily be restricted, but this will be minimal if the jugular or subclavian approach has been used. Any restrictions imposed upon activities should be carefully explained to the patient and their relatives. The availability of small, portable pacing units allows early mobilization of the patient.

The site of insertion of the pacing catheter should be regularly checked for signs of haemorrhage, haematoma or infection. Very occasionally bacterial endocarditis is a complication.

ECG monitoring will indicate whether the pacemaker is functioning properly. Observation of temperature and blood pressure are important, as is comparison of the pulse with the pacing rate. A chest X-ray will determine the position of the pacing catheter in the heart.

Routine checks on the pacing equipment, with particular attention being paid to connections and the battery charge level, are also required.

Checking the threshold   When the heart is stimulated by an electrical impulse, it either responds completely or not at all and the threshold is the term for the lowest electrical energy that will cause myocardial contraction. The threshold can be affected by the output voltage, the pulse width (duration of the stimulating pulse), the length of time the wire has been in place and any inflammatory response at the electrode tip. Patients should be lying down when the threshold is checked as they might be very sensitive to changes in pacing rate. The threshold is determined by first ensuring that the myocardium is being continuously paced (this may involve turning the rate up), then turning the output dial down until a loss of capture is seen (pacing spikes fail to produce a QRS complex), and then slowly increasing the output again until capture returns. This value is the threshold. The threshold and underlying rhythm need recording every 12 hours and setting determined for the following 12 hours. From the time of positioning, the threshold rises for about 2 weeks and then reaches a plateau. If the output of the pacemaker is less than the threshold there will be a loss of capture and absence of contraction following each pacing stimulus. Careful records of the pacing rate, threshold and pacing voltage should be made.

Although most pacing units are protected, it is advisable to switch off the pulse generator to prevent electrical damage if the patient requires defibrillation and to have the device checked afterwards. The immediate environment should also be kept as free as possible from electrical hazards. Any pacing box that has had water spilt on it or has been dropped needs to be sent to a medical electronics department for checking.

Patient education should assume prime importance. The patient should be observed for evidence of reduced cardiac output such as a fall in blood pressure, and encouraged to report any symptoms of faintness, dizziness, chest pain, shortness of breath, hiccoughs or abdominal muscle twitching. They should be informed about the pacing unit and the length of time it is expected that they will be likely to need it. The nurse should be prepared to discuss and anticipate particular fears and worries the patient may have, especially regarding pacemaker malfunction or feelings of dependency. It is vital that the family are included in such discussions and, when the time comes for discontinuing pacing or undergoing permanent pacing, that information, support and involvement in decisions are encouraged.

Analgesia may be required for pain at the insertion site. Sedation should be considered alongside nursing intervention to reduce patient anxiety which can become a problem, particularly when the temporary pacemaker is discontinued. A positive approach is required, with reassurance that the patient can return to a normal lifestyle as their heart is fully functioning.

Removal of the temporary pacemaker

Removal of the temporary pacemaker is a simple and straightforward procedure performed at the patient's bedside. The patient should be reassured that the pacemaker is no longer required and informed of the procedure to remove it. As with the removal of any central venous catheter there is a risk of air embolism and the patient should be positioned supine or lying with their head slightly downwards. Under aseptic conditions, with a defibrillator immediately available and after the pulse generator has been switched off, the dressing and retaining sutures are removed. While observing the ECG monitor for ectopic activity, the catheter should be slowly and gently withdrawn. In the case of ventricular pacing the catheter has to pass through the tricuspid valve. It is possible for it to become stuck at this point, in which case pressure should not be applied as this can damage the valve. Medical advice should be sought and the catheter removed with the aid of fluoroscopy guidance. Once the catheter has been removed a sterile air occlusive dressing should be secured in place for at least 24 hours.

It may be advisable, particularly if the patient is pyrexial, to remove the tip of the disposable pacing catheter under aseptic conditions and send it to the bacteriological laboratory. The site should be observed for leakage and the patient continued to be monitored for signs of infection.

Transcutaneous pacing

External transcutaneous, or external pacing was originally introduced over 50 years ago and was widely used as a temporary measure for the treatment of asystole and bradycardia (Zoll 1952). It is a non-invasive method of delivering electricity from an external power source which then depolarizes excitable myocardial tissue by pulsed electrical current conducted through the chest wall, between two self-adhesive electrodes stuck to the front and back of the patient's chest. The negative electrode is placed on the front of the patient's chest in the V_3 position and the positive electrode on the patient's back level with the bottom of the scapula, between the spine and the left or right scapula. Contact with bone should be avoided as it will increase the threshold. Failure to capture can occur as a result of inaccurate electrode position, poor skin contact with the electrode, failure to switch the machine on and battery failure.

Transcutaneous pacing can be a rapid, simple and safe means of maintaining cardiac output. Many defibrillators now have an external pacing facility which means more areas are able to use this method of pacing. It is particularly useful for those patients who do not require immediate pacing but are at risk of progression to AV block (ACC/AHA 1999) as active (demand) pacing electrodes can be placed in position. Transcutaneous pacing is well tolerated by patients producing little more than slight cutaneous discomfort and muscle twitching (Zoll and Zoll 1985). However, long-term transcutaneous pacing is unpleasant and high-risk patients or those requiring pacing for long periods should have a temporary endocardial wire inserted.

Permanent (implanted) pacing

In the UK, it is recommended that 550 pacemakers are inserted annually for every million of the population (British Cardiac Society 2002).

Indications

The decision to implant a permanent pacemaker is made after careful assessment of symptoms, ECG, ambulatory and intracardiac electrophysiological studies, long-term prognosis and general medical and psychological health.

For coronary patients who develop conduction problems, long-term prognosis is related to severity of the myocardial damage, not the presence or absence of heart block. Permanent pacing is seldom required following inferior infarction as those patients who do not regain permanent function seldom survive the acute infarction. However, mortality is very high in patients with conduction abnormalities following anterior infarction. It is likely that this group are at high risk of further symptomatic rhythm disturbances. Possible indications for permanent pacing in this group are shown in Table 7.6.

For those patients who recover normal AV conduction, exercise testing and 24-hour ambulatory monitoring are useful adjuncts for post-infarction assessment. Electrophysiological testing, if available, may give early indication of impaired intra-nodal conduction, thus allowing consideration for permanent pacing before problems arise (Cobbe 1986).

The permanent pacemaker

The modern pacemaker is a small metal unit weighing between 25 and 30 g, powered by a lithium battery with a life between 8 and 12 years depending on its use. Two types of pulse generator are

Table 7.6 Possible indications for permanent pacing in patients recovering from acute myocardial infarction with AV block

Infarct/block	Pace?
Inferior with transient AV block	No
Inferior with permanent second/third-degree block	Yes
Anterior with fascicular block	No?
Anterior with transient second/third-degree block	Yes?
Anterior with permanent second/third-degree block	Yes

currently available for permanent implantation:

1   single chamber pacing: an electrode placed in either the atrium or the ventricle
2   dual chamber pacing: electrodes situated in both chambers.

Most implants are now programmable using radio-frequency devices thus allowing greater flexibility in the rate, output, sensitivity and inhibitory functions, which can be altered to meet the specific needs of the patient. Usually, the pacemaker is implanted under local anaesthesia in the cardiac catheterization laboratory. After inserting the pacing catheter through a large central vein into the heart, the electrode is impacted against the endocardial surface of the chamber. It may be anchored by means of a barb, screw or clamp at the pacing electrode tip. Some electrodes are fixed with finger-like projections (tines) so that they do not actually penetrate the myocardium. The pulse generator is then implanted in a subcutaneous pocket, usually under the clavicle, axilla or abdominal wall.

Alterations in function can be accomplished by means of non-invasive transmission of information from an external programmer to the implanted generator without the need for a second operation or implementation of a different pacemaker. About one-fifth of patients will require a change in such specific requirements.

The Intersociety Commission for Heart Disease (ICHD) has devised a pacemaker coding system for differentiating the various functional capabilities of pacemakers (Table 7.7). There is a five-position code which provides a standardized means, irrespective of the pacemaker trade make or model. However, most pacemaker codes only refer to the first three positions. The first position (I) signifies the heart chamber being paced: A (atrium), V (ventricle) or D (dual, or double). The second position (II) identifies the heart chamber being sensed: A, V, D or 0 (none, or not applicable). The third position (III) indicates how the pacemaker generator responds to the sensed event: T (triggered), I (inhibited), D (double, both triggered and inhibited) or 0 (not applicable). The fourth position (IV) indicates the number of available reprogrammable functions. The fifth position (V) indicates how the pacemaker reacts to tachyarrhythmias.

The British Pacing and Electrophysiology Group (1991) and the North American Task Force (ACC/AHA 1998) have produced recommendations for the selection of pacemaker for particular patients. Wherever possible, the pacing mode that best simulates sinus rhythm should be used. The ventricle should be paced if there is actual or a risk of AV block. However, ventricular pacing alone results in about 20% reduction in cardiac output as a result of the loss of the haemodynamic

Table 7.7   Intersociety Commission for Heart Disease (ICHD) Code of Pacing Modes and Functions (after Parsonnet et al 1981)

Position				
I Chamber(s) paced	II Chamber(s) sensed	III Mode(s) of response	IV Programmable functions	V Special tachyarrhythmia function(s)
Letters used				
V: Ventricle	V: Ventricle	T: Triggered	P: Programmable (rate and/or output only)	B: Bursts
A: Atrium	A: Atrium	I: Inhibited	M: Multiprogrammable	N: Normal rate competition
D: Double	D: Double	D: Double*	C: Communicating	S: Scanning
		0: None		
	0: None	R: Reverse	0: None	E: External

*Triggered and inhibited response.

contribution of atrial systole. This may be particularly relevant in patients with poor left ventricular function who would benefit from synchronized sequential AV activity. Dual chamber pacing is becoming more common as it is able to reproduce the sequential AV contraction that occurs physiologically. This helps restore atrial transport, improve symptoms, exercise tolerance and reduces the risk of AF, emboli, stroke and heart failure.

Care of the patient with a permanent pacemaker

As soon as a decision has been made that a patient requires implantation of a permanent pacemaker, preparation for the procedure needs to be made. The procedure is usually performed on a day-case basis under local anaesthetic and this needs to be remembered during patient preparation and aftercare. Information should be tailored to individual needs and take into account existing knowledge and expectations as well as the patient's ability and motivation to learn, level of anxiety and type of lifestyle. The nurse should determine the patient's knowledge of pacemakers and clarify any misconceptions. Activities of daily living should be discussed to ascertain an appropriate site for pacemaker placement. For instance, abdominal implantation may be preferable to pectoralis muscle implantation for the enthusiastic swimmer, because of the strenuous arm activity. It is usual practice to place the pulse generator on the opposite side to the patient's dominant hand.

It is useful to give a clear explanation of the reason for the pacemaker, the actual procedure, including immediate post-insertion care, and the expected outcome. A visit from a patient who already has a permanent pacemaker may be beneficial in allaying anxiety or fear. The patient and family need to be assured that the procedure is generally very successful and that, although as with any procedure it is not without risk of complications, it will greatly aid the patient in returning to an active normal life. Some pacemaker manufacturers produce patient education literature. It is useful if the patient is shown and encouraged to examine and ask questions about a pacemaker, similar to the one to be implanted. This may help in coming to terms with alterations in body image that may accompany the thought of relying on an inanimate object being placed inside the body for maintenance of health.

Routine systemic antibiotic prophylaxis can reduce the incidence of potentially serious infective complications (DaCosta et al 1998). After the procedure, the patient should be attached to a cardiac monitor and the ECG monitored for the rhythm and the presence of pacing spikes. The patient should have a chest X-ray which is deliberately overpenetrated to observe the position of the leads. Observation of the wound site for bleeding or haematoma is important. The sutures are usually removed after 5–7 days.

If the pacemaker has been implanted in the pectoralis major muscle, passive and active range of motion exercises should be started on the affected arm 48 h after insertion to avoid the development of a 'frozen shoulder'. Such exercises should be repeated several times each day until the implantation site is free of discomfort through all ranges of arm motion. The patient should be reassured that the pacemaker will not become damaged by the performance of routine activities, including bathing, although activities that are likely to result in high impact or stress at the implantation site, such as contact sports, should be avoided. Resumption of sexual and leisure activities is encouraged, although work activities may depend on occupation. Current DVLA regulations state that the patient should refrain from driving for one week (6 weeks for HGV) after a pacemaker insertion or a box change. The patient may have to limit certain activities if their cardiac output is insufficient to meet metabolic needs. They should be taught to palpate and record their own pulse rate once daily upon waking and report a rate in excess of 5 beats per minutes slower than that at which the pacemaker is set. The patient should also report any signs or symptoms that indicate pacemaker malfunction, in other words those that indicate decreased cardiac output, such as lethargy, faintness, chest pain, shortness of breath or fluid retention (sudden weight gain or puffy ankles). Signs of infection, such as redness, swelling, drainage or increased soreness at the implantation site, should also be reported.

The patient and family should be instructed about any medication that may be prescribed and the importance of compliance with it and any other health advice. Attendance at follow-up clinics should be stressed. Instruction about the expected life of the pacemaker battery, and what replacement entails, are vital aspects of patient care. Safety measures should include informing any doctor or dentist of the pacemaker and of any medications. The patient should be advised to carry a pacemaker identification card with them at all times. This should include information regarding the brand and model of the pacemaker, the date of insertion and the rate at which it is set. It is useful to warn patients that their pacemaker may trigger off alarms on metal detector devices in airports. Microwaves are safe providing they are not leaking. Some theft control devices and metal detectors have electromagnetic fields which can alter the settings of a small proportion of pacemakers. Patients should be instructed to avoid these pieces of equipment or walk briskly away from them. Mobile phones are safe providing the phone is not placed directly over the pulse generator.

CARDIAC ARREST

Cardiac arrest may be defined as the failure of the heart to pump sufficient blood to keep the brain alive. Circulatory arrest signifies complete, or virtually complete, cessation of blood flow to vital organs. It is the immediate consequence of cardiac arrest or interruption of cardiac massage during CPR.

Cardiac arrest may be due to a number of factors as a result of problems arising within the heart or elsewhere in the body. The commonest cause is a cardiac arrhythmia secondary to coronary heart disease, of which a minority of cases will have had a recent myocardial infarction. Other common causes include trauma, drugs, massive blood loss through haemorrhage, valvular heart disease, hypoxia and pulmonary embolism. When the heart fails to maintain the cerebral circulation for about 4 minutes, the brain may become irreversibly damaged. The three main mechanisms of cardiac arrest are:

1 VF
2 ventricular asystole
3 PEA.

The majority of cardiac arrests occur outside the hospital and are 'sudden deaths', usually the result of ventricular arrhythmias.

Brain death usually occurs because of failure of oxygenation of brain cells associated either with failure in ventilation or failure of the heart to pump oxygenated blood to the brain. The vital organs such as the brain, heart, liver and kidney are very sensitive to blood flow reduction, the brain more so because it has no glycogen stores to break down for energy in the absence of oxygen. Thus, the brain can tolerate only 4–6 min of anoxia.

Cardiac arrest is not an uncommon emergency in hospital practice, and rapid diagnosis and treatment are essential. Coronary care units were originally developed primarily to treat VF and other serious arrhythmias in the first few hours following myocardial infarction. The management of cardiac arrest by the nurse requires rapid decisions (both technical and ethical) and speedy actions, based on the following considerations:

1 irreversible brain damage often occurs after about 4 min
2 the chance of restoring adequate heart rhythm and successfully resuscitating the patient diminishes rapidly with time
3 impressive survival rates can be anticipated on the coronary care unit in patients with primary VF. Both asystole and electromechanical dissociation have a much worse prognosis
4 survival rates on the ward are about 20% lower than on the coronary care unit
5 external cardiac massage can provide only a limited cardiac output (20–25% of normal).

Waiting for a second opinion, recording the blood pressure, raising the legs and lowering the head have no place in the immediate management of cardiac arrest: they are a dangerous waste of time.

The significance of location

Most episodes of cardiac arrest occur outside hospital. In fact three-quarters of all deaths from myocardial infarction occur after cardiac arrest in the community. Survival after cardiac arrest outside hospital remains low, although the development of out of hospital resuscitation has been shown to be effective in countries such as Sweden and the USA where implementation of immediate bystander resuscitation has doubled the survival rate from cardiac arrest.

The UK ambulance service aims to arrive at the scene of an emergency within 8 minutes and therefore provide defibrillation within this time frame. This is obviously a slower response than if the patient is in hospital where, particularly in high dependency areas, nurses who witness the arrest are also able to initiate advanced life support (ALS) including defibrillation. The survival rates for an in-hospital resuscitation attempt are about 1 in 8, of which only a third will be discharged from hospital (Ebell et al 1998).

A recent survey by the National Patient Safety Agency (2004) reported that there were 27 different 'crash call' telephone numbers in use in UK hospitals. The Agency has issued a Patient Safety Alert recommending standardization.

Recognition of cardiac arrest

The signs of cardiac arrest are:

- abrupt loss of consciousness
- absent carotid and femoral pulses
- absent respirations.

A rapidly developing pallor often associated with cyanosis ensues. Pupil dilatation is unreliable. Apnoea, gasping and convulsions may occur later, but are unreliable and inconsistent signs.

As speed of initiating resuscitation is crucial, and confirmation of an arrest not always straightforward, cardiac arrest must be assumed to have occurred if there is any sudden loss of consciousness, onset of seizure in a patient who is not epileptic, or sudden onset of cyanosis or respiratory distress.

Occasionally, there are warning signs preceding cardiac arrest, which experienced personnel can often recognize. Hospitals are increasingly introducing standardized 'early warning' protocols to summon expert help to prevent arrests (Hodgetts et al 2002). It is not uncommon for experienced nurses to be able to anticipate when a patient is about to arrest. A knowledge of causative and associated factors is important. In the monitored patient, R on T ectopic beats, left ventricular ectopic beats and multi-focal ectopic beats have long been associated with the onset of VF.

Nursing responsibilities

The nurse is most likely to be the first health care professional who has contact with the hospital patient who has a cardiac arrest. Nursing responsibilities include:

- accurately recognizing the occurrence of a cardiac arrest
- summoning appropriate help and initiating resuscitation
- continuing with ALS measures in accordance with competency
- maintaining patient comfort and dignity
- anticipating events and procedures
- acting as an expert role model
- giving advice and support to inexperienced colleagues
- giving care and support to the patient after the event
- giving support to relatives and fellow patients.

Most resuscitation attempts will be unsuccessful and there are consequently potential problems, such as feelings of inadequacy, guilt and self-doubt, when the patient dies. Support from peers, together with a realistic appraisal of the situation, is often invaluable.

On-going responsibilities of the nurse include checking and maintaining equipment, keeping up-to-date, encouraging and implementing new ideas on cardiopulmonary resuscitation techniques, and being aware of dilemmas and ethical considerations.

Cardiopulmonary resuscitation

CPR has three aims:

1 protection of the brain by restoring its flow of oxygenated blood, with cardiac massage and artificial ventilation
2 restoration of an adequate spontaneous cardiac output
3 correct aftercare.

There are three main phases of CPR:

- BLS (basic life support)
- ALS (advanced life support)
- ILS (intermediate life support)

Basic life support

The purpose of BLS is to maintain adequate ventilation and circulation until such time as it becomes possible to attempt to reverse the underlying cause of the arrest. The term 'basic' implies that no equipment is used. Where a simple airway or pocket face mask are used for ventilation, the procedure is termed 'BLS with airway adjuncts'. BLS is essentially a 'holding' operation as it is only in very rare situations, particularly when the underlying cause of the arrest is respiratory, that such measures will result in control of the underlying cause and precipitate a full recovery. For this reason it is vital that those finding the patient summon help from those equipped to attempt to reverse the underlying cause of the arrest, and not just focus on their own attempt at BLS.

BLS consists of:

- initial assessment (airway and breathing)
- airway maintenance (**A**)
- expired air ventilation (rescue breathing **B**)
- chest compression (circulation **C**).

The cerebral cortex can only withstand anoxia for about 4 minutes, and if effective resuscitation is not started within this time, permanent cerebral damage will occur. Thus, the critical factor in BLS is the time lapse between the onset of the arrest and the commencement of the resuscitation attempt.

Initial assessment   The assessment phase starts by ensuring the safety of the rescuer and the patient, followed by confirmation of the arrest. The collapsed patient should be shaken gently and asked if they are all right. If the patient responds at this point they should be reassessed regularly and assistance sought if needed. If the patient does not respond, the rescuer needs to shout for help, and turn the patient on to their back for further assessment and possible resuscitation.

Confirmation of the arrest involves establishing whether the patient is breathing and involves looking for chest movement, listening for breath sounds and getting close to the patient's face to feel for any expired air. This should take up to 10 seconds. If it is established that the patient is not breathing, then appropriate skilled help (i.e. the arrest team for hospital arrests) and equipment (most significantly a defibrillator), need to be summoned. This should be done before the circulation has been assessed in order to minimize any time delay in starting advanced life support. If there is no one around, it is better to leave the patient to ensure skilled help and equipment are coming.

Precordial thump   The precordial thump should be considered by professional health care workers if it can be initiated within 30 seconds or so of the onset of the arrest. It is therefore most appropriate for witnessed arrests. The thump can mechanically cardiovert VF to sinus rhythm in about 2% of cases and is significantly more successful for VT. If a defibrillator is available it should be used at once.

Airway maintenance   This involves:

- maintaining a clear airway through removal of dentures, food, sputum, vomit, or other debris
- performing the head-tilt/chin-lift or the head-tilt/jaw-thrust method (Figure 7.18) to allow maximum air entry with the patient in a supine position.

For effective resuscitation, the head and the body should be in the same plane. The head must not be

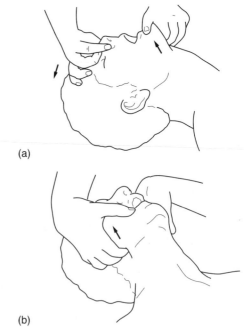

(a)

(b)

Figure 7.18   Techniques for opening the airway: (a) the head-tilt/chin-lift method; (b) the head-tilt/jaw/thrust method.

raised above the level of the thorax, or the brain will not be perfused. Immediate opening of the airway is the most important action as, in most cases, the unconscious patient will have their upper airway obstructed as the tongue falls back on to the posterior pharyngeal wall.

The head-tilt/chin lift manoeuvre involves placing firm backward pressure on the patient's forehead with the palm to tilt the head back. The fingers of the other hand being placed under the chin to lift the mandible forwards until the teeth almost close, thus supporting the lower jaw and maintaining the backward head-tilt. The neck needs to be slightly flexed and the head extended at the atlanto-occipital joint to align the oropharyngeal/laryngeal axis and thus create a straight passage from the mouth through the vocal chords to the trachea.

The head/tilt jaw-thrust method of opening the airway is technically more difficult, but it is of use if neck injury is suspected as it does not involve hyperextending the neck. The mandible is pulled forward by grasping the angle of the jaw on both sides and tilting the head back.

If positioning the head and neck fails to establish an airway, an obstruction by a foreign body, mucus or vomit needs to be considered and the mouth cleared by finger sweeps or suction with the patient lying on their side. Abdominal or chest thrusts are more efficient than the traditional back blows for dislodging foreign bodies from further down the airway.

Expired air ventilation – rescue breathing As soon as it has been established that the patient is not breathing and professional help has been summoned, rescue breathing should be commenced. If mouth-to-mouth resuscitation is the only method available, then the rescuer should pinch the patient's nostrils closed with their thumb and finger, open their mouth, take a deep breath, make an airtight seal over the mouth, and give two slow breaths into the patient's mouth. The rescuer's mouth should then be removed to allow the patient to exhale passively. Expired air contains 16% oxygen which, although less rich than that of surrounding air (21% oxygen), provides adequate oxygenation. Alternative routes are mouth-to-nose, which allows maximum head extension and jaw thrust

while usefully effecting lip closure (Simons and Howells 1986), mouth-to-mask or a self-expanding 'Ambu' bag and oxygen. Contact with vomit and saliva is reduced which makes these methods more acceptable and also reduces the risk of infection. In the hospital situation it is unlikely that rescue breathing will need to be performed without the barrier offered by a pocket mask. Although there is a theoretical risk of transmission of serum hepatitis, herpes simplex and AIDS (acquired immune deficiency syndrome) with mouth to mouth, recorded incidents of such transmission are rare.

Only a small amount of resistance to breathing should be felt during rescue breathing. Two effective breaths need to be given which make the patient's chest rise and fall. There needs to be up to five attempts to achieve this before moving on to the next steps. Each rescue breath should take two seconds. If the inflation is too quick, resistance will be greater and less air will get into the lungs. The tidal volume needs to be about 700–1000 ml, which is the amount normally required to produce visible lifting of the chest. The rescuer should wait for the chest to fall completely during expiration before next breath is given. This should normally take about 2–4 seconds so that each sequence of ten breaths takes about 40–60 seconds to complete.

Chest compression After two effective rescue breaths have been accomplished the patient is assessed for signs of circulation. This is usually done by attempting to feel the carotid pulse for a period of 10 seconds. It is acknowledged that assessing for the carotid pulse is difficult, particularly for lay rescuers (Eberle et al 1996). For this reason it is now recommended that lay rescuers check for signs of circulation, such as movement, swallowing or breathing, rather than trying to feel for a pulse. If there are no signs of circulation, then external chest compressions should be commenced.

External cardiac massage The mechanisms of external cardiac massage have not been fully determined (Peters and Ihle 1990). It was once thought that external cardiac massage led to the ejection of blood from the heart by manual compression of the ventricles between the sternum and spine, and also facilitated cyclic ventricular filling. It is now thought that blood flow may originate from an increased intrathoracic pressure rather than direct heart compression. External cardiac massage involves:

- placing the patient supine on a firm surface
- placing the heel of one hand of the rescuer on the lower half of the patient's sternum, and the other hand on top of the first (Figure 7.19).
- keeping the rescuer's arms straight and elbows locked
- kneeling level with the patient and applying firm downward pressure
- compressing the sternum at a rate of 100 per minute
- depressing the sternum 4–5 cm (one third of the chest).

External cardiac massage can provide only limited cardiac output. Cerebral blood flow is only 3–15% of normal and cardiac output about 20–25% of normal and decreases with time.

There is much controversy as to the optimum rate and timing of compressions. For example, coronary blood flow is thought to occur in the relaxation phase of the massage cycle, and so an increase in the compression rate with less time between compressions is thought to mean an increased cerebral perfusion at the expense of cardiac perfusion. The Resuscitation Council (2000) recommended that the time for compression and for relaxation during external cardiac massage should be about equal (i.e. optimal compression to relaxation ratio is 50:50), as experiments have shown that the efficacy of external cardiac massage depends on the duration of compression. Current guidelines recommend uninterrupted compressions at a rate of 100/minute. At the end of each

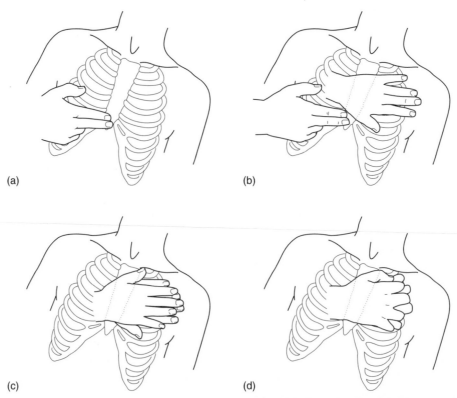

(a)
(b)
(c)
(d)

Figure 7.19 Hand positioning during external cardiac massage. (a) Middle finger locates xiphoid process; index finger positioned next to middle finger. (b) Heel of opposite hand is placed on sternum next to index finger. (c) First hand is removed from landmark position and placed on top of other hand so heels of both hands are parallel and fingers point away. (d) Fingers may be locked to avoid pressure on ribs.

compression, relaxation must be complete to allow adequate refilling of the thoracic pump. The hands, however, should remain in place in contact with the patient so as not to lose the correct placement. Studies (Maier et al 1986) have suggested that the compression rate should be even faster, approaching 120 per minute ('high impulse CPR').

Compression/ventilation intervals   The Resuscitation Council of the United Kingdom recommends a cycle of 15 compressions followed by two inflations irrespective of whether there are one or two rescuers. Resuscitation should be continuous, rhythmic and uninterrupted. Time should not be wasted in between cycles trying to establish if there is a pulse as the chances of restoring sinus rhythm without defibrillation are remote. However, if there are signs indicative of restored circulation, such as spontaneous movement, the rescuer should check for signs of circulation, but for no longer than 10 seconds.

BLS should continue until professional support and/or equipment arrives, the patient appears to recover or the rescuer becomes exhausted. If there are two rescuers it may be appropriate for them both to perform BLS or it may be more time saving for one to ensure all the necessary equipment is assembled and ready for the arrival of the emergency team. Certainly in areas where nurses can defibrillate this should not be delayed in favour of two-rescuer BLS.

An algorithm for BLS is shown in Figure 7.20.

Intermediate life support

ILS involves BLS plus the use of a defbrillator.

Advanced life support

ALS is resuscitation combining BLS with specialist care including early defibrillation, drugs and advanced airway management. Intravenous access is necessary for intravenous drug administration and continuous ECG recording allows the underlying rhythm to be monitored. Current Resuscitation Council (2000) guidelines differentiate between those rhythms that are potentially reverted to sinus rhythm with defibrillation (VF and pulseless VT) and those where defibrillation is not useful (asystole and PEA). These guidelines are summarized in the algorithm shown in Figure 7.21. This algorithm assumes that the preceding step has been unsuccessful and takes the rescuer through a sequence of treatment options. While this algorithm is useful in that it helps ensure that a resuscitation team are following a coordinated approach to the resuscitation attempt, it is still important that each patient's care is based on presenting circumstances and available skills and resources. It is difficult to determine the best treatment options in the arrest situation, as randomized controlled trials would be ethically difficult. So current guidelines offer scope for clinical judgement with less emphasis than in the past on drug administration and more on proven treatments such as defibrillation (Quinn 1998b).

Airway management

Rescue breathing using expired air delivers approximately 16–17% inspired oxygen to the patient. This reduced level of oxygenation results in a reduction in peripheral oxygen delivery which, coupled with the reduced cardiac output produced during cardiac massage, leads to tissue hypoxia with ensuing anaerobic metabolism and metabolic acidosis. Such acid base imbalance can diminish the beneficial effects of the electrical and chemical therapy options of advanced life support. Therefore 100% inspired oxygen is recommended during resuscitation attempts. Short-term therapy with 100% oxygen is beneficial for maximizing arterial blood oxygen saturation, and consequently systemic oxygen delivery, and is non-toxic. The Resuscitation Council (2000) recommends oxygen administered at 4 litres per minute by nasal cannula for the first 2–3 hours for all patients with suspected acute coronary syndromes and for up to 6 hours for those patients with continuing ischaemia, congestive heart failure or an arrhythmia.

Ventilatory devices

Airway control using an invasive airway device is essential for advanced cardiac life support. However, the training, frequency of use and monitoring

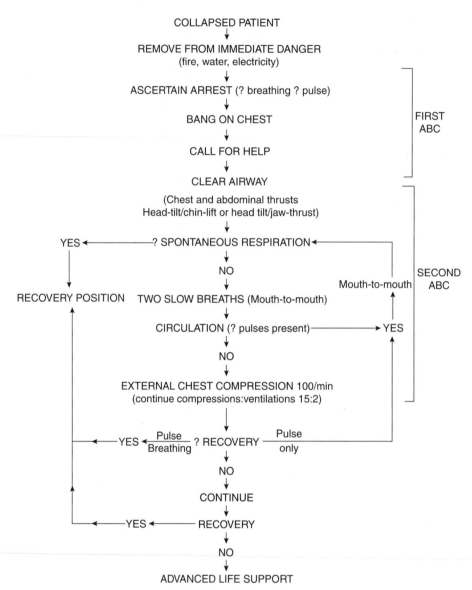

Figure 7.20 An algorithm for basic life support.

of success influence the long-term impact of any device more than the choice of any specific device (Resuscitation Council 2000).

Masks Pocket masks need to available in all clinical areas. They should be transparent to allow observation of any regurgitation, be able to form a tight seal over the mouth and nose and be fitted with an oxygen inlet. One way valves will divert the victim's exhaled gas away from the rescuer. A sufficiently tight seal is best achieved by having the rescuer positioned at the top and behind the patient's head. The mask needs to be held in place with both hands, being sure not to lose the head tilt-chin lift position in the effort to get a tight enough seal.

Bag–valve devices A bag and valve device consists of a self-inflating bag, a non-rebreathing valve and a system to deliver high concentration through

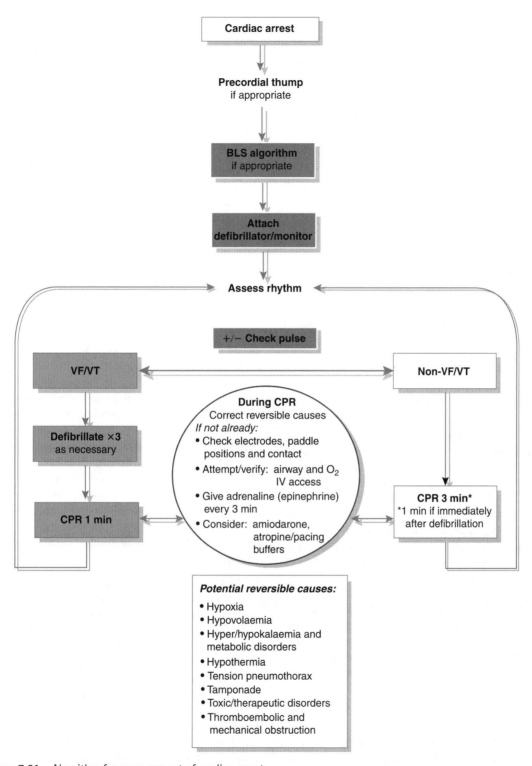

Figure 7.21   Algorithm for management of cardiac arrest.

an ancillary oxygen reservoir. This device can be used connected to a face mask, an endotracheal tube or other ventilatory devices and is able to deliver higher concentrations of oxygen if a reservoir bag is fitted to the end of the self-inflating system, as this allows oxygen (as opposed to oxygen and air) to be drawn into the system. Oxygen delivery is likely to be more effective with two rescuers; one to maintain the open airway and ensure a tight seal between the mask and the patient's skin, and the second to squeeze the bag. A tidal volume of between 700 and 1000 ml is adequate, and slow gentle inflation minimizes the risk of over-ventilation and subsequent gastric inflation which could result in regurgitation and aspiration.

Endotracheal intubation   Endotracheal intuba-tion is not an immediate requirement unless the patient cannot otherwise be ventilated, has a full stomach or has vomited. It should be preceded by preoxygenation of the patient. Intubation is a skilled procedure traditionally performed by the anaesthetist. It should only interrupt resuscitation for a few seconds to prevent brain ischaemia from occurring. Tracheal tube position should be con-firmed by observing for equal expansion of both sides of the chest and listening over the lungs with a stethoscope. Non-physical examination tech-niques, such as qualitative end-tidal CO_2 indica-tors are also useful. Ventilation should be at a rate of 12–15 inflations per minute and can be per-formed independently of chest compression. Those without appropriate training and who are unable to obtain regular clinical experience in intubation should use alternative airways such as the laryn-geal mask airway.

Suction devices   Portable and installed suction devices should be available for resuscitation emer-gencies. The equipment needs to have adjustable suction flow and have a selection of sterile suction catheters. It also needs to be easily cleaned.

Drug therapy

The evidence for the use of drugs in cardiac arrests is limited. Anti-arrhythmic drugs in particular can precipitate tachyarrhythmias and may also depress left ventricular function. The use of more than one drug in the arrest situation may compound these problems. Drugs therefore need to be selected with care with the emphasis being on defibrilla-tion and reversing the cause of the arrest if known.

Choice of route

Choice of route for drug administration depends on the skills and equipment available. Ideally, all drugs used during CPR are best administered through a central venous catheter to ensure swift distribution, as circulation time is greatly pro-longed. If a central line is not *in situ,* insertion of a cannula into a peripheral vein is usually achieved more rapidly than central venous catheterization. Drugs administered peripherally should be fol-lowed by a flush with at least 20 ml of 0.9% periph-erally administered normal saline. CPR should be continued for at least 2 min after drug administra-tion to allow circulation of the drug. Direct intrac-ardiac injections of drugs is no longer endorsed as it can be a dangerous and often difficult practice. Tracheal administration of drugs is an option when an intravenous line cannot be established. Drug absorption via this route is erratic and can be impaired by pulmonary oedema and atelectasis. Adrenaline, lignocaine, atropine and naloxone can be given in this way, although it is not an appro-priate route for amiodarone as this drug can cause local vasoconstriction. Two or three times the intra-venous dose is required, diluted in 10 ml of normal saline or water, and after installation, five infla-tions are required to facilitate distribution and absorption.

Adrenaline   Adrenaline (epinephrine) is the first drug given for all types of cardiac arrest and it may be repeated every 2–3 minutes. The recommended dose for adults is 1 mg. Adrenaline has strong alpha- and beta-adrenergic activity, with a power-ful vasoconstrictor action which diverts blood to the brain and heart and increases the likelihood of restoring cardiac action. It also raises effective coronary perfusion pressure during CPR (Waller and Robertson 1991). The beta-adrenergic activity helps myocardial stimulation following attain-ment of sinus rhythm. Adrenaline has superseded lignocaine as the first choice drug in VF. This change is based on evidence from animal models that adrenaline improves myocardial and cerebral circulation during BLS.

Lidocaine Lidocaine has traditionally been used for the control of ventricular arrhythmias complicating cardiac arrest and acute myocardial infarction. Its major action during cardiac arrest is by inhibiting the initiation of re-entry arrhythmias in the ischaemic myocardium. However, its use makes defibrillation more difficult and is not now recommended for routine use unless amiodarone is unavailable. In such an arrest situation, lidocaine should be administered as bolus therapy with the total dose not exceeding 300 mg during a one-hour period.

Atropine Atropine is used in asystolic and bradycardiac arrest. It lowers vagal tone, but its value after the first few minutes of cardiac arrest is unclear since significant vagotonia is unlikely to be present. It can also precipitate excessive increases in heart rate which can worsen ischaemia.

Amiodarone Amiodarone is effective in treating haemodynamically unstable VT and VF (Kudenchuck et al 1999) and may be considered after the initial three unsuccessful defibrillatory shocks and the first dose of adrenaline. However, amiodarone does have vasodilatory and negative inotropic properties which can destabilize haemodynamic status in the peri-arrest situation.

Magnesium Large multicentred trials have failed to demonstrate any prophylactic benefit from magnesium (ISIS:4 1995). However, it may be of benefit to patients in refractory VF who have been taking potassium-sparing diuretics and have hypomagnesia. Magnesium may also be of benefit in torsades de pointes.

Sodium bicarbonate Although intravenous sodium bicarbonate has been widely used in the past for correcting the metabolic acidosis which follows cardiac arrest, there is little evidence that this therapy improves patient outcome and it is no longer recommended. Indeed, it frequently results in harmful side effects including increased PCO_2, hyperosmolarity and hypernatraemia, extracellular alkalosis, inactivation of concurrently administered catecholamines and tissue necrosis if accidentally given extravascularly. The principal method of correcting acidosis is through establishing effective alveolar ventilation.

Defibrillation

The single most important determinant of outcome in patients with VF/pulseless VT is the time to defibrillation if available, a defibrillator should be used at once. Defibrillation involves the delivery of a current shock to the heart through the chest wall. This causes spontaneous depolarization of all the myocardial cells that are not totally refractory, thereby terminating the fibrillation and allowing, after a brief interval, the normal conducting pathways to regain control of the heart.

Spontaneous heart action can very occasionally occur without further treatment after CPR if the heart is relatively healthy and external cardiac massage is instituted quickly. However, for VF/VT arrests, the chances of successful resuscitation usually depends on the speed of defibrillation. Shocks should be given as soon as a defibrillator is available and there are staff present who are competent to use it. The ability to initiate and perform defibrillation is certainly a skill that is likely to enhance nursing practice and indeed it has become part of many nursing roles under the umbrella of the 'scope of professional practice' (UKCC 1992).

A defibrillator basically consists of a large capacitor for storing electrical energy, and two conductive paddles for delivering this energy to the heart. The energy delivered is measured in joules (volts × amps × time) which is displayed on a meter. The large electrical impulse ('shock') is delivered by two hand-held paddles which are well insulated. They have an integral discharge button so that the operator can control the timing of the delivery of the shock. In most machines the hand-held paddles can act simultaneously as electrodes for ECG monitoring. Some machines will also deliver the charge through pads attached to the skin's surface. This enables the procedure to be 'hands free' with beneficial safety implications for both the patient and the rescuer.

Preparation prior to defibrillation

Prior to defibrillation, swift preparation of the patient, environment and equipment is essential as described below.

1 Preparing the patient The patient's chest needs to be carefully prepared by the application of gel pads designed to reduce electrical resistance and prevent painful superficial skin burns. The pads need to be carefully positioned: one below the right clavicle and the other over the apex of the heart in the fifth intercostal space on the left side of the thorax. This placement ensures that a maximum mass of myocardial cells is depolarized when the defibrillator paddles are positioned and activated, thus optimizing the likelihood of successful termination of the arrhythmia (Figure 7.22a). It is unimportant which paddle is placed over which gel pad, as the polarity is insignificant and the paddles are interchangeable. Obese patients have increased transthoracic resistance and the apico-posterior position may be more useful (Figure 7.22b). Observational studies suggest that pads are often positioned incorrectly (Heames et al 2001). Self-adhesive monitor/defibrillator electrode pads are effective alternatives to the traditional gel pads and paddles and allow a hands-free shock delivery. When using defibrillator paddles at least 10 kg of pressure is needed to prevent loss of current. Gel pads need to be replaced in accordance with the manufacturers' instructions. Electrode jelly is best avoided as it carries the risk of spreading across the chest and resulting in shocks that arc across the chest wall.

2 Ensuring environmental safety Precautions should be taken to ensure that floor surfaces are dry and that all personnel are warned a shock is about to be delivered. There is a theoretical risk that the electric current being delivered could pass through the bed and reach the operator or others touching it; therefore, all personnel need to stand clear of the bed at the moment of electrical discharge. Similarly, there is a theoretical risk that current could pass from the bed to personnel standing nearby if the floor is wet due to the spillage of electrolyte fluids. Particular care is needed if the shock is being delivered by hands-free pads as it is not so obvious to those nearby that a shock is about to be discharged.

3 Preparing the equipment The defibrillator is switched on and charged initially to 200 J (or equivalent biphasic energy). Modern defibrillators are battery operated and do not have to be

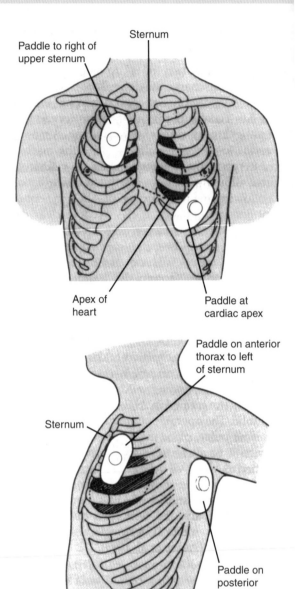

Figure 7.22 Positioning of defibrillation paddles.

plugged into the mains for use. After ensuring that all personnel are warned and well removed from the bed, the gel pads are quickly but carefully placed on the chest wall. The defibrillator paddles are positioned over the gel pads and the operator simultaneously depresses the discharge button to deliver the shock. If it is possible to coordinate defibrillation with ventilation, then the shock should ideally be delivered during expiration, as this is associated with a lower transthoracic resistance (Ewy et al 1980) and hence a higher success rate.

Energy requirements

Successful defibrillation depends on an energy level that will produce enough current flow through the heart to achieve defibrillation, while at the same time causing minimal electrical damage to the heart. The recommended energy levels for defibrillation with monophasic waveforms are:

1 an initial shock of 200 J
2 a second shock of 200 J
3 a third shock of 360 J.

These first three shocks need to be delivered rapidly, checking the monitor trace between shocks, although there is no need to perform pulse checks if the patient remains unresponsive and the trace continues to show VF/VT. BLS between shocks is also not necessary. If normal rhythm has not returned after the initial three shocks, there is a less than one in five chance of survival.

After the third unsuccessful shock, adrenaline 1 mg i.v. should be given followed by:

4 a fourth shock of 360 J within 1 minute of the third shock.

Repeated shocks, even at the same energy levels, add to the likelihood of successful defibrillation because transthoracic impedance falls with repeated shocks.

For persistent VF, different paddle positions and a change of defibrillator should be considered, together with different anti-arrhythmic agents (Chamberlain 1989). If VF is terminated by a shock, but then recurs later in the arrest, subsequent shocks should be delivered at the previously successful energy level (Resuscitation Council 2000).

BLS is continued at all times and should not be interrupted for more than 10 seconds, except when the shocks are delivered.

An oscilloscope may take up to 10 seconds to 'recover' and display an ECG after shock delivery, and so interpretation of success or failure of defibrillation is impossible during this time. If this recovery takes more than one sweep of the oscilloscope screen then BLS needs to continue to ensure that no time

is wasted without circulatory support. Cardiac massage will not seriously affect the beating heart if coordinated rhythm has returned.

Biphasic defibrillation

Biphasic waveforms deliver current that flows first in a positive direction and then in a negative direction. Although there is evidence that the lower energy biphasic shocks are safe and effective (Bardy et al 1996, Poole et al 1997), it is not yet clear what energy requirements should be used in the arrest situation.

Automated external defibrillator (AED)

The chances of successful defibrillation decline by about 7–10% with each minute delay from the onset of the arrest to defibrillation. AEDs were designed and developed for the use by out of hospital first responders including paramedics, police, firefighters, airline flight attendants and sports marshals in order to decrease defibrillation delay, and their use in this context has been shown to be effective (Auble et al 1996, O'Rourke et al 1997). AEDs are computerized devices that enable lay rescuers with minimal training to administer defibrillation quickly. Gel pads are placed on the patient's chest to determine the underlying rhythm and the computer decides whether or not a shock (at a preset energy level), should be delivered. There is a manual override facility in case of equipment rhythm interpretation error. The use of AEDs also has a place in hospital for those not trained in advanced life support techniques. It is strongly recommended that all registered nurses be trained in, and authorized to use AEDs whatever the setting (Quinn 1998b).

Success of defibrillation

The success of defibrillation depends upon a variety of factors:

● the delay in administering the first shock
● whether the fibrillation is primarily due to myocardial ischaemia or secondary to other factors

- the efficiency of the defibrillation procedure (paddle position, etc.)
- metabolic factors such as acidosis, hypoxia and duration of VF before the first shock.

Possible complications

Complications of defibrillation tend to be related to the energy levels used and include superficial burns due to poor skin preparation and transient arrhythmias immediately after the shock. These arrhythmias include asystole, complete heart block, ectopics and VF. Myocardial necrosis may occur as may transient hypotension. Systemic or pulmonary emboli rarely occur. Failure to maintain properly the defibrillator accounts for most cases of equipment malfunction and developing a culture where the equipment is checked at every change of personnel, by those who can operate the equipment, is recommended good practice (Resuscitation Council 2000). Areas which have more than one type of defibrillator need to ensure that users know the indications and use of each.

Evaluation of the effectiveness of cardiopulmonary resuscitation

Certain factors increase the likelihood of successful CPR. These are:

- arrest in a hospital environment
- a witnessed arrest
- time lapse of less than 3 min before intervention
- an electrical rather than a mechanical problem
- CPR lasting less than 15 min
- only one episode of CPR needed
- VF as the dominant arrhythmia
- the patient's underlying pathology, physical fitness and condition after the arrest.

A spontaneous palpable pulse is the best indicator of cardiac output and successful resuscitation. The femoral pulse is usually the most practical to palpate.

The electrical activity of the heart, as illustrated on the ECG, is no guide to contractile or mechanical behaviour. Ventricular complexes may be present on the ECG when the heart is mechanically asystolic, as in electromechanical dissociation.

Brain death cannot be diagnosed with certainty during CPR and apparent signs of brain death are not necessarily evidence that such death has occurred. The brain is able to survive a reduction in blood flow at a level at which all functional activity, including pupillary activity, is suppressed.

Signs of brain activity are the best indicators of effective artificial circulation with CPR, and include:

- pupils becoming smaller
- eyelash reflex
- stiffly held limbs
- struggling
- frowning
- tightly clenched jaw
- strong respiratory efforts.

However, these signs may disappear as CPR continues, making an ongoing evaluation difficult. A compression pulse, which is the pressure wave generated by chest compressions, is no guarantee of blood flow but is often the only evidence of effective CPR.

In a study of prediction of immediate survival from resuscitation, Marwick et al (1991) found the most powerful determinant of outcome was VF as the underlying cardiac rhythm. Other favourable prognostic factors included age under 60 years, presence of underlying cardiac disease, prompt CPR (within 2 min) and early defibrillation. Age over 60 years, intubation and the use of adrenaline were independent negative prognostic factors.

Initial success rates in all cases of adult resuscitation may be as low as 30%, falling to 10% in the long term (Peatfield et al 1977). The success rate is significantly higher if equipment is readily available and nursing staff are able to instigate defibrillation.

Resuscitation skills

Although the chances of resuscitation should be optimal within hospital, especially in a coronary care unit, it is clear that nurses and doctors are often deficient in the knowledge and skills of basic resuscitation (Casey 1984, Skinner et al 1985, Kaye and Mancini 1986, Wynne et al 1987, O'Donnell 1990). Kaye et al (1981) suggested that 'chaos' best described in-hospital resuscitation attempts. Experience in performing CPR appears to increase confidence but not competence (Marteau et al 1989, 1990). Thus, experience is no substitute for training, and feedback on performance during training seems to be an important factor.

Role-play sessions can be helpful in encouraging familarity with equipment and procedures in a controlled and less stressful situation. Simulated cardiac arrest may help identify deficiencies or difficulties in resuscitation (Sullivan and Guyatt 1986) and improve nurses' decision making (Baumann and Bourbonnais 1982, Thompson and Sutton 1985). Supervised simulation with a developing clinical scenario can help. This helps nurses and doctors to work together as a team, so that there is less confusion and more appropriate management at the time of a real crisis. It has been found that a year after training, the ability to perform resuscitation skills may have fallen to a level of competency similar to that before the training (Wynne et al 1999). Certainly, there is a need for 6-monthly to yearly practical updates.

There is no longer a clear distinction between which professionals perform which level of life support. Lay people with training can defibrillate and nurses are increasingly leading advanced life support attempts. The UK Resuscitation Council provides nationally recognized courses which aim to teach and assess the skills needed for basic, intermediate and advanced life support. There is evidence that nurses who undertake the advanced life support (ALS Provider) course, particularly those from general ward areas, are not always able to use these skills in practice. It has been argued that it would be more efficient for nurses to be trained and assessed specifically in the skills they are then able to use (O'Higgins et al 2001), hence, the introduction of ILS courses.

Coronary care units are distinguished by having skilled personnel and appropriate technology. Patients are monitored and have established intravenous access. Such an environment should provide an example to the rest of the hospital in the field of successful resuscitation.

Care of the patient after surviving a cardiac arrest

After successful resuscitation the patient will require skilled nursing and medical care. Full recovery from a cardiac arrest is rarely immediate and can only be said to have occurred when the patient is fully conscious, with full cardiac, cerebral and renal function. The chances of achieving this are greatly enhanced in a coronary care unit where the onset of the arrest is likely to have been witnessed and intervention achieved in less than 2–3 min.

The management of a patient following resuscitation depends on the initial outcome of the resuscitation procedure. Patients may be broadly divided into four groups (Jowett and Thompson 2003):

1 Immediate recovery with no recurrence and minimal after effects.
2 Unconscious for a few hours – these patients may suffer anxiety, confusion, delusions, and difficulty in concentrating for a few months.
3 Unconscious for more than 24 h – these patients have a variable prognosis and may show signs of uncoordination and stroke.
4 Decerebrate – these patients usually die within a few days.

Physical care

Any underlying cause of the arrest should be treated. Complications of the resuscitation procedure such as aspiration of gastric contents, pneumothorax (secondary to central venous catheterization or rib fracture) and chest soreness from defibrillation need to be dealt with.

The patient's acid–base balance needs to be assessed, together with plasma potassium levels, and any abnormalities immediately corrected. The serum potassium needs to be maintained above 4 mmol/l. Significant hyperkalaemia should be treated with a glucose-insulin infusion. Blood gas and acid–base abnormalities can be controlled initially by ventilation and restoration of renal function.

Several body systems need special attention, as described below.

1 Cardiovascular system Heart rhythm and rate should be closely monitored and a 12-lead ECG will enable an electrophysiological assessment. Prophylactic anti-arrhythmic therapy may be required. Blood pressure monitoring is required, especially if inotropic support is necessitated, and haemodynamic monitoring may be warranted. Thrombolytic therapy may be initiated in the case of acute myocardial infarction.

2   Respiratory system   Oxygen therapy needs to be continued post-arrest as ventilation–perfusion defects are common in both lungs following resuscitation. Arterial blood gas analysis is useful and artificial ventilation may be warranted. Pulse oximetry can be helpful in monitoring the ongoing situation. A reduction of the PCO_2 to about 30 mmHg (4 kPa) will decrease cerebral oedema, and control of ventilation will allow some correction of blood gas abnormalities. A chest X-ray will be needed to exclude pneumothorax.

3   Renal system   Adequate renal perfusion needs to be maintained and a low-dose dopamine infusion may help in promoting the renal blood supply and preventing acute renal failure. Urethral catheterization may be necessary to obtain accurate measurements of hourly urine output. A potent diuretic such as frusemide may be given routinely following resuscitation.

4   Central nervous system   Primary cerebral damage can occur as a result of hypoxia sustained during the cardiac arrest. Secondary damage can follow resuscitation if the injured brain becomes oedematous. Hypercapnia, hypertension and hyperglycaemia in the post-arrest period are likely to exacerbate cerebral damage.

Microthrombi may form in cerebral vessels when the blood flow is greatly diminished during arrest and resuscitation. Micro-emboli can also be ejected from the heart during cardiac massage. Occluded cerebral vessels will compromise cerebral perfusion once blood flow has been restored. Signs of lateral weakness, dysphasia and other features associated with a stroke may become apparent during assessment. Cerebral oedema may be reduced by the use of intravenous mannitol and dexamethasone and also by elevating the head to 30° to increase venous drainage. Mechanical ventilation will make adequate arterial and cerebral oxygenation easier to achieve.

5   Gastrointestinal system   Gastric distension, produced by artificial ventilation and the induction of air into the stomach, promotes vomiting and produces discomfort for the patient. The temporary insertion of a nasogastric tube will help to relieve this. Antacids and agents such as cimetidine may help control any gastric acidity. The patient may not feel like taking any diet initially, although small light meals should be made available for when they feel like eating. Cool drinks may help to relieve any throat soreness caused by irritation from the endotracheal tube or airway.

General patient comfort

Following a cardiac arrest and resuscitation, it is not uncommon for the patient to have been left lying semi-clothed in an uncomfortable bed surrounded by debris and equipment. They may have been incontinent, have a sore chest and feel exhausted and somewhat embarrassed by their current state. Having been forced to lie flat for the purpose of resuscitation, they are likely to feel more comfortable and breathe easier if they are assisted to sit upright. The application of a topical agent such as hydrocortisone to the chest wall may relieve the soreness of burns caused by defibrillation. Opiates may be required for ischaemic chest pain, and analgesics for pain produced as a result of fractured ribs.

Other considerations include offering mouthwashes, replacing dentures, combing hair and changing clothing and bedclothes.

Psychological support

The patient is likely to require assessment regarding their level of orientation, recall, fear, anxiety and general feelings of the event. Any misconceptions need to be identified and an assessment made of the patient's understanding of what has happened to them. Decisions concerning the timing and type of support needed will need to be made. The psychological support required will vary. Although nurses are usually conversant with the medical and technological management of cardiac arrest, they often lack insight into the psychological effects and their nursing management.

Although it is generally assumed that the patient is in a state of unconsciousness during the resuscitation procedure, some survivors are able to recount what happened in surprising detail (Dim et al 1974). Near-death phenomena such as the patient experiencing going down a long tunnel have been reported occasionally (Moody 1976, 1988). The patient may feel frightened of such memories and need reassurance and an opportunity to discuss the experience.

Fellow patients may wonder if the same thing is likely to happen to them. Reports of chest pain commonly increase following an arrest. Successful resuscitation may be reassuring for some patients, but they are likely still to want to discuss the matter. If the patient dies following a cardiac arrest, an honest open approach, rather than trying to conceal or deny the fact, usually seems to work best for fellow patients. Patients in adjacent beds are usually fully cognizant of the situation and often welcome the opportunity for frank discussion with the nurse. The subject of their own mortality may be more easily discussed in this sort of situation. The sudden thought of their own death being a potential reality is likely to be very frightening and elicit feelings of hostility and denial. Time should carefully be used here as an opportunity for counselling and giving an optimistic and yet realistic appraisal, clarifying issues and correcting misconceptions.

The patient's relatives will understandably be upset and require a great deal of support, whether the resuscitation is successful or not. If the patient dies, a senior doctor should discuss this with the relatives. The presence of an experienced nurse can be of great value in this situation to reinforce, explain and be a comforting presence.

Relatives will usually be initially shocked and concerned at the event, especially if the patient was improving beforehand. Some patients may arrest and die shortly after admission when the nurse has had very little time to establish a relationship with the patient's relatives. These relatives undergo a brief and traumatic experience and may have unique needs (Edwards and Shaw 1998). Relatives may display numerous reactions including anger, denial and disbelief, which require sensitive handling.

Giving bereaved relatives a barrage of information about the patient's property and death certificate is usually inappropriate, but sadly commonplace. Sensitivity and clarity are required and written information, which can be retained, may be helpful so that it can be read when the relatives are in their own environment and some time has elapsed since the initial shock of being informed of the often sudden and unexpected death.

The staff involved in the resuscitation attempt will also require support. Many resuscitation attempts will be unsuccessful and staff may experience grief reactions, stress and anxiety. Most cardiac arrest teams are made up of junior doctors who may themselves feel stressed and inadequate. The event may leave the rescuers feeling uncertain and exhausted, they may also feel guilty and experience a sense of failure that their actions did not achieve a positive outcome. After any resuscitation attempt, team members should perform a critique of events (Resuscitation Council 2000). A 'critical incident debriefing' may allow staff to discuss their thoughts, feelings and actions and it can also be used as a time for learning and support (Iserson 1999).

Family presence in the resuscitation area

It has become acceptable practice in many countries for relatives and loved ones to remain with the patient during the resuscitation attempt. The UK Resuscitation Council recommended that relatives be allowed to witness resuscitation and recommended that they be supported by appropriately trained staff at this time (Resuscitation Council 1996). Much of the evaluation of practice that supports relatives' presence during resuscitation comes from paediatrics where a reduction in post-traumatic stress and self-reports of greater resolution and fulfillment have been reported (Resuscitation Council 2000). One UK study (Robinson et al 1998), which included the relatives of adult patients, concluded that at 3 months after the witnessed resuscitation efforts, there was a trend towards lower degrees of intrusive imagery, less post-traumatic avoidance behaviour and reduced symptoms of grief in those relatives that witnessed the resuscitation. Also, three patients who survived said they felt supported by the presence of the family. However, most of the studies of witnessed resuscitation relate to A&E departments with small sample sizes and there is a need for more widespread debate and research into this area (Newton 2002). Issues in implementing witnessed resuscitation in practice include:

- being able to establish whether the relatives wish to remain during the chaos that often accompanies the start of a resuscitation attempt

- the fact that relatives may find it difficult to make a decision about a situation they know little about
- it is not always possible to have an appropriate member of staff to support relatives from the outset of the arrest
- unease and feelings of threat among members of the arrest team – being self-conscious of their comments and approach
- possible interference/disruption by the relatives during the resuscitation attempt
- making it acceptable for relatives to choose not to stay or to leave during the arrest
- relatives' presence affecting the decision to stop the resuscitation attempt.

Nurses are the professionals whom relatives are likely to approach with requests to be with a loved one during the resuscitation effort (Redley and Hood 1996) and there is a need for careful assessment and preparation of the family during and after the resuscitation. Preparation needs to include information on the patient's condition, discussion on what will be seen, heard, touched and smelled. A careful description of the patient's appearance, equipment and procedures, interpreting jargon and discussing patient responses to interventions is also important. Some hospitals have developed a specific nursing function to support relatives as part of the resuscitation team (Eichhorn et al 1996).

Teaching relatives resuscitation skills

Recognition of the problem and prompt commencement of BLS prior to the arrival of professional help is crucial to the outcome of the resuscitation attempt. The National Service Framework for CHD (Department of Health 2000) recommends that resuscitation training should be offered to family members in the early post-discharge period and many cardiac rehabilitation departments have begun to offer BLS training to relatives who wish it. Such training has been found to be associated with reduced anxiety in relatives (McLauchlan et al 1992). Training needs to be provided alongside support and tailored to the individual families so

as limit negative psychosocial states in the patients themselves (Dracup et al 1997).

The decision not to resuscitate

Registered nurses have a professional duty to act at all times in the best interests of the patient. However, unsuccessful resuscitation attempts do not enhance the dignity that is hoped for when one dies (Baskett 1986) and there are certain situations where both the patient and their relatives are subjected to what is, debatably, unnecessary stress through resuscitation procedures.

Due to the admission policies of most coronary care units, it is a likely assumption that patients admitted to them will be appropriate candidates for resuscitation. However, frail and disabled coronary patients can be admitted to a coronary care unit. Resuscitation which merely prolongs the process of dying would seem to be inappropriate in the majority of cases.

The overall responsibility for decisions regarding whether or not to attempt resuscitation rests with the responsible consultant (BMA/RCN 2001). However, the necessary discussions with the patient and family are often undertaken by junior doctors who can find this difficult (Morgan and Westmorland 2002). The decision not to attempt resuscitation centres upon many factors, including the patient's own wishes, the patient's prognosis, and the opinions of relatives, nurses and doctors. Most patients want to discuss their resuscitation status (Morgan et al 1994) and tend not to report feelings of unease or discomfort when they are able to do so (Larson 1992). They may, however, find it difficult to have to make the final decision (Liddle et al 1993). Cardiac arrests which are sudden and unexpected or take place soon after the patient's admission do not give much time for considered opinions to be formulated. Patients may be too ill to give any indication as to their own wishes.

Situations where it may be appropriate not to attempt resuscitation include (Doyal and Wilsher 1993):

- a competent, informed patient indicates that they do not wish to be resuscitated
- a patient is not legally competent to give or refuse consent to treatment and the responsible physician judges that

resuscitation would not be in the patient's best interests

- where there is almost no likelihood of a successful outcome from a resuscitation attempt.

The coronary patient who has sustained extensive myocardial damage and developed heart failure or cardiogenic shock with an extremely poor prognosis may not be suited for resuscitation attempts. Immediate, short- and long-term prognosis after in-hospital CPR has been shown to be independent of age (Di Bari et al 2000) and discrimination of older patients on the exclusive basis of their age should be avoided (Ebrahim 2000).

The decision whether or not to resuscitate should not influence the quality of other care subsequently given to the patient. At least one study has shown that having a do not attempt resuscitation order increases the likelihood of death, suggesting that the decision may result in inadequate care (Shepardson et al 1999).

Allowing a patient to die in peace and with dignity should not be considered a failure by the nurse with the expertise and technology geared to saving lives. The nurse usually knows the patient and family better than other members of the health care team, and should be prepared to act as the patient's advocate in representing the patient's best interests. An atmosphere conducive to frank open discussion will help in preventing animosity between nurses and doctors over what is an extremely sensitive and complex issue (Aarons and Beeching 1991).

See Figure 7.23 for an example of a Do Not Attempt Resuscitation Form.

When to stop the resuscitation attempt

The decision to stop CPR is traditionally a medical one and needs to be taken by the most senior physician present after consultation with the primary nurse and other staff, and if practical, the patient's relatives. Such a decision should follow a careful assessment of the patient's cerebral and cardiovascular status as well as prognosis.

Survival of an arrest of over 15 minutes duration is very low, and so a prolonged resuscitation attempt is rarely justified (exceptions being poisoning and other special circumstances).

All patients who die suddenly are potential candidates for organ donation, although organizational issues have limited this procedure. Because death diagnosis is based on cardiopulmonary criteria and cardiac arrest often occurs in a sudden manner, the key factor in this is time and it is therefore necessary for visceral perfusion and oxygenation to be maintained until a decision can be made.

Implantable cardioverter defibrillators

The National Institute for Clinical Excellence (2000) has recommended that implantable cardioverter defibrillators (ICD) should be routinely used for patients who have survived VF or VT with haemodynamic compromise for secondary prevention of arrhythmic death. The devices are also increasingly being used prophylactically for patients who are at risk from a sudden cardiac death event. This includes patients with extensive myocardial infarction (Block and Breithardt 1999) and those with cardiomyopathy or heart failure (James 1997). Suitability for the device is assessed with electrophysiological studies, coronary angiography and echocardiography.

The present day ICD system is battery operated, able to monitor the heart rate and rhythm and record the action taken. The device is implanted either into the abdomen or subcutaneously via a clavicular incision. Sensing, defibrillating and pacing electrodes are positioned via the subclavian vein with the electrodes left lying on the endocardial surface of the heart at the base of the right ventricle. The electrodes are connected to a lead wire attached to the pulse generator at the insertion site. Each device is individually programmed but is capable of providing fast pacing for overriding tachycardias, slow pacing for bradycardias, burst pacing for VT and delivering cardioversion or defibrillation shocks.

Deactivation of the device involves holding a magnet over the area of the pulse generator. The actual method for doing this varies with the device and nurses need to know the manufacturer's protocol for specific models.

It is essential that nurses preparing patients and their families for an ICD are aware of the physical, psychological and emotional problems that may occur before and after the implantation of the

University Hospitals of Leicester **NHS**
NHS trust

7. THE ORDER IS NOW CANCELLED
Doctor's name:

**DO NOT ATTEMPT RESUSCITATION
DECISION**

Grade:

Hospital
Number
Surname

**In the event of a
cardiac arrest, active
resuscitation should
not occure and 222
should not be dialled**

Signature:

First name

Date:

D.O.B.

or attach patient's
identification label

Ward/
Dept.

Hospital
Site.

1a. This decision **HAS/HAS NOT** been discussed with the patient. (please delete as appropriate)

1b. If **NOT** discussed with the patient, the reasons are:

And therefore the decision has been discussed with relatives/carers.

2a. The decision **HAS/HAS NOT** been discussed with the pateint's relatives/carers. If it **WAS** discussed

with the patient's relatives/carers, please state with whom it was discussed and where i.e. in person or

by telephone:

2b. If the decision **WAS NOT** discussed with the patient's relative/carers, please state why:

3. Date of commencement: 2 0   Time of commencement: :   am/pm

4. Doctor's Name   Grade

   Signature   Date

The decision can only be made by a Specialist Registrar/Staff Frade or consultant.

5a. Planned review date (these should be at least every 72 hours).

   /   /   /   /   /   /   /   /   /   /   /

5a. Signature

   /   /   /   /   /   /   /   /   /   /   /

6. If a regular review date is not felt to be in the patient's best interests, please stat why?

Figure 7.23   An example of a Do Not Attempt Resuscitation form.

device (James 1997). Undergoing tests prior to the implantation can be particularly stressful as patients become aware of the implications of their heart's poor condition (Dougherty 1994). Discharge home can also be a difficult time in adjusting to having an internal device. Particular concerns centre around (James 2002):

- fears about possible malfunction and failure of the device
- concern about the unpredictability of the device – particularly the lack of warning of impending shocks – leading to a feeling of loss of control
- worries about the lack of other health professionals' knowledge about the device – limiting holidays and other travel
- coming to terms with a close call with death – needing to talk this through and feeling unable to burden family with their feelings
- anger and anxiety
- changes in sexual activity – sometimes due to the incorrect assumption that if the device is activated during physical contact, the partner will be harmed.

Patients need to be advised to carry an identification card, record the details of any event requiring a shock, and to ring their regional centre for advice after each shock or if they are worried at any other time. They also need to be aware to avoid strong magnetic fields. Family members may experience stress (Pycha et al 1990) and feelings of being uncertain as to what to do if a shock happens (Dunbar et al 1993). They will need support, including preparation for witnessing and supporting the patient after a shock.

HEART FAILURE

The term heart failure is used to describe a clinical syndrome which results from an inability of the heart to provide an adequate cardiac output for the body's metabolic requirements. A variety of terminologies and descriptions have been used in an attempt further to classify the diagnosis. A simple and practical classification is (Poole-Wilson 2002):

- acute heart failure (pulmonary oedema)
- circulatory failure (cardiogenic shock)
- chronic heart failure.

Acute heart failure

Acute heart failure is a complex syndrome in which the patient's condition changes from moment to moment and it complicates between 25% and 50% of acute coronary patients. It arises from the loss of myocardial tissue and the reduced contractility of the damaged myocardium. The myocardial fibres shorten and fail to produce a forceful contraction. This situation is exacerbated by arrhythmias, or from drugs that further limit myocardial contractility or encourage the retention of salt and water.

Heart failure may develop suddenly or the symptoms may appear insidiously during the first few hours or days following infarction. Symptoms are usually due to compensatory mechanisms which the body brings about to maintain an adequate cardiac output. These compensatory mechanisms include fluid retention and increased sympathetic activity which may lead to pulmonary and peripheral oedema. In the later stages, the heart adapts to increased intraventricular tension by dilatation and hypertrophy. The failing heart may be able to cope with mild activity but be decompensated with moderate to severe exertion.

Heart failure following myocardial infarction usually presents as acute left ventricular failure (LVF), although right ventricular failure often coexists and may occasionally occur without any left ventricular involvement. Left heart failure during the acute phase of myocardial infarction is associated with poor prognosis and there is a close relationship between the degree of left ventricular dysfunction and subsequent mortality. The Killip classification (Killip and Kimball 1967) shows this relationship (Table 7.8).

Table 7.8 The Killip classification of heart failure following acute myocardial infarction

Killip class	Clinical status	Mortality (%)
1	No failure	6
2	Mild/moderate heart failure	17
3	Severe heart failure	38
4	Cardiogenic shock	81

Nursing the coronary patient who develops heart failure requires a knowledge of a pathophysiology of heart failure and how this affects the patient, both physically and emotionally. No single medical treatment is a panacea, and the overall treatment tends to become complex, with many drugs being used in varying doses at different times during the illness. An understanding of drug therapy and treatment options is therefore also important.

Compensatory mechanisms

Compensatory mechanisms are mediated through myocardial dilatation, the sympathetic nervous system, the renal response and myocardial hypertrophy. The heart depends upon these reflex activities for maintenance of its pumping activity and they come into operation sequentially as demand increases.

The first mechanism to be used is the intrinsic reflex described by Frank and Starling, whereby increased stretching of the myocardial cells, which occurs with an initial inability to expel the stroke volume, increases their contractile power and produces a reflex increase in cardiac output. This method of augmenting energy becomes increasingly limited as the failing heart continues to dilate due to an increased afterload and preload. There is an increase in myocardial oxygen demand which eventually leads to reduced contractility if the oxygen supply is inadequate.

As pumping demand increases, a second 'extrinsic' reverse mechanism is superimposed in the form of a graded increase in sympathoadrenal activity. Noradrenaline, released from the sympathetic nerve terminals, produces an increase in myocardial contractility and heart rate. Distribution of peripheral blood flow is reorganized by selective diversion to the demanding tissues through dilatation of the coronary and cerebral arterioles and constriction of the renal, splanchnic and skin arterioles. Thus, best use is made of a diminished blood supply. The secretion of renin is increased via sympathetic stimulation further enhancing vasoconstriction. However, in acute pump failure when the demand for continued sympathoadrenal support is persistent, there is eventually an increase in afterload due to increased ventricular volume, which decreases the pumping ability of the left ventricle. Also, as the heart becomes dilated the beta-adrenergic receptors lose their efficiency and so sympathetic activity becomes impaired.

If cardiac pumping failure persists despite these two compensatory mechanisms, then a third is activated resulting in retention of salt and water. Renal retention of saline is initiated as a result of the reduction in renal blood flow and decreased renin secretion, both brought about by sympathetic activity. Reduced renal blood flow causes sodium retention by activation of the renin–angiotensin system. Plasma vasopressin and aldosterone levels increase, but the role of other hormones such as atrial natriuretic hormone is unclear. Angiotensin II causes widespread vasoconstriction and secretion of aldosterone which causes sodium and water retention. Excessive retention produces an expansion of blood volume, increased stiffness of the walls of the arteries and veins, and increased capillary compression due to interstitial oedema. These compensatory mechanisms aid in the maintenance of cardiac output and support of systemic blood pressure. However, the attempt to augment the pumping function of the left ventricle is done at the expense of an increasing afterload and workload for the failing heart.

Myocardial hypertrophy is the final compensatory mechanism in an attempt to increase the contractile mass. This compensation is usually of a temporary nature and at this stage the prognosis is poor.

Clinical features

The clinical features of heart failure are caused by reduced cardiac output (sometimes referred to as forward failure) and an increased venous pressure in the lungs and peripheries caused by inadequate ventricular emptying (sometimes referred to as backward failure).

The clinical features of right and left heart failure are not mutually exclusive and frequently coexist, although they are usually divided for convenience.

The first clinical features of acute LVF are breathlessness, cyanosis, cold clammy skin, pallor, fast often irregular heart rate and a low blood pressure. As hypoxia worsens, the patient is likely to become increasingly restless and anxious, and may even become stuperous.

A chest X-ray may reveal pulmonary and venous congestion and pulmonary oedema. The ECG will not provide direct evidence of heart failure, but may illustrate increasing left ventricular hypertrophy, ischaemia and tachyarrhythmias. A prominent third heart sound, especially with a tachycardia (gallop rhythm) is usually diagnostic, particularly if it is associated with crackles at the lung bases.

Acute LVF may lead to pulmonary oedema as a result of transudation of fluid into the pulmonary alveoli. This reduces gaseous exchange within the alveoli and leads to arterial hypoxaemia. Oedema of the pulmonary membranes reduces airflow to and from the alveoli and lung compliance (stiffness) increases, making breathing more difficult. Increased production of mucus may result in a cough and a wheeze, particularly at night due to the absorption of oedema that has occurred during the day. The patient may feel increasingly short of breath at night for the same reason. The sputum may become red in colour as a result of small haemorrhages in the bronchial mucosa.

The patient is likely to be anxious and this will not be helped if a term such as heart failure is overheard. Decreased activity tolerance leads to increased dependence on the nurse, with ensuing feelings of helplessness and frustration which may lead to the patient becoming depressed.

Management

The aim of management of heart failure is to:

- reduce myocardial work (intracardiac presures and volume overload)
- increase the force and efficiency of myocardial function
- reduce the accumulation of body fluid through increasing salt and water excretion.

The underlying cause of heart failure should be treated where possible. In the acute coronary patient, meticulous attention should be paid to ventilation since hypoxaemia will further impair left ventricular function by increasing areas of critical myocardial ischaemia. The patient should be sat upright to facilitate oxygenation and given high concentrations of oxygen to breathe. General measures include monitoring for arrhythmias and checking for electrolyte imbalance.

Echocardiography is useful to assess the extent of myocardial damage, mechanical ventricular function and complications such as mitral regurgitation and ventricular septal defect.

Although positive inotropic agents such as digoxin and dopamine would seem to be the logical first-line therapy to aid the failing left ventricle, they may increase the size of the infarct by 'over-stimulation'. Treatment should therefore be primarily aimed at reducing intravascular volume which will reduce cardiac preload and, as a consequence, afterload.

Patient problems

Problems common to a patient with heart failure include:

- shortness of breath
- reduced activity
- loss of appetite
- disturbed rest and sleep patterns
- altered elimination patterns
- increased risk of pressure sore development
- increased risk of thromboembolic complications
- altered mental state
- discomfort and pain
- apathy and depression
- anxiety.

Care of the patient with heart failure

Nursing management aims to reduce myocardial work, provide a stress-free environment and observe the effects of therapy. Care plans should be devised with these objectives in mind.

The effect of interventions designed to improve outcome can be evaluated through monitoring the patient's:

- fluid balance
- daily weight
- blood pressure, heart rate, blood oxygen saturation and haemodynamic state
- subjective feelings
- level of exercise tolerance
- associated clinical features.

Heart failure is likely to resolve as myocardial functioning becomes more effective, although some patients may develop chronic heart failure. Complications of acute heart failure, such as cardiogenic shock, tend to be managed through an extension of the treatment for acute heart failure.

Rest Rest is therapeutic in that the decrease in muscular activity leads to a reduction in venous return. Filling pressure (preload) is decreased and there is greater efficiency of ventricular emptying at systole. Ventricular diastolic pressure decreases, reducing muscular distension and producing a compensated state. Thus, the heart works more effectively and cardiac output increases. Renal blood flow increases as less blood is needed to supply the muscles. Recumbency-induced diuresis also decreases intravascular volume, increases urine volume and reduces oedema.

The benefits of rest need to be weighed against the severity of heart failure and the likely incidence of complications resulting from inactivity. The patient may worry that he is unable to be as active as he would like, and needs reassurance about the probable length of time of enforced restricted activity. Discussion should be centred on strategies aimed at enabling the performance of activity which induces minimal fatigue and shortness of breath, with careful thought being given to the spacing of such activity. Sitting in a semi-recumbent position with arms supported by pillows may prove to be the most comfortable and energy-saving posture for some patients.

Control of the environment to promote an atmosphere conducive to rest will help the patient obtain the necessary amount and quality of rest and sleep. This will involve the careful coordination of activities from various health professionals involved in patient care, with thought being given to the amount and timing of interventions necessary for patient welfare.

Maximum independence should be the ultimate goal, with activity levels positively graduated as the heart failure and hence activity tolerance improves. Initially, the patient may feel too weak and short of breath to attract the nurse's attention and the nurse therefore needs to be readily available for patient communication.

Care planning should incorporate an assessment of the risk of pressure sore development. Decreased activity and a diminished blood supply to the tissues will mean an increased proneness to tissue breakdown. Passive leg exercises should be encouraged in order to prevent deep vein thrombosis.

Diet The patient may not feel like eating due to gastrointestinal congestion, ascites or lethargy, and should be encouraged to eat a small easily digestible diet followed by adequate rest. The use of nasal oxygen cannulae rather than face masks will enable the patient to eat and talk more easily.

A low sodium diet has been superseded by diuretic therapy, although it is probably advisable to encourage the patient to avoid high salt content foods. There is no need to restrict fluid intake when sodium retention is eliminated by diet and diuretics. However, in severe cases of heart failure both fluid and salt restriction is required. Drugs such as indomethacin which retain sodium in the body should be avoided.

Patients with chronic heart failure who are overweight should be advised about the benefits of weight reduction as this reduces myocardial work and enables exercise to be taken more easily, thus improving cardiac function.

Elimination The patient needs to be advised about the possible increase in volume and frequency of urine output while receiving diuretics. If possible, the timing of the administration of these drugs should be planned so as to avoid or minimize the disruption of the patient (and others) caused by passing urine during the night.

Despite feeling lethargic and short of breath, the patient is likely to find it easier to use a commode rather than a bedpan. A urinary catheter may sometimes be necessary in the acutely ill patient and will involve less energy expenditure than using a bedpan or commode and permit accurate measurement of urine output. However, the attendant risks associated with urinary catheterization should be borne in mind and careful attention to catheter care is required.

The nurse should ensure that the patient is aware of the necessity for accurate measurement of the volume of urine.

Some patients may require a mild aperient to relieve constipation caused by prolonged immobility and gastrointestinal stasis.

Drug therapy

The principles of drug therapy in the management of heart failure are to:

- retard the retention of salt and water with diuretics
- reduce the excessive preload with venodilators
- reduce myocardial work with arteriodilators
- enhance myocardial contractility with inotropes.

Nursing responsibilities towards the patient receiving drug therapy for heart failure include:

- administering the drug
- explaining its purpose
- monitoring the effect – changes in fluid balance, weight, oedema and dyspnoea
- observing for signs of dehydration and hypokalaemia – muscle weakness, arrhythmias and other side effects.

Diuretic therapy

Diuretics provide the main line of treatment for LVF though they are frequently unhelpful in pure right heart failure. By definition, a diuretic induces a diuresis of water and solutes. Diuretics also decrease preload, reduce blood volume, lower the ventricular filling pressure and resolve pulmonary and systemic congestion. The reduction in pulmonary capillary pressure will ease breathing, and the reduction in left ventricular filling pressure decreases myocardial work and oxygen requirement.

Diuretics need to be used with caution to prevent the following harmful effects:

- mild to severe electrolyte imbalance, including potassium loss, which may lead to weakness and precipitate cardiac arrhythmias
- excessive diuresis, resulting in hypovolaemia and hypotension
- cumulative effect of different types of diuretics.

The most effective diuretic needs to be selected based on an assessment of the patient's circulatory state. Ideally, diuretic therapy needs to be gauged against filling pressures and cardiac output. This is in order that the cardiac output is not decreased too far, producing an increased blood urea and increased fatigue. Haemodynamic monitoring can

facilitate accurate management of diuretic therapy in acute heart failure. The patient will need frequent assessment of potassium levels: a patient with hypokalaemia who is taking digoxin is particularly susceptible to arrhythmias, and supplementary potassium intake may be indicated.

The loop diuretic furosemide is the most widely used diuretic for acute heart failure. Loop diuretics exert their action on the ascending limb of the loop of Henle. Furosemide has the potential of increasing fractional sodium excretion by more than 25%. Administration by the intravenous route causes diuresis within 5 min, with a peak response occurring at 15–20 min. There may be a relief of dyspnoea even before diuresis as a result of venodilatation and preload reduction. In severe heart failure, the gut becomes oedematous and the absorption of orally administered diuretics is reduced. Thus, intravenous diuretics are best used in the initial management of acute heart failure. Intravenous furosemide exhibits systemic and renal vasodilating effects, producing decreased peripheral vascular resistance and increased renal blood flow.

Loop diuretics exert their effect predominantly by inhibiting active transport of chloride in the loop of Henle, and can therefore cause marked potassium depletion, alkalosis as a result of hydrogen and chloride loss, and severe hypovolaemia. Most patients with normal renal function taking furosemide will also need potassium supplements or potassium-sparing diuretics.

Angiotensin-converting-enzyme (ACE) inhibitors should be initiated within 48 hours in the absence of hypertension, hypovolaemia or significant renal failure. These drugs ultimately exert an anti-aldosterone effect and thus act as mild potassium-sparing diuretics.

Vasodilator therapy

Vasodilators are either classed as venodilators, arteriodilators, or both. The effect of this group of drugs in the patient with heart failure differs from the effect in the healthy individual. In the latter, preload is primarily affected with minimal effect on cardiac output. In the former, afterload is primarily affected and cardiac output is increased despite a fall in preload. For the coronary patient with LVF, vasodilators will reduce the filling pressure and increase cardiac output, but in patients with normal filling pressures, cardiac output will fall.

Vasodilator therapy is particularly useful when acute myocardial infarction is complicated by hypertension or sub-acute rupture. Administration of these agents is also thought to limit the size of the infarct. The reduction in afterload limits myocardial work and oxygen consumption and additionally improves efficiency of the left ventricular pump.

The haemodynamic effect of an individual vasodilator agent depends upon its ability to affect arterioles or venules.

Venodilators   Venodilators such as nitrates directly relax smooth muscle through general dilatation that affects the veins more than the arteries. They decrease the filling or preload pressure. This allows the distended ventricle to shrink, increasing the blood flow in the coronary microcirculation and subsequently improving myocardial function and cardiac output. This may also produce a reduction in cardiac workload, although this may be limited by the development of a compensatory tachycardia. Intravenous nitroglycerine is widely used but the dose needs to be titrated while monitoring blood pressure to avoid hypotension.

Arteriodilators   Arteriodilators, including nifedipine, hydralazine and minoxidil, act principally on the arteries. They reduce cardiac work by decreasing peripheral vascular resistance. They are no longer widely used for heart failure, but may be of some benefit if there is excessive arterioconstriction.

Mixed vasodilators   Mixed vasodilators, such as sodium nitroprusside and ACE inhibitors, improve cardiac output by promoting ventricular emptying, reducing vascular resistance and thus decreasing myocardial oxygen demand.

Sodium nitroprusside is a highly potent short-acting drug which, given carefully, will reduce myocardial oxygen demand and ischaemic pain by reducing arteriolar resistance, pulmonary wedge pressures and oxygen requirements while producing an increased cardiac output. Sodium nitroprusside is used for treating the coronary patient who has hypertension and severe heart failure. The drug needs to be administered under close supervision, with careful monitoring of its effect on blood pressure. Because of the increased stroke volume there may be considerable haemodynamic improvement without much hypotension but, in general, some hypotension occurs and may limit the therapeutic effect.

Sodium nitroprusside needs to be administered by the intravenous route. Its onset of action is maximal in 1–2 min and the effect dissipates rapidly when the infusion is stopped. It decomposes in the presence of light, therefore, only fresh solutions protected from light by specially designed administration sets or protective wrapping should be used. The ferrous ion in the nitroprusside molecule reacts with compounds contained in red blood cells to produce cyanide ion, but it is reduced to thiocyanate in the liver. Prolonged administration may cause thiocyanate toxicity. Adding sodium thiosulphate to the infusion prevents this problem and means that daily blood assays for cyanide levels are unnecessary.

Positive inotropic agents

Inotropes increase ventricular activity and thus minimize myocardial work. Unfortunately, many over-stimulate the heart leading to myocardial hypoxia with the possibility of ventricular arrhythmias and sudden death.

Digoxin has traditionally been the mainstay of positive inotropic treatment. It produces electrophysiological changes that decrease AV nodal conduction and increase intracellular calcium at the cell membrane. Thus the force of contraction is increased, there is a stronger systolic contraction and the heart rate is reduced. The drawback is that myocardial oxygen demand is increased. Digoxin can cause myocardial irritability if serum potassium levels are low. Digoxin toxicity is a frequent problem, particularly if there is renal impairment or hypokalaemia. Digoxin is probably best avoided unless there is evidence of AF.

Enoximone and milrinone are phosphodiesterase inhibitors. They act largely by peripheral vasodilatation, although they also have a direct inotropic effect, being inotropic dilators.

Beta-adrenergic agonists act on the vascular receptors to cause peripheral vasodilatation. Dopamine and dobutamine may owe part of their beneficial effect in heart failure to beta-mediated vasodilatation. These agents are especially useful in the coronary patient who develops heart failure or cardiogenic shock. The potentially deleterious side effect of alpha-adrenergic vasoconstriction exerted by dopamine is fortunately only present at higher doses than those required to increase contractility. Its vasodilator effect on splanchnic and renal arterioles with its positive inotropic effect generally improves cardiovascular haemodynamics and renal function.

Dobutamine is similar and, although it does not have such marked chronotropic effect, it does not specifically increase renal perfusion other than by its positive inotropic effect.

Other measures

Anticoagulant therapy Anticoagulants should perhaps be considered routine in patients with dilated or dyskinetic hearts, marked congestive cardiac failure and unstable heart rhythm, to prevent thromboembolic complications.

Diamorphine Diamorphine, may prove beneficial in relieving dyspnoea by reducing anxiety. It restores catecholamine output and causes systemic vasodilatation, thus reducing venous return and cardiac preload. Diamorphine can aggravate bradycardia and suppress ventilation and needs to be given with care.

Ventilatory support Blood gases need to be monitored and endotracheal intubation with ventilatory support may be indicated if an oxygen tension of more than 60 mmHg cannot be maintained in spite of 100% oxygen delivered at 8–10 litres per minute (Van der Werf et al 2003). However, formal ventilation with intubation can have detrimental cardiovascular effects including hypotension and reduced cardiac output as a result of the sedation. Non-invasive positive pressure ventilation may be a good alternative (Cooper and Jacob 2002).

Ultrafiltration Ultrafiltration allows controlled removal of body water without the adverse haemodynamic effects of haemodialysis, since venous access only is required. The procedure is able to provide continuous daily large volume removal to improve volume status and clinical symptoms (Sharma et al 2001).

Revascularization Patients with acute heart failure may have stunned (reperfused but with delayed contractile recovery) or hypoperfused, viable myocardium. Identification and revascularization of hypoperfused myocardium can lead to improved ventricular function.

Right heart failure

Right heart failure usually occurs secondary to left heart failure. Isolated right heart failure may result from tricuspid or pulmonary valve disease or secondary to pulmonary disease. Infarction of the right ventricular myocardium is believed to occur in about 40% of patients with transmural infarcts. Some degree of right ventricular ischaemia may be found in half of all inferior infarcts, but most will not develop clinically significant problems. In most patients the volume of right ventricular myocardium affected is small and becomes stunned, with normal function returning over a period of weeks to months. The clinical picture of hypotension, clear lung fields and elevated jugular venous pressure in the setting of an inferior myocardial infarction is characteristic of coexisting right ventricular infarction. The development of clinical features of right heart failure, without coexisting left heart failure, is rare.

Clinical features

The diagnosis of right heart failure is often overlooked because of its comparative rarity, and the clinical events caused by right heart failure are often erroneously attributed to left heart failure.

Symptoms are due to pulmonary hypertension, leading to raised systemic venous pressure and organ and tissue engorgement as blood backs up to the systemic system. As the systemic system has a comparatively large volume, clinical symptoms such as peripheral oedema, ascites or jaundice may not appear until chronic stages.

Echocardiography and radionuclide ventriculography may show abnormal right ventricular function. Confirmation may be made by right heart catheterization. Haemodynamic consequences of right ventricular infarction are primarily related to under-filling of the left ventricle. Classically, there is increased right ventricular filling pressure and increased central venous pressure (CVP), but near to normal pulmonary capillary wedge pressure. Salt and water are retained in the body, the circulation becomes overloaded and eventually fluid escapes from the circulation and accumulates in the soft tissues as oedema.

Management

Management aims to maintain right ventricular filling pressure while reducing the right ventricular afterload. Vasodilator drugs such as nitrates, diuretics, ACE inhibitors and opioids used routinely in the management of myocardial infarction, should be avoided. Volume expansion therapy alone is often successful in the treatment of low cardiac output and hypotension resulting from predominant right ventricular infarction. Therapy will need to be continued until the right atrial pressure reaches a level of 14–15 mmHg. Blind therapy with diuretics and nitrates would reduce left ventricular preload further and worsen the problem. If the condition is exacerbated by bradyarrhythmias, then atrioventricular pacing may be more successful than ventricular pacing in reversing hypotension. If hypotension persists despite correction of bradyarrhythmias and plasma volume expansion, a dopamine or dobutamine infusion is often indicated. Sodium nitroprusside has been used to unload the heart and intra-aortic balloon counterpulsation has also been recommended. Measurement of intracardiac pressures with a Swan-Ganz catheter is of significant value in balancing therapy to optimize cardiac output.

Confusion often persists in the management of patients with right ventricular failure. Amid the uncertainty of diagnosis the patient may be advised to minimize their fluid intake if LVF is suspected and then subsequently be given fluid intravenously as right ventricular involvement is confirmed. The patient and relatives may become confused as to the rationale of treatment and need particular help and support.

Cardiogenic shock

The term cardiogenic shock is used to describe a patient who is very ill with a low cardiac output, although it is often defined as the combination of:

1 a systolic blood pressure less than 100 mmHg
2 a pulse rate of more than 100 beats/min
3 a urine output of less than 20 ml/h
4 cold peripheries
5 dulled sensorium.

Cardiogenic shock occurs in some 15% of patients who subsequently die from acute myocardial infarction. Its frequency is greater in patients with anterior infarction and in patients with more than 40% loss of functional myocardium. This can be the result of one large infarct, or the cumulative effect of an acute-on-chronic infarction. Cardiogenic shock is also more likely when infarction is accompanied by recurrent arrhythmias as this reduces cardiac output and increases myocardial workload. It can also occur with mechanical complications of infarction such as a ruptured mitral valve, septum or ventricular aneurysm. Large pulmonary emboli, cardiac surgery and cardiac tamponade are other predisposing factors. The coexistence of diabetes, established cardiovascular disease and being female all place the patient at increased risk.

The clinical features of cardiogenic shock develop as a result of the compensatory mechanisms invoked by low cardiac output. This self-perpetuating process starts with an ever-increasing loss of myocardial contractility, decreasing ventricular performance and extension of necrosis. There is an associated significant rise in intracardiac pressures and critical falls in arterial pressure and cardiac output. Prolongation of this state eventually produces irreversible damage, and mortality from cardiogenic shock continues to approach 75%. The majority of deaths occur within the first 24 h following infarction, although a small proportion (15%) may die more than 7 days later.

Prevention

As cardiogenic shock is caused by massive irreversible myocardial damage, the logical therapeutic measure is to prevent or at least limit the extent of damage. The prognosis is poor once cardiogenic shock has become established. Measures to reperfuse the myocardium with thrombolysis or primary angioplasty reduce the development of cardiogenic shock in those patients presenting early enough (Fibrinolytic Therapy Trialists' Collaborative Group 1994, Hochman et al 1999). Strategies to restrict infarction size (beta-blockers and vasodilators) are also of benefit.

Early treatment of arrhythmias, autonomic disturbances and clinically apparent haemodynamic disturbances may prevent the development of cardiogenic shock over the first few hours following infarction.

Management

The outcome of cardiogenic shock is largely determined by early and effective intervention. The theoretical aim of management involves various components (Holmes 2003):

1 reducing the oxygen demands of the myocardium
2 preventing infarct expansion
3 augmenting oxygen delivery
4 removing lethal antibodies accumulating in the myocardium
5 allowing maximum development of a collateral circulation to sustain jeopardized but viable myocardium.

In reality, medical management tends to concentrate on influencing ventricular function: preload, afterload, contractility and heart rate; and limiting infarct size. Manipulation of any one parameter may result in reflex changes in another.

Reversible causes of cardiogenic shock need to be considered. The commonest, hypovolaemia, is often found in the patient with a right ventricular infarction and the patient taking diuretics or antihypertensive agents. Volume expansion is helpful in this type of shock. Haemodynamic monitoring is a necessary adjunct to management and needs to be instituted early in conjunction with clinical assessment. Thus, the insertion of a pulmonary artery flotation catheter is desirable for monitoring intracardiac pressures, pulmonary artery pressure (PAP), pulmonary arterial wedge pressure (PAWP) and cardiac output. Echocardiography is a useful technique in diagnosing the cause of cardiogenic shock. It can provide immediate information about structural problems and measures both the size and function of the ventricles. Doppler

cardiography may be indicated for detecting valvular leaks and intracardiac shunts.

Arrhythmias should be treated vigorously. The treatment of choice for tachyarrhythmias is usually DC cardioversion or overdrive pacing. This is because most anti-arrhythmic agents, with the exception of digoxin, exert a further negative inotropic effect on a usually already dysfunctioning ventricle.

Hypoxaemia and the progressive acidosis that accompanies it are common and invariably worsen myocardial function. The patient should be given oxygen via nasal cannulae with the aim of achieving an FIO_2 value of 60% or greater. With persisting hypoxaemia, and in particular a rising concentration of hydrogen ion in the blood, intubation and positive-pressure ventilation may be considered, depending on an appraisal of the patient's overall chance of survival.

Loop diuretics are useful in helping to clear pulmonary oedema. Oliguria is almost always apparent in cardiogenic shock and a diuresis is one of the first signs of recovery. Thus, careful estimation of urine output is essential, frequently necessitating insertion of a urinary catheter. The nurse therefore needs to ensure that the attendant risks such as infection are minimized by frequent aseptic catheter care.

The drugs commonly prescribed during acute myocardial infarction need to be given with care as it is possible they could exacerbate hypotension and shock (Williams et al 2000). Vasodilators are of potential value by reducing cardiac preload, afterload or both. Haemodynamic monitoring is useful in controlling the infusion rate of the chosen agent, the aim being to keep the PAWP at about 15 mmHg.

Agents such as dobutamine and adrenaline may prove useful in improving cardiac output. However, the use of catecholamine inotropes is limited by tachycardia and arrhythmias at high infusion rates. Prolonged exposure to high concentrations of these agents may exacerbate myocardial damage.

When available, emergency cardiac catheterization and angioplasty seem to improve survival and more recent developments, such as the use of coronary stents and the use of glycoprotein IIb/IIIa antagonists seem promising. In hospitals without direct angioplasty, stabilization with intra-aortic balloon counter pulsation and thrombolysis followed by transfer to a tertiary care facility may be the best option (Hollenberg et al 1999).

Patient problems

Problems the patient are likely to experience include:

- low systolic blood pressure
- tachycardia
- low urine output
- cold peripheries
- mental changes reflecting poor cerebral perfusion
- irritability
- restlessness
- coma
- fear
- anxiety
- enforced dependency
- loss of control
- personality changes
- paranoia
- poor judgement
- altered sleep patterns.

Care of the patient in cardiogenic shock

Management of the patient in cardiogenic shock will involve the close collaboration of the nurse and physician. The key to achieving a good outcome is an organized approach that includes rapid assessment and prompt initiation of therapy. Objectives include maintaining perfusion to vital organs, limiting infarction size and improving the ability of the heart to pump blood throughout the body. Care designed to increase coronary perfusion, in order to minimize myocardial ischaemia and subsequent injury, falls predominantly under the remit of the physician. However, the pharmacological, mechanical or surgical management involved necessitates effective nursing intervention in order to prepare the patient and his family for specific procedures and diagnostic tests.

Nursing intervention will be an extension of that provided for the patient with heart failure and will be aimed at minimizing the effects of impaired cardiac output, impaired gaseous exchange and impaired cerebral and peripheral blood flow on the patient. Such measures will include maintaining effective ventilation, optimizing hydration and balancing activity levels with cardiac efficiency.

An early priority will be comforting the patient and giving opiates if necessary. The patient is best nursed in a position in which they feel reasonably comfortable and which permits the frequent monitoring routines so often necessary with this condition. The nurse needs to plan and coordinate investigations and procedures to avoid the unnecessary disturbance of the patient. The patient is likely to be extremely weak and lethargic and require assistance with many daily activities.

Nutrition needs to be closely monitored, the aim being to maintain a positive nitrogen balance to avoid protein breakdown.

Great care needs to be taken to prevent the occurrence of pressure sores, as poorly perfused skin is extremely vulnerable and the patient is unable to alter their position in bed.

Psychological support The patient and family are likely to be highly anxious and fearful of the outcome. This is often exacerbated by the sight of multiple and complex items of equipment and the constant nursing and medical surveillance of the patient. Relatives require to be kept fully informed about the patient's condition and management, including a realistic appraisal of outlook, particularly in view of the extremely high mortality associated with cardiogenic shock. The patient and family should also be given every opportunity to express and discuss their worries and fears. The patient's perceptions and methods of coping may be altered and communication may be hampered because of this as well as because of factors such as oxygen masks or cannulae and the inability to change posture or attract attention.

The patient's self-concept may be altered because of helplessness and dependency on others. They may feel that the nurse is focusing a good deal of attention on monitoring systems but relatively little on them as a person. Feelings of frustration, confusion and anger may be expressed because of this helplessness or diminished cerebral function, or both. Information and support assume great importance and need to be carefully tailored for him and his family.

Family members also usually experience feelings of helplessness and frustration and will require a great deal of nursing support. They should be encouraged to become involved in the provision of patient care, provided that they appreciate this may prove stressful for them.

For some patients it will become clear that they are unlikely to recover, and careful and sensitive thought needs to be addressed towards ensuring that their final hours are spent in peace and comfort in the companionship of loved ones. Spiritual support may assume paramount importance at this time, both for the patient and his family.

Offering psychological support as well as physical care may prove stressful for the nurse who has established a close relationship with the patient and his family. The nurse may feel particularly vulnerable in discussions with medical colleagues regarding patient care issues. For example, there may be no apparent cut-off point in the physician's spiral of medical intervention, so it is vital that decisions reached are discussed sensitively and maturely between those caring for the patient. The nurse who has become emotionally involved with the patient needs to be able to offer an objective rationale to support any suggestions regarding care, otherwise there is a real danger of conflict arising between the nurse and physician regarding care issues.

Direct arterial pressure measurement

In the critically ill patient, indirect measurement of systemic blood pressure with a traditional cuff is often difficult. Thus, direct measurement by means of insertion into an artery of a catheter connected to a pressure transducer is sometimes warranted, especially if the patient is receiving vasodilator or vasopressor agents.

The radial artery is preferred for catheter insertion because it prevents immobilization of the whole arm and allows for easy observation of the catheter site. The brachial, femoral and dorsalis pedis arteries can also be used if, for example, blood flow to the hand is inadequate. A disposable cannula is inserted, under conditions of asepsis and local anaesthesia, into the artery. The cannula is attached by a fluid-filled manometer line to a transducer which converts the pressure changes into a waveform that can be seen on an oscilloscope. A continuous heparinized flush drip under pressure minimizes the risk of clot formation. The

catheter is sutured at the skin surface and covered with sterile dressing. Stopcock ports should be flushed after arterial blood sampling.

The blood pressure should be checked indirectly with cuff and stethoscope at least once a day. The direct pressure recording is expected to be 10–20 mmHg higher than the indirect reading.

Mean arterial pressure (MAP) can be derived knowing the systolic (S) and diastolic (D) arterial pressures, by the following formula:

$$MAP = \frac{S + 2D}{3}$$

Technical difficulties and complications If the direct pressure reading appears to be too low, this may be due to:

- thrombus
- air bubbles
- loose connections
- catheter kinking
- inaccurate calibration.

A too high reading may be due to:

- excessive catheter movement
- resonance in the system.

Possible complications include:

- infection
- air emboli
- ischaemia
- back flow of blood
- haematoma
- pain
- anxiety.

Blood can be rapidly lost through a disconnected arterial catheter and so the external part needs to be kept visible. If the medial artery is used for cannulation, movement of the hand should be regularly checked as nerve damage is a possibility. Aneurysm formation is a possible complication if prolonged use of a cannula causes weakness in the arterial wall.

Firm pressure should be applied to the insertion site for at least 5 min following catheter removal. The site should be observed for any inflammation, haematoma or swelling.

Haemodynamic monitoring

The ability to assess circulatory changes in the coronary patient and to evaluate therapy and predict outcome is often of major importance. In the coronary patient, hypovolaemia and LVF may coexist and contribute to significant reduction in cardiac output. It may be difficult clinically to distinguish between the two. Determining the PAP, and hence indirectly the left atrial pressure, permits distinction between hypovolaemia, which would produce a low wedge pressure, and LVF, which results in an elevated PAWP.

Haemodynamic monitoring may include measurement of the:

- central venous pressure (CVP)
- pulmonary artery pressure (PAP)
- pulmonary artery wedge pressure (PAWP)
- systemic blood pressure
- cardiac output.

Invasive haemodynamic monitoring is indicated in cases of:

- cardiogenic shock
- moderate or severe heart failure
- unexplained hypotension
- occurrence of possibility of pulmonary embolism, severe hypertension, aortic dissection, right ventricular infarction and mechanical heart defects.

Pulmonary artery and pulmonary artery wedge pressure measurement

Information about left ventricular function is often essential for complete haemodynamic evaluation. The development of the pulmonary artery flotation catheter has made it possible to plan and evaluate therapy for the acute coronary patient. This catheter was first used in clinical practice by Swan et al (1970) and Ganz et al (1971) and has since been modified but, although now produced by many manufacturers, still tends to be universally known as the Swan-Ganz catheter.

The pulmonary artery flotation catheter   The pulmonary artery flotation catheter is a thin flexible radiopaque tube about 80–110 cm in length. It has a small balloon near the tip which allows it to float through the chambers of the heart and into the pulmonary artery. The basic model has two lumens. One lumen serves to inflate the balloon and the second is for recording intracardiac pressures, infusing fluid and taking venous blood samples. A third, shorter, lumen may be present on some catheters and is used for recording right atrial pressures. A fourth, specialized, lumen may also be present which incorporates a temperature probe used to calculate cardiac output using the thermodilution technique (Figure 7.24).

Fibreoptic catheters which incorporate a manometer at the tip and which minimize the effects of external interference are available.

Uses of the pulmonary artery flotation catheter   The pulmonary artery flotation catheter is used to give constant detailed information about the patient's haemodynamic status and also in planning and evaluating therapy. It provides more detailed information than CVP monitoring, in that the CVP can only reflect the functional state of the right ventricle. However, its routine use in coronary care is now rare.

The catheter is used to obtain precise information regarding pressures in the right atrium, right ventricle and pulmonary artery and its distal branches. Pressures in the left side of the heart are inferred by measurements obtained in the right side of the circulation. This is possible because the pulmonary arteries are end arteries and the pulmonary veins contain no valves. Thus, the catheter registers the pressure transmitted retrogradely from the left atrium.

Catheter insertion   The catheter is usually inserted via a peripheral vein, usually the subclavian, and passed through the heart into the pulmonary artery. The catheter can be inserted percutaneously through the femoral vein using the modified Seldinger technique.

The procedure is performed by the bedside or in a room with fluoroscopy facilities. The patient is given a local anaesthetic, but should be warned that they may still be able to feel the catheter being inserted. Strict asepsis is essential to minimize the risk of infection associated with the technique. The procedure takes about 20–30 min during which time the patient should be prepared to lie flat, with

Figure 7.24 The Swan-Ganz thermodilution catheter and typical pressures recorded during its passage through the heart.

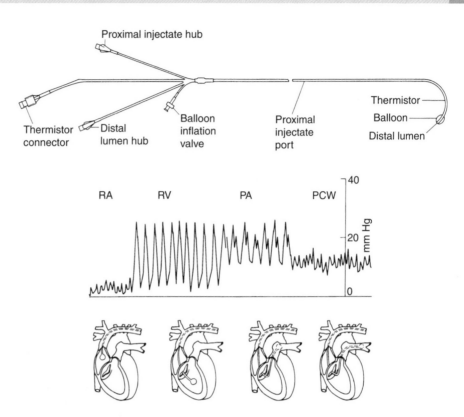

his chest covered with sterile towels and maybe with his head slightly lowered. The patient who feels short of breath while lying flat may need additional psychological support as well as oxygen therapy throughout the procedure.

Following insertion, the external end of the catheter is connected to a pressure transducer and a pressure valve display oscilloscope. The transducer senses pressure changes at the catheter tip and reflects forces produced during the cardiac cycle. The changes in pressure are transformed into weak, low-voltage electrical signals which are then amplified and displayed on the oscilloscope. The pressure waveform and the X-ray screening will indicate when the catheter enters the right atrium (see Figure 7.24). When the catheter is in the right atrium, the balloon tip is inflated with 1 ml of air. The catheter should then float with the blood flow through the tricuspid valve into the right ventricle and on into the pulmonary artery. The passage of the catheter through the heart will be reflected by pressure changes on the oscilloscope. The inflated balloon protects the endocardium and blood vessels from injury from the catheter tip.

Eventually the balloon lodges in one of the smaller distal branches of either the right or left pulmonary artery. This is described as the *wedge* position. The balloon will be deflated after initial measurements have been recorded. The catheter is sutured in position at the skin surface and a sterile dressing is applied over the insertion site.

Pressure recordings   Continuous pulmonary artery measurement can be recorded after catheter insertion. The pressures are transmitted and displayed in both wave and digital forms on the oscilloscope. The transducer contains a pressure-sensitive dome to convert the pressures to the wave and digital displays. The whole system from the catheter to the transducer needs to be airtight and filled with solution. The transducer and amplifier need to be accurately calibrated to ensure accuracy of pressure measurement. A zero reference point is obtained so that all effects of atmospheric pressure are eliminated and only internal pressures are measured. The reference point during haemodynamic monitoring is theoretically the location of the catheter tip. Provided that the transducer is readjusted to be level with the phlebostatic axis (the junction of the transverse plane of the body at the fourth intercostal space and the midline between the anterior and posterior chest), then changes in back rest position during haemodynamic monitoring are not clinically significant. Sufficiently accurate readings can be taken at 45° or less so that the patient does not have to be disturbed by changes in position. Measurements taken from patients lying on their side have proved to be inaccurate (Keating et al 1986).

When taking readings, the transducer is normally level with the patient's right atrium. The equipment needs to be calibrated between each reading and the catheter irrigated with heparinized dextrose or saline from a pressure bag to maintain patency. Results will be more accurate if all readings are taken at the same point in the respiratory cycle, usually at the end of respiration. This is because respiratory variations in the intrathoracic pressure of critically ill patients are transmitted to the pulmonary vascular bed and cardiac chambers causing corresponding variations in pulmonary capillary wedge pressures.

1 *Pulmonary artery pressure.* Normal readings are:

- systolic, 20–30 mmHg
- diastolic, 5–6 mmHg
- mean, 10–20 mmHg.

PAP increases with LVF, increased pulmonary flow and increased pulmonary arteriolar resistance, such as in pulmonary hypertension and mitral stenosis.

2 *Pulmonary artery wedge pressure.* Normal reading: 4–12 mmHg.

This is the pressure recorded when the catheter has been floated and wedged into a peripheral pulmonary artery. The balloon needs to be inflated slowly with 1 ml of air from a syringe. The balloon should not be over-inflated or left inflated, as there is a danger of pulmonary infarction. The balloon is also more likely to rupture if it is over-inflated.

In a critically ill patient there is a difference between the left atrial and right atrial pressures. PAWP is closely related to left atrial pressure. It increases in:

- left ventricular failure (>12 mmHg)
- pulmonary congestion (>18 mmHg)
- pulmonary oedema (>25 mmHg).

Cardiac output measurement The cardiac output can be calculated by what is termed the thermodilution technique. A known volume and temperature of crystalloid, usually cold, but no longer chilled, is injected at speed and emerges at an early port in the PA catheter, usually in the right atrium. The cooled blood is moved forward towards a temperature probe at the catheter tip as the heart contracts. The speed and degree of temperature change are a feature of the contractility of the heart and knowing these parameters enables a numerical value for the cardiac output to be calculated and displayed on the monitor screen. It is now possible to get continuous cardiac output readings through the use of thermal filaments which warm the blood and use the same principles of thermodilution to calculate cardiac output.

Blood gas analysis Blood gas analysis can be made on mixed blood, slowly aspirated via the port at the catheter tip. Recently developed catheters have a separate channel containing fibreoptics for light transmission. If this channel is connected to an oximeter, continuous measurement of SaO_2 is possible.

Technical difficulties and complications The measurement of PAWP is frequently associated with complications, often as a result of technical difficulties. System malfunctions that occur include:

- damped pressure trace resulting from a clot, catheter touching the vessel wall, air in the system or blood on the transducer

- unobtainable wedge pressure resulting from the balloon being over- or under-inflated, the balloon having ruptured, the catheter becoming displaced, or a problem with the monitoring system

- sudden changes in pressure or configuration of pressure waves as a result of incorrect calibration or transducer positioning, excessive catheter movement, air or blood in the system, or too long connecting tubing between the patient and the transducer.

Asking the patient to cough may reposition the catheter. Flushing the catheter may help if it has become lodged against a vessel wall. The catheter may need to be repositioned. It will need to be removed completely if it is occluded and no fluid can be aspirated back. An X-ray will show the position of the catheter.

Possible complications include:

- infection
- arrhythmias as the catheter is passed through the heart
- pulmonary infarction
- air embolism (if the balloon bursts)
- thrombophlebitis
- pneumothorax
- tamponade
- trauma.

In addition, the patient may experience pain at the insertion site, reduced mobility, increased dependency and anxiety.

Precautionary measures include:

- continuous ECG monitoring, with special attention being paid to cardiac rhythm during catheter manipulation
- suturing the catheter firmly to the skin to avoid migration of the non-sterile portion inwards causing infection
- slow, careful balloon insertion to avoid the risk of balloon rupture and possible pulmonary capillary rupture
- leaving the catheter *in situ* for the minimal time period to decrease further the likelihood of balloon rupture.

Psychological support   The patient's psychological care should not be neglected in favour of physical care and technical maintenance of equipment. Prior to the procedure the patient needs to be well prepared as to what to expect, so that the intervention and equipment will be less daunting. The patient is likely to be anxious and may perceive that the increased attention necessarily signifies a deterioration in their condition. There will be a need for individualized realistic information and support.

Physical care   This needs to be tailored to personal needs, but is likely to be similar for any patient who has restricted mobility and limited activity tolerance. Maximum independence needs to be maintained by including the patient in planning his own routine as much as is practicable. Personal hygiene, including mouth and hair care, is important together with pressure area care and encouragement of regular movement in bed to prevent complications of bed rest such as infection and thromboembolism. In order to disturb the patient as little as possible, pressure measurements should be planned to coincide with other interventions. Taking readings when the patient is being routinely assisted to change body position will avoid having to waken them unnecessarily.

Catheter removal   The pulmonary artery catheter is ideally removed after about 48 h, under aseptic conditions, with the balloon deflated, observing the patient's cardiac rhythm as the catheter is gently withdrawn through the heart chambers.

Non-invasive measurement of cardiac output

The thermodilution technique for measuring cardiac output has the major disadvantage of being invasive. It is also possible to measure cardiac output by thoracic electrical impedance techniques. The theory relies on the principle that the thorax is a volume conductor of electricity and that electrical impedance of the thoracic cavity changes with blood flow. Other non-invasive techniques for measuring cardiac output include the Doppler and the ear densitometry methods.

Intra-aortic balloon counterpulsation

Intra-aortic balloon counterpulsation is a mechanical means of supporting the acutely failing left ventricle. Essentially, it involves the insertion, percutaneously, under a local anaesthetic, of a deflated, long, sausage-shaped balloon, usually introduced via the femoral artery into the descending thoracic aorta. The procedure is commonly performed at the patient's bedside and takes about 30 min. The device has its own ECG leads which need to be attached securely to the patient. It is usually the R wave of the ECG complex which triggers the balloon to inflate and deflate within each cardiac cycle.

Following ventricular ejection, during cardiac diastole the balloon is suddenly inflated with helium, driving blood out of the aorta into the distributing arteries. At the end of diastole, just as the aortic valve is about to open, the balloon deflates causing a pressure drop in the aorta that helps to 'suck' blood out of the left ventricle. The inflation and deflation of the balloon are carefully synchronized with the ECG so there is augmentation of peak aortic pressure, reduction of left ventricular afterload and an improvement in cardiac output.

The intra-aortic balloon pump is not without problems, such as helium gas embolism, damage to the aorta, infection and haemorrhage. The patient is likely to be extremely anxious and may become psychologically dependent upon the mechanical aid. Mobility will be severely restricted, although it is possible for the patient to sit out of bed if care is taken not to dislodge the balloon and the patient's hips are not flexed more than 40°, otherwise kinking of the catheter may occur.

Diamorphine may be required for the relief of pain and anxiety. Subjectively, the patient usually feels better, although the instrumentation and constant measurement recordings can be irritating, uncomfortable and frightening.

Lower leg ischaemia is a complication caused by the presence of the balloon. Therefore, the leg pulses should be frequently palpated and the warmth and colour of the feet should be checked for comparison. If impaired circulation of the leg is suspected, the balloon should be removed immediately.

Prophylactic antibiotics are usually given at the time of catheter insertion and on a regular basis afterwards to prevent local or systemic infection. The insertion site needs to be checked for signs of infection on haemorrhage, and sterile dressings changed as necessary.

The length of time the balloon is left in position depends on the patient's condition and his response to therapy. Weaning can commence when benefit from the balloon pump has been achieved. Balloon pumping may be continued for hours or days after infarction. The rationale for stopping should be carefully explained to the patient who may feel frightened at the prospect of no longer having the assistance of the pump. The rate of inflation/deflation is gradually decreased in an attempt to wean the patient from any psychological dependency on the pump.

Intra-aortic balloon counterpulsation is indicated only when there is a good chance of remedying the underlying problem. The device is not suitable for patients with marked aortic regurgitation or damage to the aorta. Nursing the patient on an intra-aortic balloon pump is a demanding and stressful job. However, it presents a challenge to the nurse who needs to give high-quality patient-centred care in an environment crowded with technology.

Chronic heart failure

Most cases of chronic heart failure are the result of coronary heart disease. Improvements in the treatment for coronary heart disease has increased survival and the number of patients with chronic heart failure is increasing. Chronic heart failure interspersed with acute exacerbations is the most common form of heart failure seen in hospital and an average district general hospital can expect to manage over 1000 deaths and discharges related to heart failure each year (Cleland et al 2000). Almost two-thirds of those diagnosed with heart failure will die within 5 years (McMurray and Stewart 2000).

There is a poor correlation between symptoms and the severity of heart dysfunction although the New York Heart Association uses symptoms and exercise capacity to classify the severity of heart failure (Table 7.9).

The presenting symptom is usually shortness of breath, often with coughing and wheezing. Fatigue, lethargy, ankle swelling and muscle wasting are other features that contribute to a reduced quality of life. Physical signs are non-specific and include peripheral oedema, third heart sound, pulmonary crepitations, tachycardias and the raised JVP of

Table 7.9 Functional classification of patients with heart disease (Criteria Committee of the New York Heart Association 1973)

Class	
I	Heart disease with no limitation on ordinary physical activity
II	Slight limitation. Ordinary physical activity (e.g. walking) produces symptoms
III	Marked limitation. Unable to walk on the level without disability. Less than ordinary activity produces symptoms
IV	Dyspnoea at rest. Inability to carry out any physical activity

right sided heart failure. Diagnosis should include objective measures of left ventricular structure and function and accurate diagnosis can be difficult, particularly for general practitioners without access to echocardiography (Hobbs et al 2000).

Chronic heart failure requires lifelong treatment involving effective liaison between medical, nursing and other health care disciplines. Nurses have a key role in heart failure, and nurse-led intervention has been shown to reduce re-admissions (Rich et al 1995). Nurse-led heart failure clinics have developed to support, educate and monitor patients and community-based heart failure liaison nurses aim to provide seamless care between hospital and home. The aim is to empower patients in order to increase their sense of control and compliance with therapy (McMurray and Stewart 1981, Jaarsma and Stewart 2004).

Management needs to include both the prevention and treatment of heart failure and goals include (European Society of Cardiology 1997):

- improving or maintaining quality of life by improvement in symptoms or preventing symptoms getting worse
- avoidance of the side effects of treatment
- decrease in the occurrence of major morbid events
- postpone death.

Treatment of chronic heart failure is multifaceted and includes patient and family education and support, attention to dietary issues, avoidance of smoking, monitoring weight gain, regular exercise and vaccination (Gibbs et al 2000) plus optimal pharmacological management. Diuretics, ACE inhibitors, beta-blockers, calcium channel blockers, digoxin and anti-arrhythmics are all treatment options. Patients may find it difficult to retain information due to fatigue, short-term memory loss and confusion and there is a need for strategies to encourage the asking of questions and the involvement of the family (Rogers et al 2000).

Palliative care is beginning to assume the importance it deserves for heart failure patients. Shortness of breath, pain, nausea, constipation and a general low mood are common in the end stage of the disease (McCarthy et al 1996) and patient and families require support similar to that provided for cancer patients (DoH 2000).

POST-INFARCTION ANGINA

Post-infarction chest pain may be due to a variety of causes such as pericarditis, pulmonary embolism or indigestion as well as cardiac ischaemia, so a definite diagnosis is needed. Post-infarction angina may affect up to one-third of patients, and the risk of re-infarction in these patients is considerable. This is particularly the case for patients who do not originally infarct through the whole thickness of the myocardium. If flow in the infarcted artery is not fully restored there is a risk of reocclusion, particularly in the first 24 hours. Transient chest pain and response to GTN are the main confirmatory features.

Patients should be treated for unstable angina and glycoprotein IIb/IIIa antagonists are indicated prior to intervention. Patients and their family are likely to be anxious that the symptoms have recurred and individualized information and support is particularly needed at this time.

MANAGEMENT OF RAISED BLOOD SUGAR

Up to one-quarter of all patients with myocardial infarction have diabetes. A significant number will be newly diagnosed with the disorder on admission to hospital. Having to cope with frequent blood glucose monitoring and coming to terms with the significance of a second long-term diagnosis and its management can cause additional burdens for the patient and family. Mortality after myocardial infarction both in the acute phase and during long-term follow up is higher for patients with diabetes than those without with hyperglycaemia being an independent predictor of mortality. In fact, stress hyperglycaemia without underlying diabetes is also associated with an increased mortality at both 30 days and one year following acute myocardial infarction (Capes et al 2000). Elevated blood glucose levels are associated with elevated free fatty acid levels and it is thought that together they have an adverse effect on myocardial function, resulting in an increased infarct size. The DIGAMI (Diabetes and Insulin-Glucose Infusion in Acute Myocardial Infarction) study (Malberg et al 1999) showed that mortality was significantly reduced in those patients who received improved metabolic care by means of intensive insulin therapy. One life was saved for every nine patients treated and the benefit was sustained for at least 3 years. The therapy consisted of an insulin-glucose infusion for at least 24 hours followed by subcutaneous insulin for at least 3 months. This treatment has been shown to be cost effective (Almbrand et al 2000) and is recommended for myocardial infarction patients who present with a blood glucose of over 11 mmol/litre, unless a large volume of fluid is likely to be detrimental.

Potassium–insulin–glucose infusions have also been shown to reduce mortality (Fath-Ordoubadi and Beatt 1997) and may be particularly useful during reperfusion ischaemia and for those with chronic heart failure (Broomhead and Colvin 2001).

OTHER COMPLICATIONS

The nurse needs to be aware of other complications that may occur in the acute coronary patient. They are often in an ideal position to assess the patient's reported symptoms or signs and their interpretation may result in further investigations and changes in the patient's management plan. However, the general optimistic outlook conveyed to the patient may be severely disrupted if complications arise, and the potential problems may include decreased activity, increased dependency, perceived loss of control, inability to predict outcome of recovery and lack of knowledge about the complication and its management.

Thromboembolism

Following myocardial infarction, thromboembolic events may occur, including the development of left ventricular thrombi which may result in arterial embolization, and venous thrombosis with possible resulting pulmonary embolism. Likely causes include obesity, restricted activity, changes in cardiac output and flow and possible changes in the blood clotting mechanism due to elevation of some of the blood clotting factors. Some coronary patients may simply have an increased proneness to clot formation and damage to vessel walls.

Deep-vein thrombosis (DVT)

DVT is thought to complicate as many as one-third of coronary patients, but only a very small percentage produce any symptoms or have recovery clinically affected. Immobility, increasing age and heart failure make DVT a risk after myocardial infarction (THRIFT II Consensus Group 1998).

Clinical features

Clinical signs, although not always reliable, include swelling, tenderness and redness of the affected limb, usually the calf. A positive Homans' sign (occurrence of the calf pain when the foot is dorsiflexed) may also be present, as may a slight pyrexia. Venography is the ideal method of demonstrating thrombosis in the deep veins, although the benefits of the results of this invasive test need to be weighed against the risk of producing thrombophlebitis in some patients. Impedance phlebography is useful for detecting thrombosis of the great veins, but is not very sensitive for calf vein thrombosis.

^{25}I-fibrinogen scanning detects thrombi that are laying down fibrin, but this may be delayed for up to 72 h.

Management

Prevention is the first aim and subcutaneous low-dose unfractionated heparin or low molecular weight heparin should be given routinely for all patients admitted to coronary care units, with full anticoagulation usually considered for the patient with restricted mobility or heart failure. Heparin should be continued for 4–5 days, and oral anticoagulants given at the same time. The INR should be 2–3 for at least 2 days before the heparin is discontinued. Early mobility is a desirable aim for all patients, especially the elderly, provided that there are no contraindications.

The patient needs to avoid sitting for long periods as it encourages venous stasis. Elevation of the patient's legs to a level higher than the heart and the application of class II graduated compression stockings may prove helpful in aiding venous return. Explanations regarding what has happened and reinforcement that it is likely to be only a temporary setback to recovery are likely to help the patient cope with the complication.

Pulmonary embolism

Pulmonary embolism is believed to be rare, occurring in about 0.5% of coronary patients. It occurs when a venous thrombosis becomes detached from its site of origin and is carried with the blood flow through the right heart and hence the pulmonary artery. A small embolus will only block a small portion of the lung tissue, whereas a large embolus may wedge in the larger artery branches and hence deprive a greater area of the lung of its blood supply. Pulmonary emboli are considered to be *massive* if they involve more than 50% of the pulmonary arteries and *minor* if less than 50%.

Clinical features

The clinical features are related to the size of the pulmonary emboli. If the embolism is small, and only a small peripheral artery is blocked, there may be few or no symptoms. The extra work that the right ventricle incurs in order to pump blood through the lungs is minimal, and any resulting symptoms are of late onset and tend to be as a result of an area of lung becoming infarcted through a blocked blood supply. Thus, pleuritic pain, haemoptysis and a pleural rub may be present. The ECG and chest X-ray may be normal, although the latter may reveal a wedge-shaped area of shadowing, elevation of the diaphragm and a small pleural effusion. A massive pulmonary embolism will have profound and dramatic effects, since the outflow from the right ventricle through the lungs is severely obstructed. The right ventricle is unable to cope with the work necessary to pump against increased resistance, thus resulting in almost total loss of cardiac output with circulatory arrest, collapse and syncope. There is hypotension, tachycardia, a high CVP (measured by the jugular venous pressure) and a gallop heart rhythm. Rapid breathing, shortness of breath and chest pain are common. The chest pain is characteristically of sudden onset, sharp and stabbing in nature, later becoming pleuritic. The pain tends to be substernal or in the side of the back. It is not relieved by rest or glyceryl trinitrate. Recurrent episodes of weakness, sweating, coughing and the signs and symptoms of right heart failure are common.

Investigations

In order to assist the diagnosis of pulmonary embolism, a number of medical investigations may be necessary, as described below.

ECG There are no changes diagnostic of pulmonary embolism. Non-specific changes include sinus tachycardia, widespread T-wave inversion (especially in leads V_1–V_4), right axis deviation and right bundle branch block. The classical S wave in lead I and Q-wave and T-wave inversion in lead III reflect right ventricular strain and the change in electrical axis that results from it.

Arterial blood gases Blood gases are a non-specific diagnosis in pulmonary embolism, but they may be useful in assessing the severity of the disorder. Hypoxaemia and hypocapnia are usually found in massive embolism because of the ventilation–perfusion imbalance, and hyperventilation.

Lung scans Although pulmonary angiography is the definitive method for diagnosing pulmonary embolism, it is highly invasive and not without risk. The best diagnostic technique available is therefore the combined ventilation–perfusion scan. The patient is injected with technetium-labelled macroaggregates of albumin, which lodge in the pulmonary capillaries. The distribution of trapped macroaggregates is determined with a gamma-scanner. Significant perfusion defects are seen as 'cold' spots on the scan. Unfortunately, perfusion abnormalities are also produced by other conditions which may affect pulmonary flow distribution, including obstructive airways disease and pneumonia. If this is the case, a ventilation scan is additionally required to diagnose pulmonary embolism.

Ventilation should be preserved in the areas of impaired perfusion if there has been a pulmonary embolism (i.e. there is a ventilation–perfusion mismatch). If the area of malperfusion is due to primary lung disease, ventilation will also be impaired and matching ventilation–perfusion defects will be seen on the scans. The patient inhales radioactive xenon or technetium, and the gamma-camera records the distribution of the alveolar gas with a multiview series of pictures. The ventilation and perfusion scans are then compared for matching defects.

Management

Patients at risk need to be identified and preventative measures taken to minimize the likelihood of the occurrence of venous stasis and thrombosis.

Early mobility needs to be encouraged and routine anticoagulation therapy is warranted.

Medical intervention depends on the degree of haemodynamic upset. Most emboli resolve with time, and management is directed towards sustaining life and preventing recurrence. Pain and anxiety should be relieved with diamorphine, and 100% oxygen may be given. Anticoagulation is established until the patient is stable, after which warfarin can be substituted. Thrombolytic therapy via a pulmonary artery catheter has proved successful, although bleeding and allergic complications are a common problem. Embolectomy is sometimes effective but not often appropriate for the coronary patient, as it necessitates cardiopulmonary bypass and carries a high mortality.

The coronary patient who develops a pulmonary embolus is bound to be anxious and uncertain as to what the problem is. Simple explanations conveying information and realistic expectations for recovery are beneficial.

Pericarditis

Inflammation of the pericardium occurs in about 10–25% of coronary patients. It is often found in patients with epicardial or transmural infarcts and is also associated with LVF and arrhythmias. It is usually transient and benign.

Early pericarditis occurs 24–72 h after acute infarction and tends to present with characteristic pain and is recognized clinically by the presence of a pericardial friction rub. Pericardial inflammation occurring 10 days to 2 years after infarction (Dressler's syndrome) is thought to be mediated via an immunological mechanism, and is often treated with steroids.

Clinical features

The pain is often severe, usually of sudden onset, sharp and not produced by effort or relieved by rest. It is usually pleuritic, but may be overshadowed by constrictive pain resembling that of myocardial ischaemia. The pain may radiate down the arms to one or both shoulders, and the patient may find it difficult to distinguish from angina and worry they are suffering a further heart attack. The pain tends to be aggravated by deep inspiration,

coughing, swallowing, lying flat or rotating the trunk. It is often relieved by sitting up or leaning forward. A slight pyrexia and tachycardia are often apparent, with the patient reporting feeling generally unwell.

The best clinical sign is the pericardial friction rub, which is a high-pitched scratchy superficial sound heard with the stethoscope, and most commonly situated along the left sternal edge. The rub, however, is often missed as it can be transient, localized and soft.

Dressler's syndrome demonstrates clinical features similar to those of acute pericarditis, and the erythrocyte sedimentation rate (ESR) will usually be significantly raised.

Characteristically the ECG shows widespread concave ST-segment elevation in the leads directed towards the affected surface, without significant changes in the QRS complexes. The ST segments usually return to normal after several days and the T waves then become inverted. The ECG may simulate that of acute myocardial infarction, but Q waves are not seen, the ST-segment elevation is of a different configuration, and the T-wave inversion occurs only after return of the ST segment to the isoelectric line.

The chest X-ray is usually normal, but echocardiography may demonstrate a small pericardial effusion.

Management

Nursing care includes the provision of an environment conducive to patient rest and comfort through, for instance, relieving pain or discomfort, minimizing the effects of a raised temperature, assisting with activities and alleviating anxiety.

Advising the patient as to what is causing the pain and stressing that it will only be a temporary setback, with no effect on long-term recovery, is likely to help him.

Medical treatment depends on the severity of symptoms, pain relief being the main priority. Nonsteroidal anti-inflammatory (NSAI) agents, such as aspirin and indomethacin, may reduce the pain and decrease any fever, although aspirin has adverse gastrointestinal effects and indomethacin should be avoided if there is impaired renal function or the patient is in heart failure. Paracetamol, although not anti-inflammatory, does possess analgesic and antipyretic effects, and can be effective for pericarditic pain.

Anticoagulants are usually avoided in the patient with pericarditis, particularly if symptoms persist for more than a few days. A less than therapeutic range of anticoagulation is often recommended if such agents need to be used. The risk of haemopericardium (the pericardium becoming filled with blood as a result of haemorrhage) is, however, rare.

Pericardial effusion

Small effusions may complicate acute pericarditis or heart failure. They are caused by transudation in heart failure or exudation of serous fluid or pus in pericarditis. The patient is unlikely to be aware of the problem. These effusions are hard to detect clinically and are rarely of significance following acute myocardial infarction.

Cardiac tamponade

Cardiac tamponade is compression of the heart by fluid accumulating within the pericardial sac. The most common cause is intrapericardial haemorrhage caused by cardiac rupture, aortic dissection or perforation during cardiac catheterization. It is a potentially reversible cause of PEA.

Cardiac tamponade occurs when fluid collecting in the pericardial sac produces an increased intrapericardial pressure which impairs venous return to the heart. The heart is additionally unable to expand during diastole, so that filling is impaired, with a secondary decrease in stroke volume, cardiac output and blood pressure. The heart rate increases in order to attempt to maintain cardiac output, but as intrapericardial pressure exceeds $15\,cmH_2O$, the clinical signs of shock appear. There is a rise in the CVP, with a fall in systemic pressure. The pulse pressure may vary with respiration, becoming smaller on inspiration, and the neck veins may become distended on inspiration (Kussmoul's sign). The ECG will show an alteration in cardiac electrical axis from beat to beat, said to be caused by the heart swinging freely in a bag of fluid.

A pericardial tap should be performed immediately if there are signs of tamponade. Fluid is withdrawn under local anaesthesia via a needle inserted under the xiphisternum. An ECG electrode attached to the needle will show ST-segment elevation if the needle makes contact with the epicardium. If this occurs, the needle should be withdrawn a little. Fluid can be aspirated via the needle or a soft cannula. Relief of tamponade can usually be achieved by removal of about 20% of the fluid. The underlying cause of the effusion will require specific therapy.

Nursing intervention will be aimed at helping the patient overcome decreased activity tolerance, and giving appropriate information and support, especially if a pericardial tap needs to be performed.

Cardiac rupture

After arrhythmias and cardiogenic shock, the commonest cause of death following acute myocardial infarction is cardiac rupture, which complicates about 10% of cases.

The commonest site for rupture is through the free left ventricular wall. It usually occurs within the first 2 weeks following infarction, manifesting as chest pain, bradycardia, shock, increased venous pressure, shortness of breath and anxiety. Typically, chest pain is usually followed by electromechanical dissociation and rapid progression to an undetectable output. Emergency surgery or pericardiocentesis is usually indicated, although the rapid rate of haemodynamic deterioration and the practical difficulties involved mean that ventricular wall rupture is usually fatal and attempts at resuscitation are rarely successful.

Rupture of the interventricular septum tends to occur around the fifth day and is usually accompanied by sudden haemodynamic deterioration. Clinical features include chest pain, right heart failure (due to left-to-right shunting of blood), hypertension, systolic murmur, conduction defects and anxiety. Many cases probably escape detection and the patient develops severe heart failure or cardiogenic shock. Surgery is easier several weeks after infarction, but patients are seldom able to sustain an adequate cardiac output for this length of time.

The papillary muscles may become ischaemic and infarcted like any other part of the ventricular myocardium, and rupture in the healing stages. The papillary muscle affected depends on the location of the myocardial infarction. Prognosis is better than for septal rupture, and depends upon the degree of left ventricular dysfunction.

Nursing intervention involves minimizing the effects of a low cardiac output, relieving anxiety, fear and pain, easing breathing and providing comfort, information and support.

Ventricular aneurysm

Ventricular aneurysm formation occurs in 10–20% of acute coronary patients. It is often associated with anterior infarction. The infarcted area is repeatedly stretched in systole and becomes weakened, thin and bulging. There is loss of contracting muscle and left ventricular volume overload as the aneurysm becomes a pooling area for blood.

There are two types of disorder of ventricular function following aneurysm: *dyskinesis* refers to local paradoxical wall movement, and *akinesis* to local absence of wall movement. Aneurysms may develop a few days after myocardial infarction or over a period of several years. A ventricular aneurysm will produce features of LVF and increases the risk of systemic emboli and serious persistent ventricular arrhythmias. It is also likely to be associated with chest pain and anxiety.

The aneurysm may be demonstrated by echocardiography, radionuclide studies and left ventriculography. An abnormal rounded protrusion from the left ventricular wall may be apparent on the chest X-ray. ECG findings include maintained ST-segment elevation over the acute stage of infarction. Medical or surgical treatment may be indicated depending on the severity of the complications.

DISCHARGE FROM HOSPITAL

Patients' anxiety is likely to increase prior to discharge from hospital as they are faced with the uncertainty of how they will cope at home outside of the hospital environment. Realistic information and advice needs to be given so that the patient and family have guidelines about what to expect, what to do and when to call for professional help and advice. A card with the ward telephone number or some other 24-hour contact point is likely to be reassuring.

A successful discharge is the aim at the outset of the admission and planning for this stage in the patient's journey needs to be part of care planning from the start of the patient's stay in hospital. Patients may have complex support arrangements and it is easy to neglect these when care is so focused on the acute cardiac event. A comprehensive discharge plan should aim to:

- prepare the patient and family physically and psychologically for discharge home
- facilitate a smooth and safe discharge, by ensuring that all appropriate health, social care facilities and lay support arrangements are in place to support the patient at home
- provide information to the patient and family to prepare them for returning to living at home
- encouraging self-care and independence
- provide continuity and coordination of care between hospital and home through effective communication at all levels.

Education about drug treatment is particularly important as regimen are likely to have changed several times throughout the hospital stay and the cardiac pharmacist can play an important role.

There is evidence that discharge decisions can be influenced by the day of the week (higher discharge rates on Fridays) and may be dependent on organizational rather than clinical factors (Varnava et al 2002). Decisions not based on appropriate assessments of the patient's clinical status need to be avoided and nurses are in a position to influence this as advocates for care that is in the patient's best interests.

References

Aarons E, Beeching NJ (1991). Survey of 'Do not resuscitate' orders in a district general hospital. *British Medical Journal*, 303: 1504–1506.

ACC/AHA (1999). Guidelines for the management of patients with acute myocardial infarction: executive summary and recommendations. *Circulation*, 100: 1016–1030.

ACC/AHA/ESC (2001). Guidelines for the management of patients with atrial fibrillation. *Journal of the American College of Cardiology*, 38: 41–70.

ACC/AHA/NASPE (2002). Guideline update for implantation of cardiac pacemakers and antiarrhythmia devices. *Journal of Cardiovascular Electrophysiology*, 13: 1183–1199.

Achleitner Y, Rheinberger K, Futner B et al (2001). Wave form analysis of biphasic external defibrillators. *Resuscitation*, 50: 61–70.

Ahlqvist RE (1948). Study of adrenotropic receptors. *American Journal of Physiology*, 153: 586–600.

Almbrand B, Johannesson M, Sjostrand B et al (2000). Cost effectiveness of intense insulin treatment after acute myocardial infarction in patients with diabetes mellitus. Results from the DIAGMI study. *European Heart Journal*, 21: 733–739.

Antman E (2002). The Magic trial, presented at the XXIVth Scientific Sessions of the European Society of Cardiology in Berlin. September.

Auble TE, Menegazzi JJ, Paris PM (1996). Effect of out of hospital defibrillation by basic life support providers on cardiac arrest mortality: a meta-analysis. *Annals of Emergency Medicine*, 25: 642–648.

Bardy GH, Mardchlinski FE, Sharma AD et al (1996). Transthoracic investigators. Multicentre comparison of truncated biphasic shocks and standard damped sine wave monophasic shocks for transthoracic ventricular defibrillation. *Circulation*, 94: 2507–2514.

Baskett PJF (1986). The ethics of resuscitation. *British Medical Journal*, 293: 189–190.

Baumann A, Boubonnais F (1982). Nursing decision making in critical care areas. *Journal of Advanced Nursing*, 7: 435–446.

Berger M, Schweitzer P (1998). Timing of thrombo-embolic events after elective cardioversion for atrial fibrillation or atrial flutter. A retrospective analysis. *American Journal of Cardiology*, 82: 1545–1547.

Block M, Breithardt G (1999). The implantable cardioverter defibrillator and primary prevention of sudden death: the multicentre automatic defibrillator implantation trial and coronary artery bypass graft (CABG)-patch trial. *American Journal of Cardiology*, 85 (5B): 74D–78D.

BMA/RCN (2001). Decisions relating to cardiopulmonary resuscitation: a joint statement from the British Medical Association, the Resuscitation Council (UK) and the Royal College of Nursing, London.

British Cardiac Society (2002). Fifth report on the provision of services for patients with heart disease. *Heart*, 88 (suppl 3): 1–56.

British Pacing and Electrophysiology Group (1991). Recommendations for pacemaker prescriptions for symptomatic bradycardia. Report of a Working Party. *British Heart Journal*, 66: 185–191.

Broomhead CJ, Colvin MP (2001). Glucose, insulin and the cardiovascular disease. *Heart*, 85: 495–496.

Burack B, Furman S (1969). Trans-esophageal cardiac pacing. *American Journal of Cardiology*, 23: 469–472.

Capes SE, Hunt D, Malberg K et al (2000). Stress hyper-glycaemia and increased risk of death after myocardial infarction in patients with and without diabetes: a systematic overview. *Lancet*, 355: 773–778.

Casey WF (1984). Cardiopulmonary resuscitation: a survey of standards among junior hospital doctors. *Journal of the Royal Society of Medicine*, 77: 921–924.

Chamberlain DA (1989). Advanced life support. *British Medical Journal*, 299: 446–448.

Cleland JGF, Clark A, Caplin JL (2000). Taking heart failure seriously. *British Medical Journal*, 320: 1095–1096.

Cobbe SM (1986). Electrophysiological testing after acute myocardial infarction. *British Medical Journal*, 292: 1290–1291.

Cooper N, Jacob B (2002). Biphasic positive pressure ventilation in acute cardiogenic pulmonary oedema, *British Journal of Cardiology*, 9: 38–41.

DaCosta A, Kirkorian G, Chucherat M et al (1998). Antibiotic prophylaxis for permanent pacemaker implantation: a meta analysis. *Circulation*, 18: 1796–1801.

Davies W (2001). The management of atrial fibrillation. *Clinical Medicine*, 1: 190–193.

Department of Health (2000). *National Service Framework for Coronary Heart Disease*. Chapter 6, Heart failure. Department of Health, London.

Di Bari M, Chiarlone M, Fumagalli S et al (2000). Cardiopulmonary resuscitation of older, inhospital patients: immediate efficacy and long term outcome. *Critical Care Medicine*, 28: 2320–2325.

Dim BM, Stern A, Poliakoff SJ (1974). Survivors of cardiac arrest: the first few days. *Psychosomatics*, 15: 61–67.

Dougherty C (1994). Longitudinal recovery following sudden cardiac arrest: survivors and their families. *American Journal of Critical Care*, 3: 145–154.

Doyal L, Wishner D (1993). Withholding cardiopulmonary resuscitation: proposals for formal guidelines. *British Medical Journal*, 306: 1593–1596.

Dracup K, Moser DK, Taylor SE, Guzy PM (1997). The psychological consequences of cardiopulmonary resuscitation training for family members of patients at risk of sudden death. *American Journal of Public Health*, 87: 1434–1439.

Druss RG, Kornfeld DS (1967). The survivors of cardiac arrest. *Journal of the American Medical Association*, 201: 291–296.

Dunbar S, Warner C, Purcell J (1993). Internal cardioverter defibrillator device discharge: experiences of patients and family members. *Heart and Lung*, 22 (6): 494–501.

Ebell MH, Becker LA, Barry HC et al (1998). Survival after in-hospital cardio-pulmonary resuscitation: a meta-analysis. *Journal of General Internal Medicine*, 13: 805–816.

Eberle B, Dick WF, Schneider T et al (1996). Checking the carotid pulse check: diagnostic accuracy of first responders in patients with and without a pulse. *Resuscitation*, 33: 107–116.

Ebrahim S (2000). Do not resuscitate decisions: flogging dead horses or a dignified death? Editorial. *British Medical Journal*, 320: 1155–1156.

Edwards L, Shaw DG (1998). Care of the suddenly bereaved in cardiac care units: a review of the literature. *Intensive and Critical Care Nursing*, 14: 144–152.

EEC (1988). *Ionising Radiation Regulations*. EEC, Brussels.

Eichhorn D et al (1996). Opening doors: family presence during resuscitation. *Journal of Cardiovascular Nursing*, 10(4): 59–70.

European Society of Cardiology (1997). The treatment of heart failure. Task Force of the Working Group on Heart Failure. *European Heart Journal*, 18: 736–753.

Ewy GA, Hellman DA, MeClung S, Taren D (1980). The influence of ventilation phase on transthoracic impedance and defibrillation effectiveness. *Critical Care Medicine*, 8: 164–166.

Fath-Ordoubadi F, Beatt K (1997). Glucose-insulin-potassium therapy for treatment of myocardial infarction: an overview of randomised placebo controlled trials. *Circulation*, 96: 1074–1077.

Fibrinolytic Therapy Trialists' Collaborative Group (1994). Indications for fibrinolytic therapy in suspected myocardial infarction: collaborative overview of early and major mortality from all randomised trials of more than 1000 patients. *Lancet*, 343: 311–322.

Freemantle N, Cleland JG, Young P et al (2001). Beta-blockade after myocardial infarction: systematic review and meta-regression analysis. *British Medical Journal*, 318: 1349–1355.

Ganz W, Donoso R, Marcus H, Forrester JS, Swan HJC (1971). A new technique for measurement of cardiac output by thermodilution in man. *American Journal of Cardiology*, 27: 392–405.

Gibbs A, Jackson G, Lip GYH (2000). ABC of heart failure – Non-drug management. *British Medical Journal*, 320: 366–369.

Gillon R (1989). Deciding not to resuscitate. *Journal of Medical Ethics*, 15: 171–172.

Hart RG, Halpern JL (2001). Atrial fibrillation and stroke: concepts and controversies. *Stroke*, 32: 8033–8038.

Heames RM, Sado D, Deakin CD (2001). Do doctors position defibrillator paddles correctly? Observational study. *British Medical Journal*, 322: 1393–1394.

Hobbs FDR, Davies RC, Lip GYH (2000). ABC of heart failure in general practice. *British Medical Journal*, 320: 626–629.

Hochman JS, Sleeper LA, Webb JG et al (1999). Early revascularisation in acute myocardial infarction complicated by cardiogenic shock. SHOCK investigators. Should we emergently revascularize occluded coronaries for cardiogenic shock. *New England Journal of Medicine*, 341: 625–634.

Hodgetts TJ, Kenward G, Vlachorikolis IG et al (2002). The identification of risk factors for cardiac arrest and formulation of activation criteria to alert a medical emergency team. *Resuscitation*, 54: 125–131.

Hollenberg S, Kavinsky C, Parrillo J (1999). Cardiogenic shock (review). *Annals of Internal Medicine*, 131: 47–59.

Holmes DR (2003). Cardiogenic shock: a lethal complication of acute myocardial infarction. *Reviews in Cardiovascular Medicine*, 4: 131–135.

Iserson KV (1999). *Pocket Protocols for Notifying Survivors about Sudden Unexpected Deaths*. Galen Press Ltd, Tuscon, Arizona.

ISIS:4 (1995). A randomised factorial trial assessing early oral captoril, oral mononitrate and intravenous magnesium in 58 050 patients with suspected myocardial infarction. ISIS-4 (Fourth International Study of Infarct Survival) Collaborative Group. *Lancet*, 345: 669–685.

Jaarsma T, Stewart S (2004). Nurse-led management programmes in heart failure. In *Caring for the Heart Failure Patient* (S Stewart, DK Moser, DR Thompson eds). Martin Dunitz, London, pp. 161–180.

James J (1997). Living on the edge – patients with an automatic internal cardioverter defibrillator (AICD): implications for nursing practice. *Nursing in Critical Care*, 2(4): 163–167.

James J (2002). Management and support of patients with internal cardioverter defibrillators. In *Cardiac Nursing – A Comprehensive Guide* (R Hatchett, D Thompson, eds). Churchill Livingstone, Edinburgh, pp. 495–505.

Joglar JA, Hamden MH, Ramaswamy K et al (2000). Initial energy for elective external cardioversion of persistent atrial fibrillation. *American Journal of Cardiology*, 86: 348–350.

Jowett NJ, Thompson DR (2003). *Comprehensive Coronary Care*, 3rd edn. Baillière Tindall, London.

Kaye W, Linhares KC, Breault RV, Norris PA, Starnoulis CC, Kham AH (1981). The Mega code for training the advanced cardiac life support team. *Heart and Lung*, 10: 5–9.

Kaye W, Mancini ME (1986). Retention of cardiopulmonary resuscitation skills by physicians, registered nurses, and the general public. *Critical Care Medicine*, 14: 620–621.

Keating D, Bolyard K, Eichler E, Reed J (1986). Effect of sidelying position on pulmonary artery pressure. *Heart and Lung*, 15: 605–610.

Killip T, Kimball JT (1967). Treatment of myocardial infarction in a coronary care unit: two years experience with 250 patients. *American Journal of Cardiology*, 20: 457–464.

Kudenchuck PJ, Cobb LA, Copass MK et al (1999). Amiodarone for resuscitation for out of hospital cardiac arrest due to ventricular fibrillation. *New England Journal of Medicine*, 341: 871–878.

Lands GM, Arnold A, McAuliff JP, Luduera FP, Brown TG (1967). Differentiation of receptor systems activated by sympathomimetic amines. *Nature*, 214: 597–604.

Larson D (1992). Resuscitation discussion experiences of patients hospitalised in a coronary care unit. *Heart and Lung*, 21: 291–295.

Liddle J, Gilleard C, Neil A (1993). Elderly patients' and their relatives' views on CPR. *Lancet* 342: 1055.

Lund M, French JK, Johnson RN et al (2000). Serum troponins T and I after elective cardioversion. *European Heart Journal*, 21: 245–252.

Maier GW, Newton JR, Wolfe JA et al (1986). The influence of manual chest compression rate on hemodynamic support during cardiac arrest: high impulse cardiopulmonary resuscitation. *Circulation*, 74: 51–59.

Malberg K, Ryden L, Efendie S et al (1995). A randomised trial of insulin-glucose infusion followed by sub-cutaneous insulin treatment in diabetic patients with acute myocardial infarction (DIAGMI study): effects on acute mortality at 1 year. *Journal of the American College of Cardiology*, 26: 57–65.

Malberg K, Norhammer A, Wedel H et al (1999). Glycometabolic state at admission: important risk marker of mortality in conventionally treated patients with diabetes mellitus and acute myocardial infarction: long term results from the Diabetes and Insulin-Glucose

Infusion in Acute Myocardial Infarction (DIAGMI) study. *Circulation*, 99: 2626–2632.

Marteau TM, Johnston M, Wynne G, Evans TR (1989). Cognitive factors in the explanation of the mismatch between confidence and competence in performing basic life support. *Psychology and Health*, 3: 173–182.

Marteau TM, Wynne G, Kayc W, Evans TR (1990). Resuscitation: experience without feedback increases confidence but not skill. *British Medical Journal*, 300: 849–850.

Marwick TH, Case CC, Siskind V, Woodhouse SP (1991). Prediction of survival from resuscitation: a prognostic index derived from multivariate logistic model analysis. *Resuscitation*, 22: 129–137.

McCarthy M, Lay M, Addington-Hall JM (1996). Dying from heart disease. *Journal of the Royal College of Physicians*, 30: 325–328.

McLauchlan CA, Ward A, Murphy NM et al (1992). Resuscitation training for cardiac patients and their relatives – its effect on anxiety. *Resuscitation*, 24: 7–11.

McMurray JJ, Stewart S (1998). Nurse-led, multidisciplinary intervention in chronic heart failure. *Heart*, 80: 430–431.

McMurray JJ, Stewart S (2000). Epidemiology, aetiology and progress of heart failure. *Heart*, 83: 596–602.

Mitchell AR, Chalil S, Boodhoo L et al (2003). Diazepam or midazolam for external DC cardioversion (the DORM study). *Europace*, 5: 391–395.

Mittal S, Ayati S, Stein KM et al (2000). Transthoracic cardioversion of atrial fibrillation: comparison of rectilinear biphasic versus damped sine wave monophasic shocks. *Circulation*, 101: 1282–1287.

Moody RA (1976). *Life after Life*. Bantam, New York.

Moody RA (1988). *The Light Beyond*. Bantam, New York.

Morgan R, King D, Prajapati C et al (1994). Views of elderly patients and their relatives on cardiopulmonary resuscitation. *British Medical Journal*, 308: 1677–1678.

Morgan R, Westmorland C (2002). Survey of junior doctors' attitudes to cardiopulmonary resuscitation. *Postgraduate Medical Journal*, 78: 413–415.

Murphy JJ (1996). Current practice and complications of temporary pacing. *British Medical Journal*, 312: 1134.

Murphy JJ (2001). Problems with temporary cardiac pacing. (Editorial). *British Medical Journal*, 323: 527.

Murphy JJ, Frain JPJ, Stephenson CJ (1995). Training and supervision of temporary transvenous pacemaker insertion. *British Journal of Clinical Practice*, 49: 126–128.

National Institute for Clinical Excellence (2000). *Guidance on the Use of Implantable Cardioverter Defibrillators for Arrhythmias*. National Institute for Clinical Excellence, London.

National Patient Safety Agency (2004). *Differing Crash Call Numbers*. NHS Patient Safety Alert. NPSA, London.

Newton A (2002). Witnesses resuscitation in critical care: the case against. *Intensive and Critical Care Nursing*, 18: 146–150.

New York Heart Association Criteria Committee (1973). *Diseases of the Heart and Blood Vessels: Nomenclature and Criteria for Diagnosis*, 6th edn. Little, Brown and Co., Boston.

O'Donnell C (1990). A survey of opinion amongst trained nurses and junior medical staff on current practices in resuscitation. *Journal of Advanced Nursing*, 15: 1175–1180.

O'Higgins F, Ward M, Nolan J (2001). Advanced life support skills undertaken by nurses – a UK survey. *Resuscitation*, 50: 45–49.

O'Rourke MF, Donaldson E, Geddes JS (1997). An airline cardiac arrest program. *Circulation*, 96: 2849–2853.

Parker J, Cleland JGF (1993). Choice of route for insertion of temporary pacing wires: recommendations of the medical practice committee and council of the British Cardiac Society. *British Heart Journal*, 70: 294–296.

Parsonnet V, Furman S, Smyth NP (1981). A revised code for pacemaker identification. Pacemaker Study Group. *Circulation*, 64: 60A–62A.

Peatfield RC, Sillett RW, Taylor D et al (1977). Survival after cardiac arrest in hospital. *Lancet*, 1: 1223–1225.

Petch MC (1999). Temporary cardiac pacing. *Postgraduate Medical Journal*, 3: 577–578.

Peters J, Ihle P (1990). Mechanics of the circulation during cardiopulmonary resuscitation: pathophysiology and techniques. *Intensive Care Medicine*, 16: 11–27.

Pizzetti F, Tarazza FM, Franzosi MG et al on behalf of the GISSI-3 Investigators (2001). Incidence and prognosis of atrial fibrillation in acute myocardial infarction: the GISSI-3 data. *Heart*, 86: 527–532.

Poole JE, White RD, Kanz KG (1997). Low energy impedance compensating biphasic waveforms terminate ventricular fibrillation at high rates in victims of out of hospital cardiac arrest. *Journal of Cardiovascular Electrophysiology*, 8: 1373–1385.

Poole-Wilson P (2002). Treatment of acute heart failure: out with the old and in with the new. Editorial. *Journal of the American Medical Association*, 287: 1578–1580.

Pycha C, Calabrese J, Gulledge A (1990). Patient and spouse adaptation to implantable defibrillators. *Cleveland Clinic Journal of Medicine*, 57: 441–444.

Quinn T (1998a) Early experience with nurse led elective cardioversion. *Nursing in Critical Care*, 3: 59–62.

Quinn T (1998b). Cardiopulmonary resuscitation: new European guidelines. *British Journal of Nursing*, 7 (18): 1070–1077.

Redley B, Hood K (1996). Staff attitudes towards family presence during resuscitation. *Accident and Emergency Nursing*, 4: 145–151.

Resuscitation Council (UK) (1996). *Should Relatives Witness Resuscitation?* Report from a project team of the Resuscitation Council (UK). Resuscitation Council, London.

Resuscitation Council (UK) (2000). *Resuscitation Council Guidelines*. Resuscitation Council, London.

Rich MW, Beckham V, Wittering C et al (1995). A multi disciplinary intervention to prevent the readmission of elderly patients with congestive heart failure. *New England Journal of Medicine*, 333: 1190–1195.

Robinson S et al (1998). Psychological effect of witnessed resuscitation on bereaved relatives. *The Lancet*, 352: 614–617.

Rogers AE, Addington-Hall JM, Abery et al (2000). Knowledge and communication difficulties for patients with chronic heart failure: qualitative study. *British Medical Journal*, 321: 605–607.

Sharma A, Hermann DD, Mehta RL (2001). Clinical benefit and approach of ultrafiltration in acute heart failure. *Cardiology*, 96: 144–154.

Shepardson LB, Younger SJ, Speroff T et al (1999). Increased risk of death in patients with do not resuscitate orders. *Medical Care*, 37: 727–737.

Simons RS, Howells TH (1986). The airway at risk. *British Medical Journal*, 292: 1722–1726.

Skinner DV, Camm AJ, Miles S (1985). Cardiopulmonary resuscitation skills of preregistration house officers. *British Medical Journal*, 290: 1549–1550.

Sullivan MJJ, Guyatt GH (1986). Simulated cardiac arrests for monitoring the quality of in-hospital resuscitation. *Lancet*, 2: 618–620.

Swan HJC, Ganz W, Forrester J (1970). Catheterization of the heart in man with use of a flow directed balloon-tipped catheter. *New England Journal of Medicine*, 283: 447–451.

Tang W, Weil MH, Sun S et al (2001). A comparison of biphasic and monophasic waveform defibrillation after prolonged ventricular fibrillation. *Chest*, 120: 948–954.

Thompson DR, Sutton TW (1985). Nursing decision-making in a coronary care unit. *International Journal of Nursing Studies*, 22: 259–266.

THRIFT II (Thrombo-embolic risk factors) Consensus Group (1998). Risk of and prophylaxis for venous thromboembolism in hospital patients. *Phlebology*, 13: 87–97.

UKCC (1992). *The Scope of Professional Practice*. UKCC, London.

Van de Werf F, Ardissino D, Betriu A, et al: The Task Force on the Management of Acute Myocardial Infarction of the European Society of Cardiology (2003). Management of acute myocardial infarction in patients presenting with ST-segment elevation. *European Heart Journal*, 24: 28–66.

Varnava AM, Sedgwick JE, Deaner et al (2002). Restricted weekend service inappropriately delays discharge after acute myocardial infarction. *Heart*, 87: 216–219.

Vaughan-Williams FM (1984). A classification of antiarrhythmic actions reassessed after a decade of new drugs. *Journal of Clinical Pharmacology*, 24: 129–147.

Waller DG, Robertson CE (1991). Role of sympathomimetic amines during cardiopulmonary resuscitation. *Resuscitation*, 22: 181–190.

West JA, Miller NH, Parker KM et al (1997). A comprehensive management system for heart failure improves clinical outcomes and reduces medical resource utilisation. *American Journal of Cardiology*, 79: 58–63.

Williams G, Wright DJ, Tan LB (2000). Management of cardiogenic shock complicating myocardial infarction: towards evidence based medical practice. *Heart*, 83: 621–626.

Wynne G, Marteau TM, Johnston M, Whiteley CA, Evans TR (1987). Inability of trained nurses to perform basic life support. *British Medical Journal*, 294: 1198–1199.

Wynne GA, Gwinnutt C, Bingham B, Van Someru V et al (1999). Teaching resuscitation. In *ABC of Resuscitation* (MC Colquhoun, AJ Handley, TR Evans, eds.), BMJ books, London, pp. 54–60.

Zoll PM (1952). Resuscitation of heart in ventricular standstill by external electrical stimulation. *New England Journal of Medicine*, 247: 768–771.

Zoll PM, Zoll RH (1985). Noninvasive temporary cardiac stimulation. *Critical Care Medicine*, 13: 925–926.

Chapter 8

Rehabilitation

INTRODUCTION

Cardiac rehabilitation is defined by the World Health Organization (1993) as 'The sum of activities required to influence favourably the underlying cause of the disease, as well as to ensure the patients the best possible physical, mental and social conditions so that they may, by their own efforts, preserve, or resume when lost, as normal a place as possible in the life of the community. Rehabilitation cannot be regarded as an isolated form of therapy, but must be integrated with the whole treatment, of which it forms only one facet' (p. 5). In essence, therefore, it is the process by which patients with coronary heart disease are helped to achieve their optimal level of recovery (physical, emotional, social, economic and vocational) and thus improve and extend their quality of life.

Cardiac rehabilitation has often been offered as a comprehensive package of services for patients whether or not they need all the components (Ades 2001). This seems to contradict the individualized approach to care. Programmes should offer a menu of available services, based on an assessment of individual need, which are selected in conjunction with the patient and which define the desired outcomes of each component (Thompson et al 1996b). Using this approach, patient outcomes can be measured against their own specific goals for each component of rehabilitation, making evaluation more relevant and reflective of achievement.

HISTORICAL PERSPECTIVE

The concept of cardiac rehabilitation has developed over the past five decades. In the first half of the last century coronary heart disease was relatively rare and tended to be confined to the elderly. Also, there was no visible handicap following the acute coronary attack. There was little objective knowledge available on which to base advice; return to work was considered ill-advised and there were many obstacles to a resumption of an active life. Prescribed treatment tended to comprise prolonged bed-rest for a period of 6 weeks in order to give the scarred heart muscle a chance to heal and allow the collateral circulation to develop. Levine (1944) advocated an easing of enforced bed-rest, citing its deleterious effect on patient morale and psychosocial recovery. However, despite mounting evidence to support early mobilization, clinical practice lagged behind and, as recently as the 1970s, some hospitals continued to keep patients in hospital for 6 weeks following an uncomplicated heart attack.

In the 1950s it became clear that the proportion of patients who could return to work was higher than expected and that subsequent progress was good. This led to the idea that it might be possible to improve an individual's physical capacity by designing training programmes. The next few years saw the development of various types of exercise training programmes and testing to evaluate their effect. These formed the basis of cardiac rehabilitation programmes, the focus of which was almost exclusively on exercise.

For many years, only the physical aspects of rehabilitation received attention, an attitude that still persists today in some quarters, with many rehabilitation programmes being referred to as exercise programmes. As a result, psychosocial rehabilitation has lagged behind physical rehabilitation, although it is now receiving more prominent attention. There is now an impressive body of knowledge pertaining to the effects of angina, myocardial infarction, heart failure and coronary revascularization on the family, work and economic status as well as on psychological state, and there is a need to incorporate such information into patient rehabilitation.

The early 1990s saw a significant growth in the number of cardiac rehabilitation programmes, and in 1992 the British Association for Cardiac Rehabilitation was launched. The importance of cardiac rehabilitation was emphasized in the National Service Framework for CHD (DoH 2000). National standards contained within it state that 'National Health Service (NHS) Trusts should put in place agreed protocols/systems of care so that, prior to leaving hospital, people admitted to hospital suffering from coronary heart disease have been invited to participate in a multidisciplinary programme of secondary prevention and cardiac rehabilitation. The aim of the programme will be to reduce their risk of subsequent cardiac problems and to promote their return to a full and normal life'.

EVIDENCE FOR EFFECTIVENESS

There is growing evidence attesting to the benefit of cardiac rehabilitation (Wenger et al 1995, NHS Centre for Reviews and Dissemination 1998, Dinnes et al 1999). These benefits include improvements in exercise tolerance, symptoms, blood lipid levels and psychosocial well-being as well as reductions in tobacco use and stress. Because cardiac rehabilitation is often a multifaceted intervention, with input from a range of health care professionals, it is often difficult to ascertain whether benefits, if they accrue, are due to a single component or a combination of them. However, exercise-based programmes certainly reduce all cause mortality (Jolliffe et al 2004).

Despite the evidence for the effectiveness of cardiac rehabilitation, referral to and uptake of services is variable, and only about a quarter of patients with myocardial infarction are enrolled into programmes (Bethell et al 2001). Most centres tend to restrict access to young, male, white patients who have suffered a (usually first, uncomplicated) myocardial infarction (Thompson et al 1997a, Lewin et al 1998), and certain groups are under-represented, including women, elderly people, ethnic minority groups and individuals who live in rural areas. Thus, there is a need to develop acceptable and accessible rehabilitation services (Tod et al 2002).

GUIDELINES, STANDARDS AND AUDIT

Clinical guidelines are aids to, not substitutes for, clinical judgement and are powerful tools for helping to put research evidence into practice and as such are an important part of any clinical effectiveness initiative. Guidelines for cardiac rehabilitation have been available in the USA for some years and are updated regularly (AACVPR 2002). National guidelines and audit standards in the UK have been produced (Thompson et al 1996a, 1996b, 1997b) with the aim of ensuring that cardiac rehabilitation is offered to all who are likely to benefit, based on an individual assessment of need, and followed by a later menu of options. Auditing and individual monitoring of the patient's progress should also accompany this.

Interventions that should be offered at each stage of the rehabilitation process include:

- a comprehensive assessment of risk
- a written, individualized plan
- lifestyle advice
- psychological interventions
- use of effective medications
- involvement of carers
- access to cardiac support groups
- aftercare and follow up.

Where appropriate, individuals may need:

- health promotion
- vocational advice
- structured exercise
- referral to specialist services.

SECONDARY PREVENTION

It is now recognized that comprehensive cardiac rehabilitation should be linked with secondary prevention. Indeed, the former is often an ideal vehicle for delivering the latter (Thompson and de Bono 1999). Correction of at least some of the risk factors associated with coronary heart disease seems likely to improve the patient's prognosis. Secondary prevention aims to stop or slow down the progression of disease or its consequences at any stage after its first occurrence. The rationale for secondary prevention is based on the assumption that even in the presence of coronary heart disease the progression of vascular lesions, arterial thrombosis and the occurrence of arrhythmias can favourably be influenced by a variety of metabolic and cardiovascular factors. Thus, for example, trials of exercise combined with nutritional counselling have shown a slowing of the atherosclerotic process

and decreased rates of subsequent coronary events and admission to hospital (Ades 2001).

Secondary prevention needs to be planned to cater for the individual's clinical and psychological state, lifestyle, health beliefs and future goals and expectations. Cardiovascular factors considered to be related to a poor prognosis, including extent of myocardial damage, increased cardiac volume, arrhythmias and conduction disturbances, unstable angina and increased likelihood of thrombus formation, require specific intervention. Diseases such as hypertension, diabetes mellitus and hyperlipidaemia need to be monitored and regulated. Obesity, nicotine abuse, stress, socioeconomic problems and a sedentary lifestyle are other modifiable factors. However, the implementation of secondary prevention and cardiac rehabilitation remains sub-optimal (Dalal et al 2004).

COMPONENTS OF REHABILITATION

The major components of rehabilitation of patients with acute coronary syndrome are the early ambulation, education and support of the patient and family, especially the partner. Medication, surgery and angioplasty also have an important role to play for some patients. In theory, the rehabilitation process should begin the moment the patient enters the hospital; in practice, it rarely does.

Few doubt the need for an organized and supervised programme of rehabilitation that incorporates a multidisciplinary approach. Although the nurse is, potentially, the key person to the programme, cardiac rehabilitation involves the use of a wide range of skills from different health professionals, including the cardiologist, physiotherapist, occupational therapist, dietician, clinical psychologist and social worker. The nurse assumes a central role in this process and is responsible, directly and indirectly, for coordinating interventions, referring to and liaising with other health professionals and controlling the many factors that influence the patient's recovery and welfare. The nurse is ideally placed for patient and family education and support because of the frequent contact and availability. The nurse is also responsible for assessing, planning, delivering, implementing and evaluating care for the patient and family.

PROCESS OF REHABILITATION

The process of rehabilitation should contain the following elements (Thompson et al 1996b):

- explanation and understanding
- specific rehabilitation interventions
- re-adaptation.

The phases and the elements contained within them should be flexible and tailored to suit the needs of the patient and family. This means that the timing and location of sessions need to be flexible and the length of participation in a programme sufficient to cater for the patient.

Rehabilitation should be viewed as a continuous and seamless process, though in many instances it is fragmented into phases. Using phases is outmoded and can be mechanistic, impose artificial boundaries and fragment care, although the following terms are still used in some settings:

Phase 1 (inpatient stay)
Phase 2 (immediate post-discharge period, up to 6 weeks)
Phase 3 (intermediate post-discharge period, 6–12 weeks)
Phase 4 (long-term maintenance period, indefinite).

Assessment

This involves determining the patient's needs, problems, desired health state, educational readiness, motivation, support structures, and physical and psychological suitability. All patients are likely to benefit from a rehabilitation plan that is tailored to suit them. A patient's self-assessment is likely to be helpful.

Planning

This involves using the information obtained in the assessment, together with knowledge of the resources available, to weigh alternatives, propose interventions and predict the realistic outcomes. It is essential that goals are realistic and achievable with plans being defined and agreed upon by the patient, family and health care professionals.

Implementation

This involves carrying out the strategies that have been planned. This stage needs to be flexible, as the patient's problems and goals may change. Unexpected problems may occur on discharge and priorities may change as the patient experiences the reality of having a cardiac problem. The personality of both the patient and the nurse and the interaction between them is likely to be an important factor in the rehabilitation process. Other factors such as family members, friends, fellow patients, health care workers, the media, culture, and past experience, will also be important.

The main function of the nurse is to enable the patient and family to understand, accept and adapt to the acute coronary event and any necessary limitations this entails; to stimulate them to take an active part in recovery and rehabilitation; to assist them in making realistic plans for the future; and to provide support, understanding and guidance. It is essential that the coronary care unit staff adopt an attitude of optimism and realism. From early convalescence in hospital the patient and family should be encouraged that a return to normal functioning within a matter of a few weeks is not only expected, but is also safe and beneficial. Individualized cardiac rehabilitation that starts early and is based on guidelines seems to be effective, with improvements in quality of life, more confidence about returning to activities and fewer treatment needs (Thompson et al 1996a, Mayou et al 2002).

Successful rehabilitation should not be viewed narrowly in terms of economic or vocational outcomes, but rather as the achievement of a lifestyle which enables the patient and family to enjoy a full and active life, with some allowance for impairment. Initially, the cardiac rehabilitation programme consists of patient education, often coupled with counselling, and exercise. The education component consists of teaching the patient and family better to understand the illness, including the factors that may have caused it, and its management, to enable them to assume responsibility for care. It is also necessary for the nurse to offer emotional support, correct misperceptions, instil hope and provide optimism. The exercise component involves a graduated and progressive approach, beginning with passive and low-level activities.

Evaluation

The outcome of rehabilitation needs to be evaluated by determining whether the aims of the rehabilitation process for that individual have been achieved. The lack of agreement about a successful recovery, a lack of standardized interventions, and an inconsistency in the use of outcome measurement tools for evaluation, make it difficult to ascertain objectively the effectiveness of rehabilitation programmes.

For each patient, the following questions could to be asked:

1 Is the patient back to normal activities of living?
2 Are the demands of living within the limits of the patient's functional capacity?
3 Is the patient psychologically stable?
4 Have measures against risk been implemented?
5 Has the patient's quality of life improved?

COMPLIANCE, ADHERENCE AND CONCORDANCE

One way of evaluating rehabilitation is to determine patient concordance. The term compliance assumes that behaviour change will automatically follow the delivery of expert information. This is clearly not the case in many instances. A more accurate term is concordance, which takes into account the patient's context and encourages him or her to be an active decision maker.

The factors affecting compliance, adherence and concordance are complex, and theories and models have been developed in an attempt to clarify and explain them. However, no single theory explains why some individuals comply, adhere or concord and others do not. Various strategies may help but they are likely to be influenced by individual circumstances. Difficulties in adhering to health advice may occur at any stage of the health-illness continuum, ranging from keeping outpatient clinic appointments to following dietary advice and taking medications. Denial, for instance, may present an obstacle and patients first have to recognize and accept that they have a serious problem before accepting the need for any lifestyle modification. The stress of modifying and constantly monitoring behaviour has to be weighed against the predicted benefits of such changes.

Non-adherence or non-concordance may be manifested in a number of forms such as delay in seeking help, not participating in health-check programmes, breaking appointments and failing to follow advice. However, this is often notoriously difficult to measure and it is likely that, in relation to rehabilitation, it will be related to an amalgamation of heeding suggestions, compromising and choosing not to follow advice.

LIFESTYLE CHANGE

In practice, changing an individual's behaviour is notoriously difficult and is fraught with problems. Efforts are more likely to be successful in those patients who are willing and able to make changes to their lifestyle. It is important to acknowledge that many patients make spontaneous changes to their lifestyle when confronted with the knowledge that they have heart disease. Many others respond to brief advice or behaviour change counselling (Rollnick et al 1999) and it is only in the more 'resistant' instances that one needs to resort to other more specialized techniques, such as motivational interviewing (Miller and Rollnick 2002).

Brief advice consists of:

- asking permission
- using open questions
- demonstrating respect
- providing clear information
- encouraging responsibility.

Behaviour change counselling is more complex but consists of:

- establishing rapport
- using empathy
- setting the agenda
- exchanging information
- using open questions
- listening with empathy
- rolling with resistance.

Thus, there will be issues such as assessing motivation and brainstorming solutions. The former can be assessed by questions such as:

- How important is it for you ...?
- How confident are you that you will succeed?

Whereas, the latter can be aided by statements such as:

- I have a number of ideas
- I know about what worked with others.

However, there are numerous factors that inhibit patients and carers from making changes to their lifestyle, or result in lapses, and these should be acknowledged. It is difficult to change the behaviour of individuals through advice alone; there must be an incentive for change. Concordance to any measures instituted is much more likely to be accomplished if health care professionals understand the principles of behaviour change and apply, where appropriate, such strategies. There are some notable examples of where such strategies have been successful in accomplishing lifestyle change, notably the multiple risk factor intervention (MULTIFIT) programme (Miller and Taylor 1995). This programme is designed to facilitate patients' recovery in the first year following a myocardial infarction. However, many of the principles can be applied to all acute coronary syndrome patients. Some of the key elements are described below.

Individuals are likely to change behaviour when they believe they are at risk of developing a problem, when they believe the recommended change will improve their condition or reduce their risk, and when they have the ability to accomplish the desired changes (Becker 1974). It is, therefore, important to discuss the following with each patient (and carer) for each behaviour to be changed (Miller and Taylor 1995):

- why the patient is at risk
- how the recommended changes will improve the patient's condition or reduce his/her risk
- whether the patient has the confidence and resources to accomplish the change.

Individuals may be at differing stages of readiness to change (Prochaska and DiClemente 1983):

- pre-contemplation: considering change but not strongly committed
- contemplation: willing to change and can be influenced to do so
- action: highly committed to change and has begun process.

This can be assessed fairly easily by simply asking the patient if he or she intends to adopt a particular behaviour.

The following principles are adopted by the MULTIFIT programme (Miller and Taylor 1995) in guiding lifestyle intervention:

1   Build positive and accurate expectations
2   Define the behaviour to be changed
3   Help patients set realistic goals
4   Use contracts to enhance commitment
5   Prepare for lapses/relapses
6   Model the desired behaviour
7   Use prompts to remind the patient of the desired behaviour
8   Provide feedback about the patient's progress
9   Teach problem solving
10   Reward achievement
11   Enlist appropriate social support as needed.

Accomplishing behaviour change is difficult but maintaining it is even more difficult. Behaviour strategies that are likely to affect this include:

- contracting: written agreements about setting goals (which are well-defined)
- social support: partner, family, friend or health care professional
- self-monitoring and feedback: activity log, feedback in the form of praise
- relapse prevention: warning signals/high risk situations indicating relapse may occur.

Lack of skills, time, organizational support and educational materials have presented obstacles in maintaining behaviour strategies. Novel approaches will need to be considered. One promising avenue is the use of a computerized telephone conversation system (telephone-linked care) designed to offer nutrition and exercise counselling (Glanz et al 2003). This has been rated well in terms of satisfaction and helpfulness.

EDUCATION, COUNSELLING AND SOCIAL SUPPORT

The terms education, teaching and counselling are often used interchangeably. They are used to give blanket coverage for processes that share certain principles and strategies. It is important to make distinctions between them if one is to select the most appropriate approach for the patient. Patient education is the process of influencing behaviour, producing changes in knowledge and attitudes and the skills required to maintain and improve health, whereas patient teaching is only one component of the education process: the actual imparting of information. Counselling is largely concerned with helping patients cope with their situation by leading them to the discovery and utilization of their own coping mechanisms. Most patients are likely to need information, some modification in behaviour and/or attitude, and some reassurance and psychological support.

In terms of chronic disease management programmes, patient education is the most commonly used intervention (Weingarten et al 2002). Education, feedback and reminders are associated with significant improvement in patient disease control.

Patient education

Patient education plays a major role in compliance and successful rehabilitation. Providing information to assist patient understanding is fundamental in helping the patient cope with his illness and treatment. Patient teaching can be seen as the systematic provision of relevant information and knowledge for those with a health problem.

Traditionally, patient education has been a key component of nursing (Redman 1997), although in relation to acute coronary patients nurses seem to be unclear about their actual role in this activity, what they should teach and the precise nature and content of the information given (Scott and Thompson 2003). Lack of preparation, peer support, time and positive feedback are all reasons why nurses may not fulfill this aspect of their role. This is compounded by patients being in hospital for shorter periods and in some instances being discharged before full recovery. For patients to care successfully for themselves after discharge, they often must gain essential knowledge and skills before returning home.

Patients often report that their need for information is unsatisfied and they remain anxious, ignorant and uncertain about what they should do. Specific barriers to the education of acute coronary patients include their short length of hospital stay, especially in the coronary c[...] of drugs, especially narcotic a[...] for adequate rest and the empha[...] on the technical aspects of patient care. [...] care unit nurse may consider that patient [...] tion is best accomplished when the patient is stable and ought, therefore, to be postponed until patients are on the ward. The nurse in the medical ward may assume that the experts in the coronary care unit have already provided necessary information.

Major obstacles to the provision of effective patient education include:

1 insufficient time to prepare and carry out teaching
2 inadequate knowledge of the content to be taught
3 insufficient time to document all aspects of teaching.

There appears to be a difference between nurses' and patients' perceptions of the nurse's role in patient education. In a systematic review, Scott and Thompson (2003) found that nurses identified the role of the nurse as being the most suitable for patient teaching for coronary patients, whereas patients most frequently chose a physician to teach them specific information related to their condition, and also that patients expressed greater preference for physicians to teach them cardiac information, and noted that this implied that patients view physicians as being the more credible authority for giving information needed to restore and maintain health. Such findings suggest that coronary care nurses need to develop a clear definition of their role in patient education and implement strategies to improve patients' perceptions of nurses as authoritative patient educators.

The nature of education

Education involves instruction, advice, explanation, listening, leading discussion and helping the patient make decisions. A brief chat and supplying a booklet to the coronary patient is not a substitute for detailed nurse–patient discussion. Many patients and their families are poorly informed and have little idea of what is happening. They therefore need useful and relevant information to explain what has happened and what is expected.

Much patient teaching is based on nurses' assumptions of patient learning needs rather than individualized learning needs assessments and the evaluation of patient learning is often limited. Education programmes should emphasize: the assessment of individual learning needs and learning styles; the identification of patient-specific content; the selection of appropriate teaching methods; and the evaluation of learning (Barber-Parker 2002).

The process of patient education should include an assessment of the patient's characteristics in relation to learning, planning behavioural objectives and selecting a method of achieving them, intervention based on learning principles and evaluation of the products of teaching to determine if goals have been achieved.

Assessment needs to involve an appraisal of the patient's motivation, physical and emotional state, knowledge deficit, learning readiness and level of comprehension. Planned learning objectives, set in conjunction with the patient, need to include cognitive, affective and psychomotor components. The understanding of new information will be at its best when the patient is motivated and when the information is presented clearly, concisely, in small doses and is considered relevant (Redman 1997). Advice and information needs to be tailored to individual needs and should be given early, systematically and consistently.

The lack of information patients and family members receive about their stay in hospital, treatment and subsequent recovery is well documented. Yet it is the responsibility of all health professionals, especially the nurse, to ensure the patient and family understand the illness, the purpose of treatment and how to cope outside hospital.

Objectives of education

The main objective of education is to give the patient and family a basic understanding of the illness and recovery process. However, during the patient's stay in hospital, the goals are essentially to reduce the feeling of helplessness, help restore self-esteem and bolster confidence in terms of a successful outcome, enhancing the patient's ability to cope with the coronary event. Patients who understand the cause and likely outcome of their illness and its management are likely to have an improved ability and motivation to adhere to advice and treatment, and cope with the problems of illness.

It seems likely that patients and their families do benefit from being given information, which results in less anxiety, more participation and an increased sense of control. Patients particularly need information about their condition, treatment and hospital stay, and about returning home, because they seem to lack knowledge of how they can expect to feel, how much they can expect to be able to do, and how long recovery will take. It is important that those potential events that are likely to occur when professional help is unavailable are discussed.

Planning education

Contemporary approaches to patient teaching are numerous and varied, but information needs to be given in a consistent and structured fashion. Advice must be realistic, practical and very specific about what should be done (Thompson 2002). Certainly nurses should avoid vague and useless advice such as 'take it easy' and 'don't worry', which is often responsible for the delayed return to normal functioning. An education programme is designed to provide the patient and family with enough information about the coronary event and its management to enable them to assume increasing responsibility for their future health.

Subject matter

Scott and Thompson (2003) found that patients rated their perceived information needs as:

- personal risk factors and modification
- structure and function of the heart
- medications
- physical activity
- diet
- psychological factors.

Changes in the ranking of these information categories occur over the illness trajectory and are congruent with decreasing levels of patient dependency. The nurse, physician and patient generally agree upon certain topics which should be included for discussion, including, most importantly, those just outlined and the nature of the disease, emergency measures, resumption of activities, and physical, psychosocial and financial problems encountered on return to home and work. Neglected topics include instruction on recording the pulse, resuming sexual activity and convalescing after the coronary event.

In hospital
- Acceptance of the illness
- understanding the reasons for early mobility
- understanding the reasons for stopping smoking
- how to recognize possible limiting factors in physical activity
- understanding existing residual symptoms
- advice on diet, social activities and sexual life
- advice on resuming work.

During convalescence
- Understanding the importance of regular, graduated physical training
- accepting long-term control of possible risk factors
- understanding prescribed drug treatment and possible adverse reactions
- understanding about the optimal time to resume sexual activity, leisure pursuits and hobbies
- resumption of travel
- preparing for return to work
- understanding significance of symptoms and action to be taken.

After rehabilitation
- Reinforcing secondary preventative measures.

Information in hospital

Information in hospital is given to increase the patient's and family's understanding of what has happened, what is being done and what they can do to help themselves. The information should be practical and relevant to the individuals concerned and should not be vague or ambiguous.

Brief explanations regarding the staff, equipment, layout, procedures and routines of the coronary care unit will reduce the likelihood of worry and misunderstanding and help the patient and family adjust to the crisis. The nurse should be careful to avoid bombarding patients with information

during the acute phase of the coronary event, as they are unlikely to retain much of it during the crisis stage when readiness for learning is impaired by fear, anxiety, pain and fatigue. They are, however, likely to benefit from answers to specific questions.

Information should be clear, simple and repeated frequently. The type of information to be imparted needs to be considered. For instance, if the patient has to undergo a painful invasive procedure, information regarding the likely experiences and sensations will be more effective in alleviating anxiety than details about the procedure alone. Certainly, psychological factors and the level of cardiac information are important considerations that may affect the amount of information patients gain during hospital and influence their rate of recovery (Thompson and Lewin 2000). When the patient's mental and physical condition permits the assimilation of more detailed and complex information, the nurse can provide information about the medical condition and the limitations, possible problems and likely outcome associated with it.

Structure and function of the heart

A general discussion of the normal cardiac structure and function and the disturbances that result from atheroma, leading to a heart attack, should be presented so that the patient and family understand the disease process and its effect on functioning.

Visual presentation is usually best using a variety of illustrations, audiovisual aids, literature and models. A plastic model of the heart is a useful adjunct for demonstrating the coronary arteries and explaining about the blood supply and oxygenation of the heart. This helps correct the common myth that the heart receives its nourishment from blood flowing through the four chambers. The patient can then be taught how myocardial oxygen extraction results in increased oxygen demand requiring increased flow. The atherosclerotic process then follows, including plaque formation and progressive narrowing and obstruction, often consequently resulting in myocardial infarction. The discussion should include an explanation of pain and other symptoms that the patient may have such as sweating, palpitations and shortness of breath. The role of coronary artery spasm can be briefly discussed if the patient has a history of variant angina. The healing process of the heart and the meanings of the ECG and laboratory findings should also be briefly explained.

The nurse needs to correct any misconceptions patients may have. For instance, that they understand that the underlying problem is in the coronary arteries and not in the heart itself, and that the heart is a muscle and able to adapt and recover its function (Thompson and Lewin 2000).

Information for convalescence

It is not uncommon for the patient and family to be left to cope by themselves with vague instructions about increasing activity, resulting in uncertainty that leads to distress and maladjustment. Therefore, a well-planned programme is essential for anticipating the homecoming, with specific and individual instructions concerning activity levels, lifestyle and medications.

Patients and partners often have specific information needs during the period of convalescence, including resumption of leisure, sexual and work activities and guidelines on drinking, driving, smoking and weight. General health recommendations for all coronary patients and their families should include:

- a varied diet with appropriate caloric intake to achieve or maintain an ideal body weight
- the cessation of smoking
- a programme of regular physical activity
- a regular health examination, including measurement of blood pressure, and control if necessary.

Discussion and counselling regarding the psychological problems that may confront the patient and partner after discharge is essential, as these are often more disabling than the physical illness. They should be warned about common physical and psychological sequelae, such as moodiness, tearfulness, disturbed sleep, irritability, acute awareness of minor somatic sensations, and poor concentration and memory (Thompson and Lewin 2000). It should be further explained that these symptoms are normal, and universal, and that they are part of the natural course of recovery after a potentially life-threatening event. The partner may have

specific needs that they may want to discuss in privacy. Giving adequate information and support to the partner is likely to affect the patient indirectly. The partner's reaction and response may be a source of worry for the patient.

What to expect during recovery

The patient and family need information on what to expect during the first few weeks and months following recovery. Common issues are:

- uncertainty about what constitutes a safe level of exercise
- over-protectiveness by spouse and family
- conflicting advice from hospital and family doctor
- when to return to work and strenuous activity
- boredom and irritability at home
- concern over angina and breathlessness
- the reason for the acute cardiac event
- uncertainty about informing insurance company and dealing with benefits
- concern regarding the use of drugs
- unsuitable housing
- the need for definite guidelines about resuming work, sexual relations, driving, drinking and leisure activities
- the need for definite guidelines about the amount of weight to lose and how to stop smoking.

The patient and family are likely to be unable to foresee many of these potential problems or areas of concern and so the nurse needs to be able to anticipate them.

When to seek professional advice

During the first months of recovery the patient is likely to be seen by the physician in the outpatient department and by the family doctor. Patients need to be advised to inform them if they experience an increase in severity or number of episodes of angina, shortness of breath, palpitations, weakness, side effects of medications or emotional problems. Such matters can usually be dealt with by a visit to the family doctor. Keeping a diary of symptoms, which gives a record of the timing, duration and associated factors, will help the patient present accurate information. Writing down any questions that come to mind and making a list of points to cover at visits to the doctor will ensure that the visits are productive.

It should be stressed to the patient and family that they must promptly summon an ambulance in the event of the occurrence of symptoms suggesting a heart attack.

Timing of patient education

Formal teaching needs to begin once the individual displays a readiness to learn. Prior to this, informal sessions explaining immediate care, answering specific questions and setting the scene for future sessions are likely to help establish a relationship with the patient that will facilitate later teaching. Formal teaching sessions need to be of short duration; 20 minutes has been acknowledged as the maximum attention span by many educationalists. Privacy is essential yet difficult to achieve in a busy unit or ward: a side room, day room or office may be a suitable place. It is important not to overwhelm the patient with information, as this may be tiring and precipitate stress and possible cardiac symptoms. Teaching needs to be carried out at a time suitable for the patient, family, especially partner, and the nurse. Setting a fixed time for teaching sessions serves to emphasize the importance that is attached to the activity.

Methods of providing information

Instructional aids for the nurse exist in three formats: printed, audiovisual and physical. When evaluating these materials the nurse needs carefully to consider vocabulary, sentence construction and length, illustrations, type size and readability, and correctness of the information presented. Certainly, oral discussions should be supplemented by written material, and perhaps by a variety of audiovisual aids and models, which make the presentation more attractive and varied and helps improve retention. Written and taped information should complement the verbal communication and if required be available in appropriate languages. Educational impact can be maximized by using a variety of formats, such as education classes or group discussions. Treatment plans should be discussed with the patient and partner and a copy of the plan given to them.

Teaching should not be totally confined to structured formal teaching sessions. The patient and family need to feel that they can ask questions mulling over in their minds. Encouraging patients to write down any questions they may have, for example after a medical round, is likely to reduce misconceptions and anxiety.

Teaching and learning are a two-way process and the patient's knowledge, desires and goals must be incorporated into all aspects of it. Certainly, learning will vary between patients because of differences in general educational background and intellectual ability.

The nurse needs to assess the patient and family before beginning the teaching. The assessment includes demographic variables, including family composition, ethnic and religious background and educational level; the patient's and family's pre-existing knowledge and misconceptions; the patient's lifestyle and habits; and the patient's readiness to learn. Specific instructions provide important individualized information and give the patient and family a framework on which to build. Verbal information is more effective when simple language is used. Earlier statements are remembered better than later ones. Repetition also increases recall, as does specific rather than general advice.

Evaluation of education

Questionnaires and tests devised for evaluating the patient's needs and levels of knowledge and learning are useful adjuncts. In assessing the efficacy of an educational programme, it is important to differentiate between what the patients learn and what they may do about it. The acquisition of new information does not necessarily result in a change of behaviour. It is difficult to measure the specific effects of education on the outcome of rehabilitation programmes. Counselling, social support, exercise training and family involvement may all contribute towards rehabilitation success.

The goals of health education are the desired outcome behaviours, i.e. the patient understanding the level of activity that places the least demand on the heart. These goals have to be clear and precise and need to be written so that they may be evaluated. Evaluation serves to provide a measure of the patient's knowledge and understanding, a basis for further teaching, feedback for the nurse on the effectiveness of the teaching and reinforcement of successful behaviours in the patient. Evaluation of the outcome of education will vary with patient goals and therefore needs to incorporate feedback from the patient, family and nurse. The education needs of various groups such as women, elderly people and ethnic minority groups appear not to have been assessed systematically and patients have often not been involved in the design of evaluation instruments.

Education goals can include:

- changes in health consciousness
- changes in knowledge
- changes in self-awareness and attitude
- decision making
- behaviour change
- social change.

Counselling

Counselling, which has been variously defined, essentially involves one person helping another through purposeful conversation in an understanding atmosphere. It is linked with education and forms an intrinsic part of the nurse's role in rehabilitation.

There are various models of counselling, but none needs to be adhered to rigidly because counselling should be a dynamic flexible process. The patient sets the style and pace of the counselling process, although the nurse needs to be an active partner in the interaction. Posture, gesture, touch and facial expression will contribute to the communication. A hurried approach is likely to limit the effectiveness of the interaction, and therefore adequate planned time should be given specifically for such sessions to give credence and increase the patient's feeling of self-worth.

Unlike many counselling sessions, the acute coronary patient in hospital is rarely actively seeking the skills of a counsellor. The nurse needs to ensure that patients are aware that it is appropriate for them to be approached with problems and concerns and to ask questions. It may help initially if

the nurse approaches the patient. Looking after the patient from admission means that a relationship that can be developed, will already exist between the nurse and the patient. Asking questions such as 'Tell me how you feel?' will initiate conversation and begin the interaction, which needs to be purposeful and not dissolve into aimless chit-chat.

The aims of counselling are to make the situation safe (without threat to the patient), to enable patients to express their feelings, to communicate understanding and empathy and acceptance of patients, and to share personal feelings with them as well as to support them. It is also an opportunity to explore attributions and correct misconceptions (Furze et al 2001).

The nurse uses a mixture of *open questions,* which encourage expression about thoughts and feelings (e.g. 'How do you think you are going to cope at home?') and *closed questions,* which are useful for obtaining information and facts (e.g. 'Does your wife go out to work?'). *Leading questions,* which suggest the expected answer in the question (e.g. 'You wouldn't want to go back to work too soon, would you?') and *statements that sound like questions,* which leave the patient uncertain as to whether to respond (e.g. 'You quarrel with your wife don't you?') should be avoided.

Skills involved in counselling are multiple and complex. They include rapport, empathy, a non-judgemental attitude, understanding and responding appropriately. To be successful nurses need to have an understanding of the information they are likely to be asked to provide and the confidence to present it to the patient in a way that is understood and relevant. On some occasions the patient may not want specific answers but just welcome the opportunity to express worries and talk through problems. The appropriate use of silence during interactions may give the patient an opportunity to work out problems and answers for himself. The nurse may be able to make the best use of the interaction for the patient by reflecting, paraphrasing and summarizing the topics covered to give clarity and structure.

Resistance represents an important signal of dissonance within the counselling process and it is important that this is recognized and addressed (Miller and Rollnick 2002). Resistance can mean that it is less likely that behaviour change will occur.

Motivational interviewing

Motivational interviewing (Miller and Rollnick 2002) has assumed increasing interest and importance in the field of health care, especially in public health and medical settings. Although it has its roots in addiction counselling, it is used to address a range of health behaviours, such as smoking, diet, physical activity, pain management, sexual behaviour and adherence (Resnicow et al 2002). In contrast to addiction counselling, where the client often has been referred to or has sought treatment for their condition, the acute coronary patient has not sought to do this, and it is usually the nurse that raises issues such as smoking, diet or exercise. However, perhaps the most limiting factor in using motivational interviewing is time. The nurse's contact with the patient is limited in terms of frequency and duration, usually typified to around four contact sessions, each lasting perhaps 15 minutes or so. Thus, there is a need to adapt it into a briefer format suited to limited contact. Motivational interviewing-based techniques tailored to brief encounters have been developed by Rollnick et al (1999). One example of this approach, described earlier, is the 0–10 importance/confidence strategy, which allows the nurse to assess motivation and facilitate patient movement along the change continuum (Rollnick et al 1999).

Evaluation of counselling

There is a growing body of evidence from primary and secondary research showing that counselling is an effective intervention not only for patients but for partners too, especially if combined with education (Linden et al 1996, Dusseldorp et al 1999). In-hospital counselling improves knowledge and satisfaction and reduces psychological distress in patients and partners (Thompson and Meddis 1990a,b) and these effects are maintained with extended forms of counselling (Johnston et al 1999). There is evidence that psychoeducational counselling can also reduce morbidity and even mortality (Linden et al 1996, Dusseldorp et al 1999).

It is difficult to determine which of the components of the psychological support are responsible for the effect. For instance, is it the education,

counselling or just attention, or is it a combination? Further research is needed to determine which techniques are superior. Clearly, however, such interventions are useful and have substantial benefits over conventional nursing and medical care.

MODIFICATION OF RISK FACTORS AND HEALTH PROMOTION

Risk factors

Studies have shown that coronary patients consider information on risk factors and their modification to be their most important learning need (Scott and Thompson 2003).

The teaching programme should include those risk factors relevant to the patient, particularly those that may result in an increased risk of reinfarction. The potential benefits of changing them should be carefully considered. Teaching patients about risk factors presumes that they will change them when informed about the relative risks involved. However, health education, be it on an individual or mass media basis, is not sufficient by itself to produce desired changes in health behaviour. Scant attention has been paid by nurses and other health professionals to functional behaviour and the strategies which are effective in changing behaviour. There is also a paucity of evidence available to demonstrate that long-term changes with risk factors result from behaviour therapy.

Lifestyle modification does not occur easily. Denial frequently has to be overcome, and motivation and belief in the change are necessary. The patient needs time to consider and reappraise the situation. Change is then introduced gradually, with the patient's full consent and cooperation. Modifying behaviour is a long-term process and this needs to be appreciated by all concerned.

The concept of risk factors currently dominates thinking about the aetiology and pathogenesis of coronary heart disease. These so-called risk factors have been identified from epidemiological evidence: a person with a given risk factor associates positively with the risk of the disease. However, it by no means follows that risk factors are causal. Even a positive association does not necessarily imply causation – a maxim that is often disregarded.

In the context of public heath, modifiable risk factors, such as certain dietary factors, are distinguishable from immutable or non-modifiable risk factors, such as sex. The main risk factors are generally believed to be hypercholesterolaemia, hypertension, cigarette smoking, obesity, lack of voluntary physical exercise, personality, diabetes mellitus and a family history of coronary heart disease.

Although the hospital setting provides an ideal environment for discussing and motivating the patient to adopt a healthier lifestyle, educational opportunities are constrained by the anxiety and general crisis of the situation. Therefore, such advice needs to be reinforced over a long period of time. Nevertheless, the latter part of the patient's stay in hospital affords an ideal opportunity for founding patient and family education.

Blood cholesterol

The risk of coronary heart disease is directly related to blood cholesterol levels. Blood cholesterol levels can be reduced by drugs, physical activity and dietary changes, in particular a reduction in the consumption of saturated fat. It is estimated that 45% of deaths from coronary heart disease in men and 47% of deaths from coronary heart disease in women are due to a raised blood cholesterol level (in this case greater than 5.2 mmol/l) and that 10% of deaths from coronary heart disease in the UK could be avoided if everyone in the population had a blood cholesterol of less than 6.5 mmol/l (National Heart Forum 2002).

Lipid is a general term that is used to refer to animal and plant fats and oils. The main lipids are cholesterol and triglycerides. The link between cholesterol and atherosclerosis is strong, whereas that between triglycerides and atherosclerosis is more tenuous. *Cholesterol* is essential for cell membrane function and synthesizing myelin sheaths and steroid hormones.

Triglycerides are the principal components of lipid and are composed of fatty acids and glycerol. They are broken into free fatty acids and provide an important source of energy.

Saturated fats are fatty acids that have no double bonds between the carbon atoms in their molecules. Animal fats are usually considered to be saturated fats, although their unsaturated fatty acid content may be quite high. Fats containing predominantly saturated fatty acids tend to be solid at room temperature.

Unsaturated fats are found in vegetable and fish oils, most nuts, fruit and corn oil. They contain double bonds in their carbon chain and tend to be liquid at room temperature.

Hyperlipidaemia is a general term that refers to abnormally raised levels of total blood lipids and can mean an excess of cholesterol, triglyceride or both.

Hypercholesterolaemia is common with over half the British population having cholesterol levels exceeding the 'optimal' 5.0 mmol/l. *Cholesterol* is not water soluble and it is transported attached to a protein to form a lipoprotein.

Lipoproteins are complex compounds consisting of various densities. Although a high total plasma cholesterol concentration is a very strong risk factor for coronary heart disease, the risk actually depends on the concentration of low-density lipoprotein (LDL) cholesterol. It is estimated that up to 30% of deaths from coronary heart disease are due to unhealthy diets (National Heart Forum 2002). However, it is unlikely that diet alone will achieve target cholesterol concentrations, and a pragmatic approach is recommended with all patients suffering an acute coronary syndrome being prescribed hypolipidaemic therapy before discharge from hospital. Statins are the preferred drugs for secondary prevention, but the choice and starting dose is contentious (Jowett and Thompson 2003).

Despite excellent evidence of cholesterol-lowering in post-infarct patients around 80% of British patients surveyed in 1996 still had a cholesterol of 5 mmol/l or more following myocardial infarction (Bowker et al 1996).

Alcohol consumption

Observational studies consistently show an inverse (U-shaped) relationship between alcohol intake and death from coronary heart disease (Thun et al 1997). Moderate drinking of 1–2 units per day, particularly of wine, is associated with a 20% reduction in coronary events, which is lower than those who do not drink alcohol (Department of Health 1995).

For men, the upper limit is around 20 units of alcohol per week, and for women, 15 units per week. One unit is equivalent to half a pint of beer, a glass of wine or sherry or a single whisky or other spirit.

Beer is very fattening and the patient trying to lose weight will benefit from drinking alternatives. If the patient does drink excessively, rehabilitation may be an ideal opportunity to tackle the problem. Discussing why the patient feels he needs to drink heavily, how this need has become a habit, and then working out a plan for breaking the habit, are ways in which the nurse can be involved.

Caffeine consumption

Coffee, tea, cocoa and cola contain methylxanthines of which caffeine is one. There is about 65 mg of caffeine in an average cup of instant coffee. In high doses, caffeine acts as a stimulant and produces a tachycardia due to decreased vagal stimulation. There is some controversy in regard to whether there is a relationship between coffee and tea drinking and the incidence of myocardial infarction. It seems unrealistic to advise patients to cut down on consumption unless it is excessive or there is a history of palpitations.

Obesity

Overweight and obesity increase the risk of coronary heart disease. It is estimated that about 5% of deaths from coronary heart disease in men and that 6% of such deaths in women are due to obesity and that 2% of deaths from coronary heart disease in the UK could be avoided if targets for the prevalence of obesity (6% for men and 8% for women) were to be achieved (National Heart Forum 2002).

In Western countries, in particular, there is an increase in the prevalence of obesity. Obesity occurs when energy intake exceeds energy output and the excess is stored as fat, mainly in the abdomen and known as central obesity. This can be identified by a high waist to hip ratio. The effect of obesity in general is to increase blood pressure, blood volume, resting cardiac output, left ventricular filling pressure and vascular resistance. All these factors will result in increased cardiac work. Obesity also impairs glucose tolerance and slightly increases plasma uric acid. It is, therefore, desirable for obese

Table 8.1 BMI ranges defining degrees of obesity (WHO 1998)

WHO classification	BMI (kg/m^2)	Health risk
Underweight	<18.5	Low (but may indicate other health problems)
Normal	18.5–24.9	Average ('ideal' weight)
Overweight	25.0–29.9	Mild increase
Obese	>30.0	
Class I	30.0–34.9	Moderate
Class II	35.0–39.9	Severe
Class III	>40.0	Very severe

patients to lose weight by decreasing caloric intake and increasing energy expenditure. The goal is to achieve a body weight appropriate to age, height and sex. A distinction should be made between 'average' weights and 'ideal' weights. The former are always higher in the West, where people overeat. The latter are based on the pooled experience of life assurance companies, who have calculated desirable weight based on excess mortality figures. Obesity may be assessed by the *body mass index* (BMI) that adjusts the weight for height:

$$BMI = \frac{Weight\ (kg)}{Height^2\ (m)}$$

Internationally accepted ranges of BMI used to define degrees of obesity are shown in Table 8.1. Since abdominal fat relates more strongly to coronary heart disease than does fat on the limbs or hips, the waist:hip ratio may be a better predictor of cardiovascular mortality than the BMI (Royal College of Physicians of London 1998).

Losing weight

There are several causes of obesity, including affluence, obesity in the family (role modelling and eating habits within the family) and lifestyle (an increase in sedentary lifestyle with ageing). Psychological factors such as boredom, stress and poor self-image may also contribute. The nurse needs to try to ascertain the cause when counselling and establish with the patient and family a realistic, agreeable goal for weight reduction, and assist in planning a reward system. A regular record, such as a graph, should be kept which gives a quick and effective indication of progress. The hospital is an ideal setting for launching the plan, which must be relevant to the patient's lifestyle, culture and socioeconomic status. Practical advice should consist of calorie intake versus calorie expenditure, eating foods slowly and in small amounts, regular physical activity, regular meal times, and attempting to resolve any underlying psychological problems.

The patient needs to be aware that when caloric intake is reduced there is an initial rapid loss of weight that is due primarily to water loss. As reduction in caloric intake continues, the basal metabolic rate will decline. Therefore, further weight loss may not occur unless the metabolic rate is increased (e.g. through exercise). Too frequent weighing may produce disillusionment and decreased motivation. The problem of being overweight needs to be taken in the context of other risk factors. The patient who is struggling to give up smoking may benefit initially from being advised against gaining weight. The positive aspects of losing weight, such as increased vitality, improved physical appearance and self-esteem, need to be emphasized.

The priority is weight control plus risk factor reduction, not major weight loss (Hooper 2001). However, it will be more difficult to influence the patient credibly if family members or those counselling the patient are themselves overweight.

GENERAL DIETARY ADVICE

Dietary advice for the acute coronary patient must take into account personal preferences, socioeconomic and cultural factors. An infinite variety of foods is now available and it should be possible to advise a diet which is nutritious, balanced, varied, affordable and enjoyable.

When teaching the patient and family about diet, nurses should be confident that they possess the necessary knowledge and skills to meet their nutritional requirements. Advice certainly needs to be truthful and based on sound scientific evidence if it is to be considered credible. One of the major problems is not in the giving of advice to patients and their relatives, but in achieving appropriate behavioural responses which are in their own best interests. For most patients it is better to emphasize an alteration in general eating habits, rather than the necessity for adhering to a specific dietary plan.

Nutrition is an area that nurses frequently neglect. In hospital the patient's diet is often seen as a minor concern that can be left to the most junior nurse or ancillary staff. In the coronary care unit the responsibility is often given over entirely to the dietician. This is unfortunate, because the nurse has an important role with regards to the activity of eating and drinking. The nurse is usually present at the patient's mealtime when the partner may also be visiting, and can discuss relevant issues pertaining to diet with both of them. The relationship between the patient's knowledge about diet, attitude to healthy eating and existing eating behaviour needs to be incorporated into the rehabilitation plan. If dietary advice is inadequate, the patient may implement choices based on information from the family, neighbours and media. This may be inaccurate and produce misconceptions and inappropriate behaviour.

The patient and family should be presented with factual information, objectively and in a fashion that can be easily understood. Dietary restrictions must be realistic and thoroughly understood by all concerned if they are to be adhered to. A rationale for and suggestion of how to accomplish changes in diet will be required. Such advice needs to be as simple and as practical as possible in order to maximize adherence. Referral to the dietician may be useful if expert advice regarding more complex changes is sought. Alternative diets (vegetarian and vegan) are increasingly popular and they need to be discussed.

In planning dietary changes with the patient and family, the nurse must take into account their cultural preferences. If the patient is male, then the partner needs to be influenced if she normally does the cooking. Cookbooks and sample menus may be provided if guidelines are needed. Factors such as the availability of food, the patient's financial resources, attitudes to food and current media and promotion issues need to be considered. Before advocating any change in eating habits, the nurse needs to balance the stress of changing diet against the likely benefits.

The most sensible general dietary advice that can be given by the nurse is the reduction of excess weight and sugar intake and an increase in dietary fibre intake. A greater use of fish, poultry, vegetables, grains, cereals and fruit should be encouraged. Moderate consumption of a wide variety of foods and the maintenance of an ideal body weight, accompanied by proper physical exercise, are logical recommendations.

Tobacco smoking

It is estimated that about 20% of deaths from coronary heart disease in men and 17% of deaths from coronary heart disease in women are due to smoking (National Heart Forum 2002). The risk of death from coronary heart disease increases proportionally with the number of cigarettes smoked, and appears to be greater for women (Prescott et al 1998).

The cardiovascular risks of pipe and cigar smokers are variable and may not be the same risk as cigarette smokers because most do not inhale. However, former cigarette smokers who change to cigars and pipes do tend to inhale smoke, thus maintaining the risk. Similarly 'weaker' brands of cigarettes may cause more intense inhalation and thus counteract the purpose of switching brands. There is no evidence that filters reduce the risk of coronary heart disease.

There is overwhelming evidence that cardiovascular disease is substantially reduced in quitters, with a significant reduction in risk becoming apparent within 2–3 years and continuing to decline over the next decade, although, in heavy smokers, it may never reach the non-smoker's level (Wilhelmsen 1998).

The habit of smoking is a complex addiction with strong dependence. It exerts its addictive influence by satisfying a physical need, providing stimulation and pleasure, as well as relieving anxiety and tension. Stopping patients smoking is not easy, and the best approach is encouragement with support (Van Berkel et al 1999). Simple advice has a small effect on cessation rates, and more intensive interventions are marginally more effective than minimal interventions (Silagy and Stead 2001).

Patients should, ideally, be advised to stop all forms of smoking, noting that ex-smokers (among coronary patients) have only half the subsequent mortality of those who continue to smoke. The aim of cigarette smoking cessation involves the nurse obtaining help from the family, especially the partner. Stopping abruptly rather than gradually is probably best, but often extremely difficult. It is important to be aware that the habit of smoking is a complex issue that appears to serve multiple functions. It can exert a great influence by satisfying a need to create a certain image, and to provide stimulation, pleasure and good taste. It can reduce anxiety and tension, or it can be a state of addiction. The nurse needs to try and ascertain what need it serves for the patient.

The nursing history should include information as to whether patients have tried to give up smoking before, and if so how they planned to stop, how long they were able to stop, what support they received and why they started smoking again. Discussing these issues with them, together with their beliefs and knowledge about the effects of smoking and their intentions for the future, will mean that subsequent attempts at stopping smoking can be based on experience gained in conjunction with new information and advice given. The shock and fear of having a coronary event may be itself sufficient to stop people smoking. Others may feel more inclined to smoke during the period of stress that their condition brings.

A realistic practicable plan can be drawn up between the nurse, patient and family with the ultimate aim of stopping smoking.

The benefits of stopping smoking

Some of the benefits of smoking cessation are as follows:

- improvement in sense of taste and smell
- avoidance of nicotine stains on fingers
- fresher smelling clothes
- fresher home environment
- improved lung function and easier breathing
- improvement in cough
- not setting a bad example to others, especially children
- increased self-esteem
- financial advantages
- free from feelings of guilt
- preventing indirect harm to others, especially children.

These benefits should be made explicit. If the patient's family do not smoke, the task is made easier. The nurse who is a non-smoker will be more credible as a role model. Other methods of stopping smoking include watching a film about lung cancer or emphysema and the pathological changes that occur, hypnosis or substitution. The former is dramatic and may have short-term benefits only. The latter involves substituting a pleasurable task for a cigarette when smoking is heaviest and related more to habit than enjoyment.

Practical suggestions for the patient

Positive advice regarding smoking cessation includes the following:

- set a firm date to start giving up smoking
- throw away cigarettes and matches left
- try to break the association between pleasure and smoking; e.g. carry a book to occupy oneself
- carry something else in hands, such as a pen, to doodle with
- collect the money saved
- leave cigarette lighter at home
- reward oneself if successful
- relax and use other stress-reducing techniques
- join a self-help group/give up with a friend.

Many other techniques, such as acupuncture, aversion therapy, rapid smoking and group therapy, have been tried, although there is no scientific evidence that any of these is better than the others. Particular methods can be targeted towards different subgroups of smokers who have different obstacles to overcome in smoking cessation, such as psychological dependence, nicotine dependence or social pressure.

It is important to ensure that the patient avoids succumbing to the common temptation of 'just one more cigarette'. The family should be informed that distraction is useful when the patient has a craving for a cigarette. During the initial period of smoking cessation, the patient and family should be warned to expect episodes of irritability and inability to concentrate. Mood swings, gastrointestinal upsets and even an initial bad cough are not uncommon. However, these side effects are temporary.

Although the hospital is an ideal setting for commencing smoking cessation, it is necessary for the nurse to check on compliance with advice periodically after discharge. A diary of cigarette consumption is useful, although this relies on the patient's memory and honesty. A great improvement is the use of a carbon monoxide monitor that is a relatively inexpensive item of equipment and is very accurate.

Hypertension

The risk of coronary heart disease is directly related to both systolic and diastolic blood pressure levels. The aim is to maintain a systolic blood pressure of less than 140 mmHg and/or diastolic of less than 85 mmHg (Williams et al 2004). Non-pharmacological intervention is helpful regardless of the need for medication, and includes advice on exercise, weight reduction and dietary restriction of salt and alcohol. Control can be achieved in many cases by maintenance of an ideal body weight, regular physical activity and the avoidance of stressful situations and smoking. Adequate rest and sleep are essential, and various behavioural techniques and relaxation procedures, such as yoga, transcendental meditation and biofeedback, are useful adjuncts.

If drugs have been prescribed they should be carefully explained to the patient and family, and the need to take them, often for many years or even a lifetime, should be reiterated. It is important that they notify any symptoms of dizziness, headache, blurred vision, oedema, shortness of breath or nocturia to their family doctor. These symptoms may be a result of a rise in blood pressure or iatrogenesis.

Diabetes mellitus

Diagnosis may be based on a fasting or random blood glucose, but may need a formal glucose tolerance test. It is possible that admission to hospital with an acute cardiac event leads to the diagnosis of diabetes. This means that the patient will need to come to terms with two chronic disease processes, including coping with the day-to-day management which may include self-injections of insulin. Most diabetic patients are overweight and therefore weight reduction is important. The patient, family and nurse need to identify the appropriate caloric intake for the patient and encourage regular physical activity, maintain an ideal body weight, avoid cigarette smoking and comply with diet and medication.

Physical activity

People who are physically active have a lower risk of coronary heart disease. It is estimated that about 36% of deaths from coronary heart disease in men and 38% of deaths from coronary heart disease in women are due to a lack of physical activity and that 9% of deaths from coronary heart disease in the UK could be avoided if people who are currently sedentary or have a light level of physical activity increased their level of physical activity to a moderate level (National Heart Forum 2002). It is recommended that adults should participate in a minimum of 30 minutes of accumulated moderate intensity activity (such as brisk walking, cycling or climbing the stairs) on at least 5 days every week (Britton and McPherson 2000). Moderate intensity is defined as energy expenditure of 5–7.5 kcal/min, and equates to a brisk walk for half an hour.

Information regarding physical activity will depend upon the stage of recovery the patient has reached. Initially, the reasons for temporary restriction of activity and relating the progressive resumption of activity to healing of the myocardium will need to be discussed. It is important to discuss exercise in terms of individualized and gradually progressive behaviour, otherwise patients may overdo the activity. They should be prepared for the feelings of weakness that often occur as activity increases which is a result of prolonged bedrest and inactivity. They should be encouraged to resume physical activity, which will be on a gradual basis to allow cardiac output to meet the needs of the body. Restrictions should be explained in a positive fashion, otherwise patients might become irritated and frustrated with progress.

The most beneficial activity is walking, with later progression to jogging, swimming or cycling. Age needs to be taken into account, but the benefits should be stressed, for example, ideal blood pressure and body weight, and a general feeling of well-being. In some patients such a plan of activity will involve a major change in a sedentary lifestyle. They may need to be discouraged from sitting or watching television for long periods, and a change in posture which results in improved breathing is often indicated. Practical advice to the patient and his family (who could positively help by engaging in the activity themselves) includes the avoidance of alcohol or a heavy meal before exercising, and to exercise in sensible conditions, such as wearing appropriate clothing and footwear and choosing the coolest time of the day in summer and the warmest part of the day in winter. The avoidance of cigarettes is essential, as are the hazards of adverse environmental conditions, intense competition, and emotional or stress-provoking situations.

Psychosocial well-being

Although many patients believe stress to have played a part in their illness, its precise role is unclear. It may help to draw up a list of events which regularly make the patient feel tensed and stressed. Strategies such as getting up 10 minutes earlier than normal to avoid driving to work in the rush hour, travelling to work by bus or train rather than driving, avoiding doing more than one thing at a time and allocating extra time for activities may help. Consciously taking more time at meals to enjoy the food and socialize can be used as a starting point to practise control of time pressure three times a day. Planned periods of rest and relaxation are most beneficial for the majority of patients and are more productive if the spouse participates. Methods of relaxation are numerous and varied, and one that is suitable to the individual should be chosen. Relaxation on a regular basis should be encouraged, otherwise many patients cease the practice once they feel they have recovered.

The role of frequent moderate exercise is often underplayed, but it is ideal for returning general body stress and giving the patient an opportunity for privacy and self-appraisal. Perhaps the best practical advice is to emphasize the avoidance of engaging in polyphasic activities (engaging in multiple activities, such as watching television, eating and reading the newspaper, more or less simultaneously). Some patients may require modifications or reappraisal of some presently held beliefs and attributions, and instruction in self-recognition of the causes underlying any emotional reactions such as anger, impatience and irritation.

RELAXATION TECHNIQUES

Some individuals seem to be constantly active and will display physical tension such as tapping the foot or clenching the fist even when sitting still. For some, being (or at least appearing) busy is part of their image and is seen as creating a positive impression. Relaxation techniques of various kinds can be used to help reduce stress, including progressive muscle relaxation, meditation, biofeedback, yoga, self-hypnosis and prayer. Relaxation therapy, coupled with a conscious avoidance or reduction of stress and planned periods of rest or sleep, should be beneficial not only for the patient but for the partner also. Thus, both should be encouraged to participate. The patient needs to be advised that relaxation is not synonymous with having nothing to do or just being asleep. If relaxation is practised regularly, it eventually becomes habit-forming and may aid in promoting sleep, reducing pain, increasing sense of control and reducing fears and anxieties. Most people do not realize how tense they have been until they learn to relax.

Methods of relaxation are numerous and varied, and the choice will depend on the individual. Most involve the person selecting a comfortable sitting or reclining position. A quiet, peaceful environment, often with the light subdued, is ideal for performing the therapy, otherwise the patient may become distracted and have difficulty in concentrating or relaxing. Most methods of relaxation help focus attention on various parts of the body and then relaxing the muscles in that area. Relaxation techniques may not be appropriate for all patients, and a lack of commitment, feelings of embarrassment and a too dogmatic approach may limit its effectiveness.

An example of a relaxation exercise

Choose a comfortable sitting or reclining position in which your head, arms and legs are supported; close your eyes and relax:

1   Take a deep breath ... and relax. Concentrate on your breathing. (Pause for 10–15 seconds between instructions.)
2   Again, take a deep breath ... and relax.
3   Now, focus your attention on the muscles in your right arm. Tense them for 10 seconds ... and relax.
4   Now, focus your attention on the muscles in your left arm. Tense them for 10 seconds ... and relax.
5   Now, focus your attention on the muscles in your right leg. Tense them for 10 seconds ... and relax.
6   Now, focus your attention on the muscles in your left leg. Tense them for 10 seconds ... and relax.
7   Now, focus your attention on the muscles in your right arm and left leg. Tense them for 10 seconds ... and relax.
8   Now, focus your attention on the muscles in your left arm and right leg. Tense them for 10 seconds ... and relax.

Unmodifiable risk factors

Patients should be aware of the possible effects of age, sex and hereditary factors. This may help explain the heart attack to patients who feel they have no modifiable risk factors.

PSYCHOLOGICAL ASPECTS

Many patients with acute coronary syndromes when discharged home are confronted by various uncertainties and minor physical symptoms that provoke anxiety and depression. Anxiety is a universal and generally adaptive response to a threat, but can become maladaptive in certain circumstances (House and Stark 2002). Depression describes a spectrum of mood disturbance ranging from mild to severe and from transient to persistent (Peveler et al 2002). Two cardinal symptoms are present: persistent and pervasive low mood and loss of interest or pleasure in usual activities. Such reactions are responsible for poor recovery in a significant proportion of these patients. Certainly, psychological factors are stronger determinants of maladjustment than physical state. Such responses are influenced by various factors, including the extent and severity of the infarct, and the physical, emotional, social, financial and vocational circumstances of the patient. The partner, as well as the patient, also reports a low level of understanding and considerable distress (Thompson 2002).

The majority of patients who do develop problems will have transient disturbances of mood lasting no more than a few weeks (Thompson and Lewin 2000). The lack of structure in the lives of those accustomed to a busy existence may result in boredom, frustration and a loss of confidence. Insomnia is common, and as a result of decreased sleep individuals may become irritable, quick to take offence and may seek to prolong their invalid role by imposing excessive demands on the family.

Anxiety is a very common initial response to myocardial infarction, especially in women (Kim et al 2000). Many patients report high levels of anxiety during their stay in hospital and a peak during convalescence (Thompson et al 1987). Specific worries reported by these patients concern the effect of their heart attack on return to work, leisure and sexual activities; the receipt of inadequate information about their illness and subsequent recovery; and possible complications and the necessary action required should symptoms recur. The threat of sudden cardiac death is also a further source of continued anxiety. Anxiety can be assessed by the use of a measure such as the Hospital Anxiety and Depression Scale (Zigmond and Snaith 1983).

If anxiety is unrelieved, depression usually supervenes, and both may persist for long periods of time in many patients (Lane et al 2002). Depression is common in coronary heart disease with one in five patients having major depression, a prevalence rate similar in patients recovering from myocardial infarction (Carney et al 2002). It is associated with increased risk for cardiac mortality and morbidity in patients with coronary heart disease, especially following acute myocardial infarction. It is often felt as a sense of isolation, sadness or resentment. The depression that begins in hospital often becomes manifest when the patient goes home and finds the positive aspects of being there becoming replaced by negative aspects such as tiredness, weakness and the perceived prospect of a life with restrictions and limitations. Loss of libido, irritability, insomnia and inattentiveness may all have their roots in underlying depression, as may generalized pessimism, hopelessness and withdrawal. Depression in cardiac patients can be assessed by the use of the Hospital Anxiety and Depression Scale or a specific instrument, the Cardiac Depression Scale (Hare and Davis 1996) validated in the UK (Birks et al 2004).

It is important to intervene if anxiety or depression are identified in order to reduce disability and use of health service resources and improve quality of life. Giving information tailored to the wishes of the individual is an important first step. Effective communication is essential to the process. This means using open questions, discussing issues and summarizing. Simple reassurance is important and can often be effective in most cases. For severe anxiety or depression referral to specialists may be warranted and brief psychological treatments such as cognitive behavioural therapy may be of value.

It is important that pre-discharge education and support is adequately provided. An optimistic and realistic outlook is necessary otherwise patients will be less likely to achieve a high level of morale and a successful return to work and family and social involvement. They need to be prepared for the problems that are frequently encountered during convalescence, including anxiety, depression, poor concentration, irritability, sleeplessness and fear of complications, especially of dying during sleep. The partner often experiences more trauma than the patient and will require supportive counselling and be warned against being over-protective towards the patient.

The transition from hospital to home is a traumatic event for the patient and family, and a frequently neglected aspect of care planning. It is a vital time for the nurse to ensure continuity of care. Periodic checks, such as telephoning the couple at home, may be useful in some instances to bridge the gap and reassure them if they have any worries or concerns. Liaison with the community nurse ensures that continuity is maintained in providing resources and assistance. Communication between the primary and secondary care sectors needs to be consistent, accurate, free and openended. The community nurse, for example, is the best-equipped source for providing information about community resources, including counselling services, home helps, rehabilitation facilities and coronary clubs, as well as being in regular contact with the patient's general practitioner.

It is difficult to identify in the early stages those acute coronary syndrome patients who are likely to require special support, and therefore an appropriate time to assess the patient for extra psychological help needs to be determined. Certainly, before discharge, there should be an assessment made of the rehabilitation and aftercare needs of patients and partners, with appropriate referral where necessary (Thompson et al 1996b). Patients who are distressed in hospital are at high risk of adverse psychological and quality of life outcomes during the ensuing year (Mayou et al 2000). There is a need, therefore, for more critical evaluation of the effectiveness of concentrating rehabilitation in such subgroups and for examining criteria for selecting those patients most likely to benefit (Mayou et al 2002).

Early in-hospital counselling reduces anxiety and depression for patients and partners (Thompson and Meddis 1990a,b) and these effects are maintained by continued counselling (Johnston et al 1999). Individualized educational and behavioural treatment delivered by cardiac nurses in hospital also appears efficacious in terms of reduced psychological consequences and improved quality of life (Mayou et al 2002).

A number of measures specific for quality of life in cardiac patients are now available (Lewin et al 2002, Thompson et al 1998, 2002, Thompson and Roebuck 2001).

The partner

During the early phase of the patient's illness, the partner is also often distressed and needs a good deal of support (Thompson 2002). The partner is faced with the difficult task of developing a support role to assist the patient's recovery but is often ill-equipped to do this. Thus, the partner will need guidelines regarding the level of activities the patient will be expected to perform, and answers to specific questions such as whether to leave the patient unattended, when to call the doctor, when to resume a normal daily routine, and what is the likelihood of another coronary event.

The major threats associated with distress during the early recovery phase include the loss of a healthy partner, fear of another heart attack, and uncertainty over treatment and care (Thompson 2002). Specifying how the partner may help the patient in recovery will help provide a clearer role and may prevent feelings of inadequacy in fulfilling the new role.

Partners need to be prepared for the effect the patient's illness will have on them both as individuals and on their relationship; to anticipate mood changes in the patient, particularly anxiety and depression, and understand that they may become the scapegoat for the patient's frustrations. Partners also need to develop strategies to minimize this stress, including support from other family members, continuing with outside interests and activities and maintaining open communication.

DRUG THERAPY

The acute coronary syndrome patient may be taking drugs on a regular basis for the first time, and compliance is likely to rest upon four main factors:

1 The ability of the patient to understand, accept and comply with instructions.
2 The maintenance of a good relationship between the clinician and the patient.
3 The awareness of the patient that symptoms might regress with effective treatment.
4 Treatment with an easily used drug formulation in a simple regimen, preferably once daily.

Patients' factual knowledge of medication is generally low and many patients do not take the medications according to the regimen prescribed, with about half occasionally forgetting to take them (Haugbolle et al 2002). It is likely that a reduction in the number of drugs prescribed, simplification of both the packaging and dispensing, and verbal and written instruction and the use of simple aids to monitor drug usage, such as diaries, will help to increase compliance. Compliance is difficult to evaluate, but does include certain measurable factors such as:

1 Knowledge of the name, purpose and side effects of the medication.
2 Knowledge of the correct action in the event of side effects.
3 Taking the correct dose at suitable times.
4 Knowledge of correct action in the event of a missed dose.
5 Correct number of tablets taken between discharge and follow up.
6 Knowledge that the treatment needs to be continued.

Patients' knowledge about prescribed medication is very limited, possibly because of confusion by technical jargon and a poor memory for medical information. Information about medications should be brief, concise and comprehensible. It should include details of the medication, how to take it, possible side effects and what to do about them; and precautions such as possible side effects on driving, sexuality and interaction with alcohol or other drugs. Also, the patient needs to know what to do when a dose is missed, how to store the medicine, what to do when the course is completed, and how to dispose of any unused medications. A patient may have difficulty in understanding medications for a variety of reasons, including fear of dependency or effect of the drug.

Family participation in patient teaching may exert a strong influence on the patient's learning and long-term behaviour. A useful method involves the use of a small file or index with a sample of the patient's tablet(s) affixed. Details of the drug name, dose, time to be taken, action, possible side effects and storage are written on the card. This is then given to the patient for storage with medications at home, thus serving as a reminder and teaching aid.

Prescription information leaflets

Information leaflets have advantages and benefits for patients. They increase knowledge, compliance, satisfaction and therapeutic outcomes. Leaflets should be checked for readability, as the average Briton has a reading age of only 9 years. Special leaflets should be produced for those who do not speak English and for the blind. Information leaflets require careful preparation and the support of oral information at the point of delivery.

PHYSICAL ACTIVITY

Prolonged immobilization is associated with a reduction in physical work capacity due to a comparable reduction in stroke volume. Resumption of activity after a period of bedrest results in a tachycardia and orthostatic hypotension, which is partly due to hypovolaemia in which the plasma volume decreases more than the red cell mass, thus increasing blood viscosity. Other effects of immobilization include a decrease in maximum oxygen uptake, a negative balance of nitrogen and protein, and a decrease in skeletal muscle mass and contractile strength.

An early graduated programme of physical activity is designed to avert or minimize these undesirable effects. Besides reducing the risk of venous stasis and its complications (the possible formation of thrombi and pulmonary emboli), such a programme is likely to improve physical work capacity and cardiac performance, improve mood and morale and facilitate an early return to work.

A normal response to an early exercise test reliably identifies the patient at low risk of future cardiac events. It may also help to identify patients in need of further evaluation.

Activity planning

The functional classification of the New York Heart Association provides a crude guide for determining appropriate activities as well as expected symptoms for acute coronary syndrome patients (Table 8.2).

Advice about specific activities should be individualized and take into account the extent and severity of the disease process, its limitations, the patient's previous level of activity, the extent of recovery and stability of the current condition, as well as the patient's usual living environment.

Progress in early rehabilitation can be greatly assisted by the use of metabolic equivalents (METs) for prescribing specific physical activities. One MET is defined as the oxygen consumption by the patient at rest and is roughly equivalent to 3.5 ml of oxygen per kilogram of body weight per minute.

Table 8.2 Functional classification of patients with heart disease (Criteria Committee of the New York Heart Association 1973)

Class	
I	Heart disease with no limitation on ordinary physical activity
II	Slight limitation. Ordinary physical activity (e.g. walking) produces symptoms
III	Marked limitation. Unable to walk on the level without disability. Less than ordinary activity produces symptoms
IV	Dyspnoea at rest. Inability to carry out any physical activity

Physical activity on the coronary care unit

Early ambulation in uncomplicated myocardial infarction is essential to avert or minimize the deleterious effects of prolonged bedrest, including the decrease in physical work capacity. It also reduces the anxiety and depression that often occur. In some coronary care units patients are encouraged to sit out of bed on the day of admission, provided that they are free of pain and significant arrhythmias. Where there has been a prolonged period of bedrest, resumption of activity results in the occurrence of a moderate tachycardia and orthostatic hypotension. Physical activities should therefore be of low-level intensity (1–2 METs), such as eating, dressing/undressing, washing hands and face, using a bedside commode, doing simple active and passive arm and leg exercises, or sitting in a bedside chair.

Observation of patients as they perform these activities is useful to ensure that they can cope and that no harmful effects ensue. Early rehabilitation should not be associated with chest pain, dyspnoea, sweating, palpitations or excessive fatigue. Arrhythmias and ST-segment displacement on the ECG should not occur, and systolic blood pressure should not fall more than 10–15 mmHg.

Patients are usually the best judge of how much they can do, but they should be prepared for any feelings of weakness that may accompany increases of activity.

Physical activity on the ward

Once patients leave the coronary care unit, the aim is for them to attain a level of cardiac functioning that permits personal care and independence (or at least semi-independence) by the time of discharge.

The ward activity plan should consist of warm-up isotonic (dynamic) exercises, which allow the heart rate to increase proportionally to the intensity of the activity, the systolic blood pressure to increase slowly and the diastolic blood pressure to remain unchanged or decrease slightly. Isometric exercises should be avoided. These result in a minimal increase in heart rate and a significant and steep increase in systolic blood pressure, which cause a sudden increase in afterload which is poorly tolerated by an ischaemic left ventricle, and which may result in angina and lethal arrhythmias.

Walking, gradually and progressively increasing pace and distance, should be the major component of the activity plan. The aim is to achieve full and rapid mobility and return home. It is advisable for most patients who will have to climb stairs at home to do so under supervision before leaving hospital. This results in increased confidence and reduced worry for the patient and family. At the time of discharge from hospital, the patient should be able to perform activities at peak levels of 3.5–4.0 METs for short periods, to simulate usual activities at home.

References

Ades PA (2001). Cardiac rehabilitation and secondary prevention of coronary heart disease. *New England Journal of Medicine*, 345: 892–902.

American Association of Cardiovascular and Pulmonary Rehabilitation (2002). *Guidelines for Cardiac Rehabilitation Programs*, 4th edn. Human Kinetics, Champaign, IL.

Barber-Parker ED (2002). Integrating patient teaching into bedside patient care: a participant-observation study of hospital nurses. *Patient Education and Counseling*, 48: 107–113.

Becker MH (1974). The health belief model and personal health behavior. *Health Education Monographs*, 2: 236–508.

Bethell HJN, Turner SC, Evans JA et al (2001). Cardiac rehabilitation in the United Kingdom. How complete is the provision? *Journal of Cardiopulmonary Rehabilitation*, 21: 111–115.

Birks Y, Roebuck A, Thompson DR (2004). A validation study of the Cardiac Depression Scale (CDS) in a UK population. *British Journal of Health Psychology*, 9: 15–24.

Bowker TJ, Clayton TC, Ingham J (1996). A British Cardiac Society survey of potential for the secondary prevention of coronary disease. ASPIRE (Action on Secondary Prevention through Intervention to Reduce Events). *Heart*, 4: 334–342.

Britton A, McPherson K (2000). *Monitoring the Progress of the 2010 Target for Coronary Heart Disease Mortality: Estimated Consequences on CHD Incidence and Mortality from Changing Prevalence of Risk Factors*. National Heart Forum, London.

Carney RM, Freedland KE, Miller GE, Jaffe AS (2002). Depression as a risk factor for cardiac mortality and morbidity. A review of potential mechanisms. *Journal of Psychosomatic Research*, 53: 897–902.

Criteria Committeee of the New York Heart Association (1973) *Nomenclature and Criteria for the Diagnosis of the Heart and Great Vessels*. Little, Brown, Boston.

Dalal H, Evans PH, Campbell JL (2004). Recent developments in secondary prevention and cardiac rehabilitation after acute myocardial infarction. *British Medical Journal*, 328: 693–697.

Department of Health (1995). *Sensible Drinking*. The report of an inter-departmental working group. The Stationery Office, London.

Department of Health (2000). *National Service Framework for Coronary Heart Disease*. The Stationery Office, London.

Dinnes J, Kleijnen J, Leitner M, Thompson DR (1999). Cardiac rehabilitation. *Quality in Health Care*, 8: 65–71.

Dusseldorp E, van Elderen T, Maes S, Meulman J, Kraaij V (1999). A meta-analysis of psychoeducational programs for coronary heart disease patients. *Health Psychology*, 18: 506–519.

Furze G, Lewin RJP, Roebuck A, Thompson DR, Bull P (2001). Attributions and misconceptions in angina: an exploratory study. *Journal of Health Psychology*, 6: 501–510.

Glanz K, Shigaki D, Farzanfar R, Pinto B, Kaplan B, Friedman RH (2003). Participant reactions to a computerized telephone system for nutrition and exercise counseling. *Patient Education and Counseling*, 49: 157–163.

Hare DL, Davis CR (1996). Cardiac depression scale: validation of a new depression scale for cardiac patients. *Journal of Psychosomatic Research*, 40: 379–386.

Haugbolle LS, Sorensen EW, Henriksen HH (2002). Medication- and illness-related factual knowledge, perceptions and behaviour in angina pectoris patients. *Patient Education and Counseling*, 47: 281–289.

Hooper L (2001). Dietetic guidelines: diet in secondary prevention of cardiovascular disease. *Journal of Human Nutrition and Dietetics*, 14: 297–305.

House A, Stark D (2002). Anxiety in medical patients. *British Medical Journal*, 325: 207–209.

Johnston M, Foulkes J, Johnston D, Pollard B, Gudmundsdottir H (1999). Impact on patients and partners of inpatient and extended cardiac counseling and rehabilitation: a controlled trial. *Psychosomatic Medicine*, 61: 225–233.

Jolliffe JA, Rees K, Taylor RS et al (2004). Exercise-based rehabilitation for coronary heart disease. (Cochrane Review). In *The Cochrane Library* Issue 1. Wiley, Chichester.

Jowett NI, Thompson DR (2003). *Comprehensive Coronary Care*, 3rd edn. Baillière Tindall, London.

Kim KA, Moser DK, Garvin BJ et al (2000). Differences between men and women in anxiety early after acute myocardial infarction. *American Journal of Critical Care*, 9: 245–253.

Lane D, Carroll D, Ring C et al (2002). The prevalence and persistence of depression and anxiety following myocardial infarction. *British Journal of Health Psychology*, 7: 11–21.

Levine SA (1944). Some harmful effects of recumbency in the treatment of heart disease. *Journal of the American Medical Association*, 148: 80–85.

Lewin RJP, Ingleton R, Newens A, Thompson DR (1998). Adherence to cardiac rehabilitation guidelines: a survey of rehabilitation programmes in the United Kingdom. *British Medical Journal*, 316: 1354–1355.

Lewin RJP, Thompson DR, Martin CR et al (2002b) Validation of the Cardiovascular Limitations and Symptoms Profile (CLASP) in chronic stable angina. *Journal of Cardiopulmonary Rehabilitation*, 22: 184–191.

Linden W, Stossel C, Maurice J (1996). Psychosocial interventions for patients with coronary artery disease: a meta-analysis. *Archives of Internal Medicine*, 156: 745–752.

Mayou R, Gill D, Thompson DR et al (2000). Depression and anxiety as predictors of outcome after myocardial infarction. *Psychosomatic Medicine*, 62: 212–219.

Mayou RA, Thompson DR, Clements A, et al (2002). Guideline-based early rehabilitation after myocardial infarction. A pragmatic randomized controlled trial. *Journal of Psychosomatic Research*, 52: 89–95.

Miller NH, Taylor CB (1995). *Lifestyle Management for Patients with Coronary Heart Disease*. Human Kinetics, Champaign, IL.

Miller WR, Rollnick S (2002). *Motivational interviewing: preparing people for change*. Guilford Press, New York.

National Heart Forum (2002). *Coronary Heart Disease: Estimating the Impact of Changes in Risk Factors*. The Stationery Office, London.

NHS Centre for Reviews and Dissemination (1998). Cardiac rehabilitation. *Effective Health Care*, 4: 1–12.

Peveler R, Carson A, Rodin G (2002). Depression in medical patients. *British Medical Journal*, 325: 149–152.

Prescott E, Hippe M, Schnohr P et al (1998). Smoking and the risk of myocardial infarction in women and men: longitudinal population study. *British Medical Journal*, 316: 1043–1047.

Prochaska JO, DiClemente CC (1983). Stages and processes of self-change of smoking: towards an integrative model of change. *Journal of Consulting and Clinical Psychology*, 51: 390–395.

Redman BK (1997). *The Process of Patient Education*, 8th edn. CV Mosby, St Louis.

Resnicow K, DiIorio C, Soet JE et al (2002). Motivational interviewing in medical and public health settings. In *Motivational Interviewing: Preparing People for Change*, (WR Miller, S Rollnick, eds). Guilford Press, New York, pp. 251–269.

Rollnick S, Mason P, Butler C (1999). *Health Behavior Change: a Guide for Practitioners*. Churchill Livingstone, London.

Royal College of Physicians of London (1998). *Clinical Management of Overweight and Obese Patients*. Royal College of Physicians, London.

Scott JT, Thompson DR (2003). Assessing the information needs of post-myocardial infarction patients: a systematic review. *Patient Education and Counseling*.

Silagy C, Stead CF (2001). *Physician Advice for Smoking Cessation*. Cochrane Library Issue 4. Update Software, Oxford.

Thompson DR (2002). Involvement of the partner in rehabilitation. In *Advancing the Frontiers of Cardiopulmonary Rehabilitation*. (J Jobin, F Maltais, P Poirier, P LeBlanc, C Simard, eds). Human Kinetics, Champaign, IL. pp. 211–215.

Thompson DR, Bowman GS, de Bono DP, Hopkins A (1996a). The development and testing of a cardiac rehabilitation audit tool. *Journal of the Royal College of Physicians of London*, 31: 317–320.

Thompson DR, Bowman GS, Kitson AL, de Bono DP, Hopkins A (1996b). Cardiac rehabilitation in the

United Kingdom: guidelines and audit standards. *Heart,* 75: 89–93.

Thompson DR, Bowman GS, Kitson AL, de Bono DP, Hopkins A (1997a). Cardiac rehabilitation services in England and Wales: a national survey. *International Journal of Cardiology,* 59: 299–304.

Thompson DR, Bowman GS, de Bono DP, Hopkins A (1997b). *Cardiac Rehabilitation: Guidelines and Audit Standards.* Royal College of Physicians, London.

Thompson DR, de Bono DP (1999). How valuable is cardiac rehabilitation and who should get it? *Heart,* 82: 545–546.

Thompson DR, Jenkinson C, Roebuck A et al (2002). Development and validation of a short measure of health status for individuals with acute myocardial infarction: the myocardial infarction dimensional assessment scale (MIDAS). *Quality of Life Research,* 11: 535–543.

Thompson DR, Lewin RJP (2000). Management of the post-myocardial infarction patient: rehabilitation and cardiac neurosis. *Heart,* 75: 89–93.

Thompson DR, Meadows KA, Lewin RJP (1998). Measuring quality of life in patients with coronary heart disease. *European Heart Journal,* 19: 693–695.

Thompson DR, Meddis R (1990a). A prospective evaluation of in-hospital counselling for first time myocardial infarction men. *Journal of Psychosomatic Research,* 34: 237–248.

Thompson DR, Meddis R (1990b). Wives' responses to counselling early after myocardial infarction. *Journal of Psychosomatic Research,* 34: 249–258.

Thompson DR, Roebuck A (2001). The measurement of health-related quality of life in patients with coronary heart disease. *Journal of Cardiovascular Nursing,* 16: 28–33.

Thompson DR, Webster RA, Cordle CJ, Sutton TW (1987). Specific sources and patterns of anxiety in male patients with first myocardial infarction. *British Journal of Medical Psychology,* 60: 343–348.

Thun MJ, Peto R, Lopez AD et al (1997). Alcohol consumption and mortality amongst middle aged and elderly US adults. *New England Journal of Medicine,* 337: 1705–1714.

Tod AM, Lacey EA, McNeill F (2002) 'I'm still waiting …': barriers to accessing cardiac rehabilitation services. *Journal of Advanced Nursing,* 40: 421–431.

Van Berkel TF, Boersma H, Roos-Hesselink JW et al (1999). Impact of smoking cessation and smoking interventions with coronary heart disease. *European Heart Journal,* 20: 1773–1782.

Weingarten SR, Henning JM, Badamgarav E et al (2002). Interventions used in disease management programmes for patients with chronic illness – which ones work? Meta-analysis of published reports. *British Medical Journal,* 325: 925–933.

Wenger NK, Froelicher ES, Smith LK et al (1995). Cardiac rehabilitation. *Clinical Practice Guideline No. 17.* Agency for Health Care Policy and Research and National Heart, Lung, and Blood Institute, Rockville, MD.

Wilhelmsen L (1998). Effects of cessation of smoking after myocardial infarction. *Journal of Cardiovascular Risk,* 5: 173–176.

Williams B, Poulter NR, Brown MJ et al (2004). British Hypertension Society guidelines for hypertension management 2004 (BHS-IV): summary. *British Medical Journal,* 328: 634–640.

World Health Organization (1993). *Needs and Action Priorities in Cardiac Rehabilitation and Secondary Prevention in Patients with CHD.* WHO Regional Office for Europe, Copenhagen.

World Health Organization (1998) *Obesity: Preventing and Managing the Global Epidemic.* WHO, Geneva.

Zigmond AS, Snaith RP (1983). The hospital anxiety and depression scale. *Acta Psychiatrica Scandinavica,* 67: 361–370.

Further reading

Hatchett R, Thompson DR (eds) (2002). *Cardiac Nursing: A Comprehensive Guide.* Harcourt, London.

Jobin J, Maltais F, Poirier P, LeBlanc P, Simard C (eds) (2002). *Advancing the Frontiers of Cardiopulmonary Rehabilitation.* Human Kinetics, Champaign, IL.

Jowett NI, Thompson DR (2003). *Comprehensive Coronary Care,* 3rd edn. Baillière Tindall, London.

Index

W

X